APPLIED ASPECTS OF ULTRASONOGRAPHY IN HUMANS

Edited by **Philip Ainslie**

Applied Aspects of Ultrasonography in Humans
Edited by Philip Ainslie

Published by InTech
Janeza Trdine 9, 51000 Rijeka, Croatia

Publishing Process Manager Oliver Kurelic

Technical Editor Teodora Smiljanic

Cover Designer InTech Design Team

Additional hard copies can be obtained from orders@intechopen.com

Applied Aspects of Ultrasonography in Humans, Edited by Philip Ainslie
p. cm.
ISBN 978-953-51-0522-0

For EU product safety concerns:
IN TECH d.o.o., Prolaz Marije Krucifikse Kozulić 3, 51000 Rijeka, Croatia,
info@intechopen.com or visit our website at intechopen.com.

Meet the editor

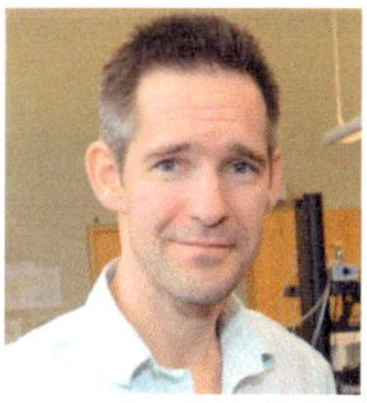

Professor Ainslie is based at the School of Health and Exercise Sciences at the University of British Columbia, Okanagan, Canada. Since completing his PhD in 2002, Dr Ainslie has published >100 peer-reviewed manuscripts and >14 major book chapters. The majority of these publications have resulted from his independent research program, principally focusing on various aspects of vascular regulation, in particular the interactions between the systemic and cerebrovascular systems. Recently, he was awarded Canada Research Chair in Cerebrovascular Physiology. He has also been the recipient of the young investigator award (Canadian Society of Exercise Physiology) and University of British Columbia researcher of the year.

Contents

Preface

This book is devoted to some novel and applied aspects of ultrasound, which has shown rapid developments in the last decade. Written by international experts, this publication provides the reader with the present knowledge and future research directions of diagnostic and therapeutic ultrasound and spectroscopy. Focused topics include Duplex ultrasound, transcranial color Duplex, MRA- guided Doppler ultrasonography and near-infrared spectroscopy. New directions in the use and application of transcranial and color Duplex ultrasound are provided, as well as the use of ultrasound and arterial stiffness for measuring human vascular health and circulatory control. Novel use of ultrasound for the detection of intra-cardiac and intra-pulmonary shunts is also described along with its utility for the assessment of gastric emptying.

I hope this edition will be useful and stimulate further use and research in applied aspects of ultrasonography.

Philip N. Ainslie, PhD
The University of British Columbia,
Faculty of Health and Social Development,
Canada

1

New Directions in the Dynamic Assessment of Brain Blood Flow Regulation

Christopher K. Willie, Lindsay K. Eller and Philip N. Ainslie
School of Health and Exercise Sciences, Faculty of Health and Social Development, University of British Columbia Okanagan, Canada

1. Introduction

The principal aim of this book chapter is to provide an overview of the utilities of transcranial Doppler ultrasound (TCD), and high resolution vascular ultrasound for the assessment of human cerebrovascular function with respect to other common measurement tools. Specifically, we aim to: (1) examine the advantages and disadvantages of TCD in the context of other imaging metrics; (2) highlight the optimum approaches for insonation of the basal intra-cerebral arteries; (3) provide a detailed summary of the utility of TCD for assessing cerebrovascular reactivity, autoregulation and neurovascular coupling and the clinical application of these measures; (4) give detailed guidelines for the appropriate use and caveats of neck artery flow measures for the assessment of regional cerebral blood flow distribution; and (5) provide recommendations on the integrative assessment of cerebrovascular function. Finally, we provide an overview of new directions for the optimization of TCD and vascular ultrasound. Future research directions - both physiological and methodological - are outlined.

2. Background

Maintenance of adequate cerebral blood flow (CBF) is necessary for normal brain function and survival. That the brain receives ~15% of total cardiac output and is responsible for ~20% of the body's oxygen consumption, despite being 2-3% of total body weight, is testament to its high energetic cost. This, combined with a very limited ability to store energy (the brain's total energy pool would theoretically allow it to function for ~12 minutes were energy substrate supply abolished) requires effective regulation of blood supply. Numerous pathologies such as head trauma, carotid artery disease, subarachnoid haemorrhage and stroke result in disturbances to the regulatory mechanisms controlling CBF (Hossmann, 1994; Panerai, 2009). However, the skull makes it difficult to measure parameters such as blood flow and blood velocity. Many approaches such as radio-opaque tracers, radioactive markers and similar methods are inadequate because of poor temporal resolution (see See Table (appendix) for a summary of the advantages and disadvantages of other methods). Key factors that determine adequate CBF for maintenance of cerebral oxygen delivery are: (1) sensitivity to changes in arterial PO_2 and PCO_2 (cerebrovascular reactivity) and the unique ability to extract a large amount of available oxygen; (2) effective cerebral autoregulation (CA) that assists maintenance of CBF over a wide range of perfusion pressures, helping to prevent over/under perfusion and consequent risk of hemorrhage or ischemia; and, (3) matching of local flow to localized metabolic needs (neurovascular coupling; NVC). The high temporal resolution and non-invasive nature of transcranial Doppler ultrasound (TCD) make it a useful tool in the assessment of integrative cerebrovascular function in terms of cerebral reactivity, autoregulation, and NVC. New technologies are further increasing the utility of TCD. For example, combining TCD with microbubble contrasting agents allow for quantification of local changes in perfusion for measuring absolute volumetric flow (Powers *et al.*, 2009). However, the interaction of ultrasound with microbubble contrast agents is complex and beyond the scope of this review; the reader is referred to (Powers *et al.*, 2009) for a detailed review of the current state of contrast TCD technology. With or without contrast, a TCD machine is relatively inexpensive ($20,000 to $50,000 USD); moreover, TCD is easy to use and it is safe in healthy and disease states alike. For these reasons TCD is practical in the clinical setting, where it is used to assess a variety of different cerebrovascular pathologies.

The principal aim of this chapter is to summarize the utilities of TCD in the assessment of cerebrovascular function with respect to other common measurement tools. Specifically, we aim to: (1) examine the advantages and disadvantages of TCD in the context of other imaging metrics; (2) highlight the optimum approaches for insonation of the basal intra-cerebral arteries; (3) provide a detailed summary of the utility of TCD for assessing cerebrovascular reactivity, autoregulation and neurovascular coupling and the clinical application of these measures; and (4) provide recommendations on the integrative assessment of cerebrovascular function and avenues for future research.

2.1 Techniques for the measurement of cerebral blood flow and velocity

Kety and Schmidt (1945) were the first to quantify CBF using an inert tracer (e.g., nitrous oxide, N_2O). The reference method for the measurement of global CBF, the Kety-Schmidt method is based on the Fick principle, whereby the arterio-venous difference of an inert tracer is proportional to the volume of blood flow through the brain (Kety & Schmidt, 1948). The tracer is infused until tension equilibrium is attained (the saturation phase) and then terminated, after which the concentration falls toward zero (the desaturation phase). Simultaneous arterio-jugular venous samples are withdrawn during either phase and CBF calculated by the Kety-Schmidt equation:

$$CBF = 100 \times \lambda \times \frac{C_{jv}(\text{equilibrium})}{\int_{t=0}^{t=\infty} (C_{jv}(t) \times dt) - \int_{t=0}^{t=\infty} (Ca(t) \times dt)},$$

where Cjv(t) and Ca(t) are the jugular-venous and arterial concentration, respectively, of the tracer at time t (in minutes), and λ is the brain-blood partition coefficient (in ml g^{-1}). The global cerebral metabolic rate (CMR) of substance *x* is given by the Fick principle as:

$$CMR = CBF \text{ x a-jv } D(x) = CBF \text{ x } (Ca(x) - Cv(x)),$$

where a-jv D (x) is the arterial to jugular-venous concentration of x. This provides a valid CMR due to the identical sampling sites (regions of interest) for the CBF measurement and the a-v D(x) (See Figure 1).

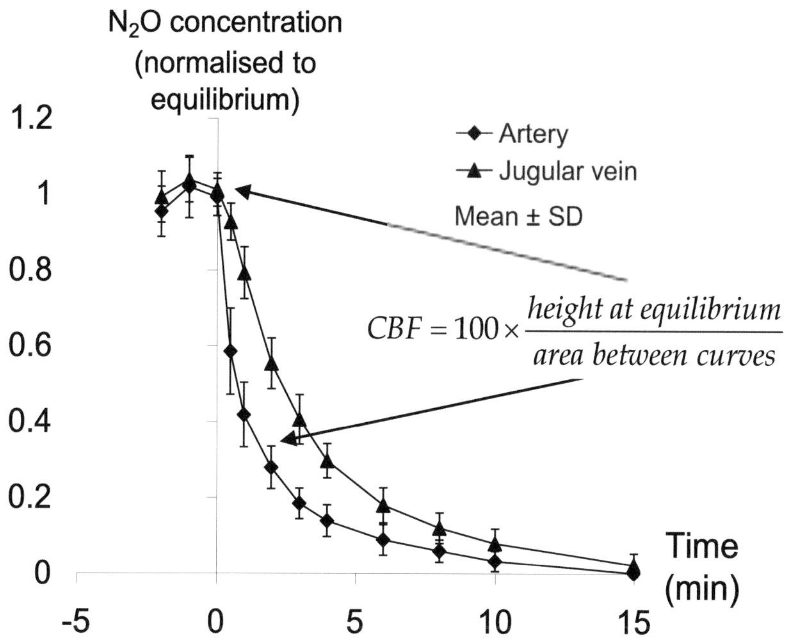

Fig. 1. The Kety-Schmidt method using N_2O. N_2O concentration is given on the y-axis as the percent of equilibrium concentration (mean ± SD) versus time, by discontinuous blood sampling in the desaturation phase during normocapnia.

Theoretically, this principle can be exploited using any freely diffusible tracer; indeed N_2O, ^{133}Xe, hydrogen, and iodoantipyrine have all been utilized (Edvinsson & Krause, 2002). While this method did stimulate seminal research in cerebrovascular physiology (Kety, 1999), there are several important limitations: measurements are taken over the course of minutes, making it impossible to assess dynamic changes in CBF; only a global, but not regional, measure of CBF, cerebral metabolic rate, or blood-brain substrate exchange is possible; internal jugular and peripheral arterial lines are necessary making it quite invasive; and, finally, the value of cerebral oxygen consumption must be assumed (Kety & Schmidt, 1948). Furthermore, venous outflow from the brain may not be symmetrical, with 50% of individuals exhibiting cortical drainage of venous blood mainly through the right internal jugular vein, and subcortical largely through the left. Two decades later, the measurement of cerebral oxygen consumption was improved using radioactive inert gases ^{85}Kr (Lassen *et al.*, 1963)] and ^{133}Xe (Harper & Glass, 1965) that allow extracranial imaging of gamma emission from the cerebral cortex. However, the aforementioned temporal resolution combined with potential problems of extra-cranial tissue sampling and inadequate desaturation are limitations that remain with these approaches.

The use of Doppler ultrasound was first described as early as 1959 for assessing blood velocity in the extracranial vessels (Miyazaki & Kato, 1965). The thickness of the skull bones greatly attenuates the penetration of ultrasonic waves making noninvasive use of the technique difficult. Ultrasound was therefore limited to surgical procedures, or to use in children with open fontanels. However, Aaslid *et al* (1982) demonstrated that the attenuation of sound by bone within the frequency range of 1-2MHz was far less than conventional frequencies of 3-12MHz. Indeed, insonation is possible through thinner regions of the skull, termed "acoustic" windows, making it feasible to measure static and dynamic blood velocities within the major cerebral arteries. For the first time, a non-invasive measure of beat-to-beat changes in blood velocity in the vessels of the brain with superior temporal resolution than indicator-dilution techniques was available. However, it is imperative to note that TCD cannot measure CBF *per se*. Rather, TCD measures the *velocity* of red blood cells within the insonated vessel. Moreover, only the larger basal arteries provide an adequate signal for measurement of cerebral blood velocity with TCD. Because these arteries tend to deliver oxygenated blood to large regional areas of the brain, TCD gives an index of global, rather than local, stimulus-response. This is an important distinction given that local changes in CBF likely differ (Hendrikse *et al.*, 2004; Nöth *et al.*, 2008; Piechnik *et al.*, 2008). Certainly, there is a notable dissimilarity in vasoreactivity across the cerebrovasculature. At least in hypercapnia, small vessels and capillaries possess much higher reactivity to CO_2 (Mandell *et al.*, 2008), and vasculature residing within gray matter show higher reactivity than vasculature within white matter (Nöth *et al.*, 2008; Piechnik *et al.*, 2008). This lack of spatial resolution in brain hemodynamics is the principal limitation of TCD. There are a variety of modern imaging techniques that allow sufficient spatial resolution to discern localized brain perfusion [see See Table (appendix) for a summary and (Wintermark *et al.*, 2005) for a detailed review].

3. The cerebrovascular exam

3.1 Recording principles

The principles of TCD are the same as extracranial Doppler ultrasound: the Doppler probe emits sound waves that are reflected off moving red blood cells, which are subsequently detected by the transducer. The resultant Doppler-shift is proportional to the velocity of the blood (DeWitt & Wechsler, 1988; Aaslid, 1986a). Duplex ultrasound (simultaneous two dimensional B-mode and pulse-wave velocity) typically used in vascular ultrasound to measure both vessel luminal diameter and blood velocity (and therefore volumetric flow; see Section VI) is not possible with current TCD systems due to lack of resolution. Because the diameter of the insonated vessel is unknown, TCD only measures cerebral blood velocity (CBV) *not* absolute volumetric flow. The velocity of blood through a vessel is proportional to the fourth power of vessel radius; the measurement of CBV by TCD assumes constant diameter of the insonated vessel - this assumption has been found to be valid in various studies (Serrador *et al.*, 2000; Bishop *et al.*, 1986; Nuttall *et al.*, 1996; Peebles *et al.*, 2008; ter Minassian *et al.*, 1998; Valdueza *et al.*, 1997). Despite these validations, however, it remains possible that the cerebral conduit vessels do, in fact, change diameter, and as such, any TCD data should be openly interpreted with this possibility in mind. In addition, other problems remain for meaningful velocity quantification. For example, the velocity of blood through a vessel - in the presence of laminar flow - is approximately parabolic in shape, with the fastest velocity in the center of the vessel. The Doppler signal consequently represents not a single value but rather a distribution of velocities, therefore requiring mathematical manipulation to extract meaningful velocity values. Typically, a power spectrum distribution is produced from segments of ~5 seconds using a Fast Fourier transform, and maximum or mean velocity is calculated from the maximum or intensity weighted mean, respectively (see Figure 2; Lohmann *et al.*, 2006; Aaslid, 1986b).

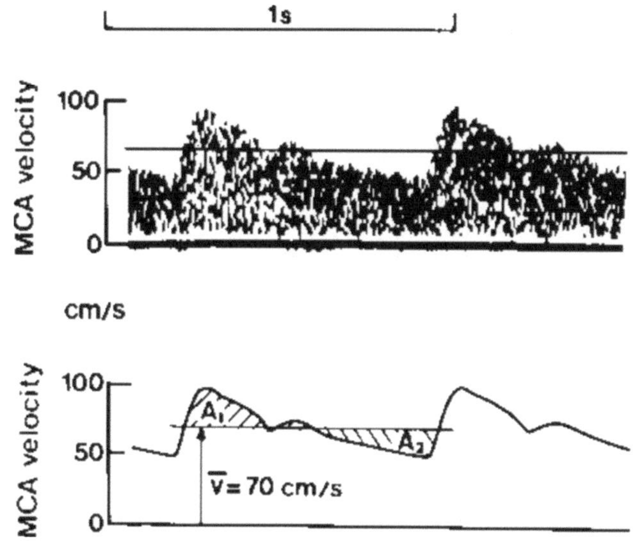

Fig. 2. (A) Spectral display of middle cerebral artery Doppler signal. (B) Maximal velocity outline of Doppler spectrum with the horizontal line representing the mean velocity and systolic and diastolic velocities above and below, respectively. Modified from Aaslid et al. J Neurosurg (1982) vol. 57 (6).

A frequency of 2MHz is typically used for TCD because higher frequencies do not sufficiently penetrate the bones of the skull (DeWitt & Wechsler, 1988; Aaslid *et al.*, 1982). Despite the increased penetration of TCD, an acoustic window in the skull is necessary for adequate insonation of intracerebral arteries. The choice of window, however, can dramatically affect the type of recording possible. For example, insonation through the transtemporal or foramen magnum windows allow use of a headpiece for securing the Doppler probe, whereas this is not possible when insonating through the optic canal.

Imaging modalities such as colour-coded Doppler and power Doppler, significantly increase the reliability of TCD as direct visualization of the target vessel facilitates better insonation angle correction (Martin *et al.*, 1995). Studies have demonstrated that the use of colour-coded and/or power TCD facilitates: (1) an improved signal-to-noise ratio with transcranial insonation (Postert *et al.*, 1997); (2) insonation in the presence of poor acoustic windows, particularly when combined with the use of contrast (Nabavi *et al.*, 1999; Gerriets *et al.*, 2000); (3) the measurement of arterial diameter threshold for collateral flow in the circle of Willis (Hoksbergen *et al.*, 2000); and, (4) an increase in the diagnostic sensitivity for cerebral vasospasm (Sloan *et al.*, 2004). Readers are referred to Willie et al., (2011b) for a detailed review of general TCD principles.

4. Regulation of cerebrovascular function

The cerebral vasculature rapidly adapts to changes in perfusion pressure (cerebral autoregulation; CA), regional metabolic requirements of the brain (neurovascular coupling), autonomic neural activity (Cassaglia *et al.*, 2009; Cassaglia *et al.*, 2008), and humoral factors (cerebrovascular reactivity). Regulation of CBF is highly controlled and involves a wide spectrum of regulatory mechanisms that together work to provide adequate oxygen and nutrient supply (Ainslie & Duffin, 2009; Ogoh & Ainslie, 2009a; Edvinsson & Krause, 2002; Panerai *et al.*, 1999a; Querido & Sheel, 2007); (Ainslie & Tzeng, 2010; Lucas *et al.*, 2010a). Indeed, the cerebral vasculature is highly sensitive to changes in arterial blood gases, in particular the partial pressure of arterial carbon dioxide ($PaCO_2$) (Ainslie & Duffin, 2009). It is thought that CA acts to change cerebral vascular resistance via vasomotor effectors, principally at the level of the cerebral arterioles and pial vessels (Edvinsson & Krause, 2002). Additionally, neuronal metabolism elicits an effect on CBF as necessitated by changes to regional oxygen consumption, with the sympathetic nervous system possibly playing a protective role in preventing over-perfusion in the cerebral vasculature ((Ainslie & Tzeng, 2010; Tzeng *et al.*, 2010a; Tzeng *et al.*, 2010b; Tzeng *et al.*, 2010c; Wilson *et al.*, 2010; Cassaglia *et al.*, 2009; Cassaglia *et al.*, 2008).

4.1 Regulation by arterial PCO_2

The cerebral vasculature is highly sensitive to changes in arterial blood gas pressures, in particular $PaCO_2$, which exerts a pronounced effect on CBF. Alveolar ventilation, by virtue of its direct effect on $PaCO_2$, is consequently tightly coupled to CBF. The response of CBF to $PaCO_2$ is of vital homeostatic importance as it directly influences central CO_2/pH, which is the central chemoreceptor stimulus (Chapman *et al.*, 1979). In response to increases in $PaCO_2$, vasodilation of downstream arterioles increases CBF. This, in turn, lowers $PaCO_2$ by increasing tissue washout, resulting in vessel constriction, and a subsequent decrease in CBF. Functional modulation of CBF by $PaCO_2$ influences pH at the level of the central chemoreceptors and directly implicates CBF in the central drive to breath (reviewed by Ainslie & Duffin, 2009; also see (Fan *et al.*, 2010a; Fan *et al.*, 2010b; Lucas *et al.*, 2010b). Indeed, previous studies have found a correlative link between blunted cerebrovascular CO_2 reactivity and the occurrence of central sleep apnea in patients with congestive heart failure (Xie *et al.*, 2005), and also in the pathophysiology of obstructive sleep apnea (Burgess *et al.*, 2010; Reichmuth *et al.*, 2009).

4.2 Regulation by arterial PO_2

Hypoxia is a cerebral vasodilator as reflected by a proportional increase in CBF with decreasing PaO_2 in conditions of isocapnia (Reviewed in (Ainslie & Ogoh, 2010). However, the resultant hyperventilation that accompanies hypoxic exposure yields hypocapnia that induces a counteracting cerebral vasoconstriction and decreased CBF. Indeed, a threshold of <40mmHg PO_2 is required in the face of prevailing hypocapnia for cerebral vasodilation to occur (Ainslie & Ogoh, 2010). This minor sensitivity is clinically relevant given the arterial hypoxemia encountered during exercise in elite athletes (Ogoh & Ainslie, 2009a; Ogoh & Ainslie, 2009b) and at high altitude (Ainslie & Ogoh, 2010) as well as in certain pathologies such as chronic lung disease and heart failure (reviewed in Ainslie & Ogoh, 2010 and Ainslie

& Duffin, 2009; See also: (Galvin *et al.*, 2010). The extent to which changes in cerebrovascular reactivity to hypoxia are related to pathological outcome is unknown. Moreover, unlike the CO_2 reactivity test, complex feedback (Kolb *et al.*, 2004; Ito *et al.*, 2008; Robbins *et al.*, 1982) or feed-forward (Slessarev *et al.*, 2007) gas manipulation techniques are needed to independently control $PaCO_2$ and PaO_2.

4.3 Neuronal metabolism and coupling

The effect of neural activity on CBF was demonstrated approximately 130 years ago in patients with skull defects (Mosso, 1880). Neurovascular coupling can be utilized as a sensitive method to test the function of cerebral vasculature. This activation–flow coupling describes a mechanism that adapts local CBF in accordance with the underlying neuronal activity (Girouard & Iadecola, 2006). The adaptation of regional CBF is based on local vasodilation evoked by neuronal activation, but the cellular mechanisms underlying neurovascular coupling are not fully understood. Synaptic activity has been shown to trigger an increase in the intracellular calcium concentration of adjacent astrocytes, which can lead to secretion of vasodilatory substances - such as epoxyeicosatrienoic acid, adenosine, nitric oxide, and cyclooxygenase-2 metabolites - from perivascular end-feet, resulting in increased local CBF (reviewed by Jakovcevic & Harder, 2007). Thus, astrocytes, via release of vasoactive molecules, may mediate the neuron-astrocyte-endothelial signaling pathway and play a profound role in coupling blood flow to neuronal activity (reviewed by (Iadecola & Nedergaard, 2007). Indeed, the 10-20% increase in CBF observed during aerobic exercise is likely due to combined elevations in cortical neuronal activity in addition to elevations in mean arterial pressure (MAP) and $PaCO_2$ (reviewed by (Ogoh & Ainslie, 2009a). Yet, even during exercise neurometabolic coupling with visual stimulation remains intact (Willie *et al.*, 2011a). The relative contribution of neurometabolic factors (i.e., neurovascular coupling) and systemic factors (i.e., increased $PaCO_2$ and blood pressure) is currently unknown.

4.4 Cerebral autoregulation

CBF is traditionally thought to remain relatively constant within a large range of blood pressures (60 to 150 mm Hg), at least in non-pathological situations (Lassen, 1959). This unique characteristic of the mammalian brain is known as cerebral autoregulation (CA). If CA fails, the brain is at risk of ischemic damage at low blood pressures or hemorrhage at high blood pressure. Preceding the advent of technologies with temporal resolution capable of measuring changes in CBF over the course of seconds, CA was measured under steady-state conditions (*See Section 2.1*). This "static" CA is a measure of cerebrovascular regulation of gradual changes in perfusion pressure. Traditionally, static CA was believed to hold CBF constant through a MAP range of ~60-150 mmHg (Lassen, 1959), but this concept has been recently challenged with evidence to support CBF closely paralleling changes in blood pressure (Lucas *et al.*, 2010a). Furthermore, static CA through this supposed autoregulatory range is difficult to assess because the upper range of blood pressures can only be achieved in healthy individuals using relatively high-dose pharmacological intervention. Indeed, we and others, have found that induction of hypertension using continuous phenylephrine infusion produces cardiotoxic effects on ECG, limiting MAP increases to <120 mmHg. Moreover, pharmacologically induced changes in BP also cause marked changes in ventilation; thus, the confounding influence of arterial PCO_2 needs to be considered. The extent to which a normal healthy human can cope with extreme static changes in BP is unknown for obvious reasons. Regardless, even within the "autoregulatory range", static autoregulation appears to be influenced by blood pressure (Immink *et al.*, 2008; Lucas *et al.*, 2010a).

Dynamic CA (*d*CA) describes the ability of the cerebral vasculature to resist *acute* changes in perfusion pressure, (due to changes in arterial blood pressure) over a short time-course of less than five seconds (Zhang *et al.*, 1998). *d*CA can be quantified from either spontaneous fluctuations in MAP, or from stimulus-induced changes in MAP. With increased utilization of TCD a number of methods of MAP perturbation and *d*CA quantification have been developed.

That CBF appears to vary directly with MAP, suggests that arterial baroreflex regulation of peripheral blood pressure likely plays a more significant role in CBF control than previously thought (Lucas *et al.* (2010a). Moreover, Tzeng *et al* (2010a) showed an inverse relationship between cardiac baroreflex sensitivity and *d*CA, suggesting the presence of compensatory interactions between peripheral blood pressure and central CBF control mechanisms, directed to optimizing CBF control. Such interactions may account for the divergent changes in CA and baroreflex sensitivity seen with normal aging, and in clinical conditions such as spontaneous hypertension (Serrador *et al.*, 2005), autonomic failure (Hetzel *et al.*, 2003), and chronic hypotension (Duschek *et al.*, 2009). Some evidence also suggests that free radicals - particularly superoxide anion observed in pathologies such as ischemic and traumatic brain injury - causes impaired CA and increased basal CBF through activation of potassium channels within vascular smooth muscle cells (Zagorac *et al.*, 2005).

5. Assessment of cerebrovascular function

In this section we provide a practical overview of methods used to assess cerebral autoregulation (CA) including the use of suprasystolic thigh cuff, postural alterations, lower body negative or oscillatory pressure, the Valsalva maneuver, the Oxford technique and transfer function analysis.

5.1 Suprasystolic thigh cuffs

The rapid release of thigh cuffs inflated to suprasystolic pressures for ≥2 minutes elicits a transient hypotension (Aaslid *et al.*, 1989; Mahony *et al.*, 2000; Tiecks *et al.*, 1995a). The rate of regulation (RoR), quantifies the rate at which cerebrovascular resistance (CVR), or conductance changes in response to a perturbation in MAP and can be given by Equation 1:

$$\text{RoR} = (\Delta\text{CVR}/\Delta t)/\Delta\text{MAP}$$

where ΔCVR is given by $\text{MCAv}_{\text{mean}}/\text{MAP}$, and ΔMAP by control $\text{MAP-MAP}_{\text{mean}}$. Δt is taken as the 2.5 second period one second following thigh cuff release (Figure 3).

This time interval was originally put forth by Aaslid *et al* (Aaslid *et al.*, 1989) based on two factors: (1) the change in CVR is relatively linear during this period, allowing a slope of the response to be taken; and, (2) it was thought that the latency of the baroreflex response was such that within the first 3.5 seconds of the cerebrovascular response to a hypotensive

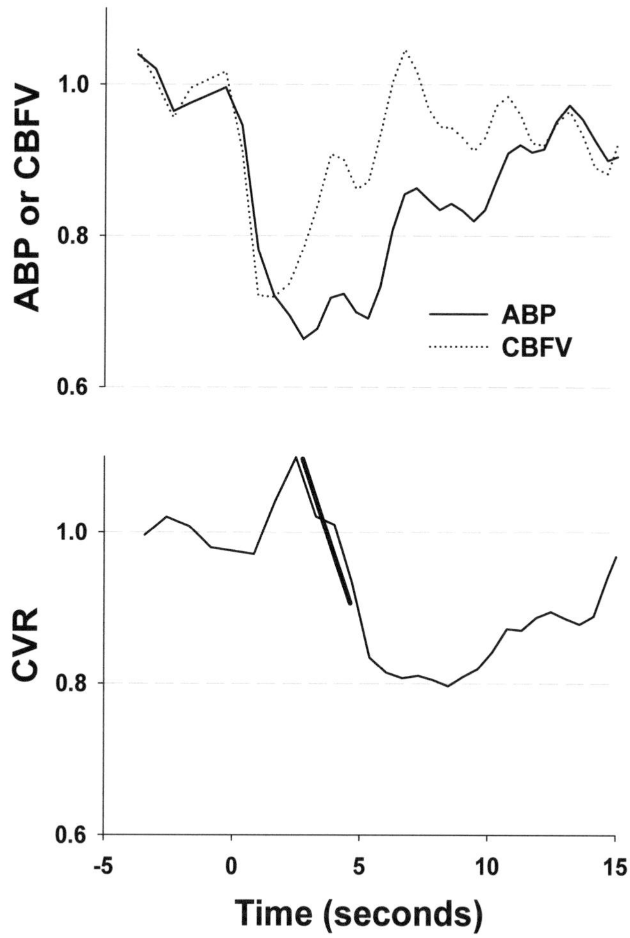

Fig. 3. Typical changes in arterial blood pressure (ABP), cerebral blood flow-velocity (CBFV) and cerebrovascular reactivity (CVR) in response to thigh cuff deflation, for determining dynamic cerebral autoregulation (CA). All tracings are shown in normalized units relative to control pre-release values from -4 to 0 seconds. Straight line (bold line) through CVR (bottom figure) curve is determined by regression analysis of data obtained in the interval from 1 to 3.5 seconds after thigh cuff release and is used for calculating rate of regulation (RoR).

challenge, only cerebrovascular mechanisms (i.e., *d*CA) would be involved in regulation of CBF. However, the drop in arterial pressure following thigh cuff deflation engages the arterial baroreflex within 0.44 seconds of baroreceptor unloading by neck pressure (Eckberg, 1980) causing transient tachycardia. Although unilateral thigh cuff deflation was reported to not alter central venous pressure (Fadel *et al.*, 2001), unpublished observations from our laboratory indicate this may not be the case for bilateral thigh-cuff release. It is unclear, consequently, how cardiac output is affected following bilateral thigh-cuff release. Some authors (Ogoh *et al.*, 2003; Ogoh *et al.*, 2007), but not all (Deegan *et al.*, 2010), have reported that increases in cardiac output can augment CBF; thus, it is plausible that baroreflex function may exert a modulating influence on dynamic CBF regulation such that RoR reflects the integrated response of both the baroreflex and *d*CA (Ogoh *et al.*, 2009). The thigh cuff technique is also somewhat painful, with inflation often associated with an increase in MAP that is maintained until cuff release. The influence of sympathetic nervous system activity in response to discomfort is not known, but a minimum 8-minute recovery period has been recommended following cuff deflation (Mahony *et al.*, 2000).

Another prevalent method to quantify the *d*CA response to thigh cuff release, termed the autoregulatory index, was proffered by Tiecks *et al* (1995a). This approach uses a second order differential equation to relate changes in MAP and three predefined model parameters (T: time constant; D: damping factor; and *k*: autoregulatory gain) to generate ten templates of CBV-response to a non-pharmacologically induced transient hypotension (Figure 4). Typically, rapid thigh-cuff deflation is used to induce a transient hypotension. According to the Tiecks model, the autoregulatory index assigns an integer value to each of ten template curves (0-9). These coefficients are generated using a second-order linear differential equation:

$$dP_n = \frac{\text{MAP} - \text{MAP}_{\text{base}}}{\text{MAP}_{\text{base}} - \text{CCP}}$$

$$x2_n = x2_{n-1} + \frac{(x1_n - 2D \cdot x2_{n-1})}{f \cdot T}$$

$$x1_n = x1_{n-1} + \frac{(dP_n - x2_{n-1})}{f \cdot T}$$

$$mV_n = \text{MCAv}_{\text{base}} \cdot (1 + dP_n - k \cdot x2_n)$$

where dP_n is the normalized change in mean arterial blood pressure (MAP) relative to baseline MAP (MAP_{base}) and adjusted for estimated critical closing pressure (CCP); $x2_n$ and

A

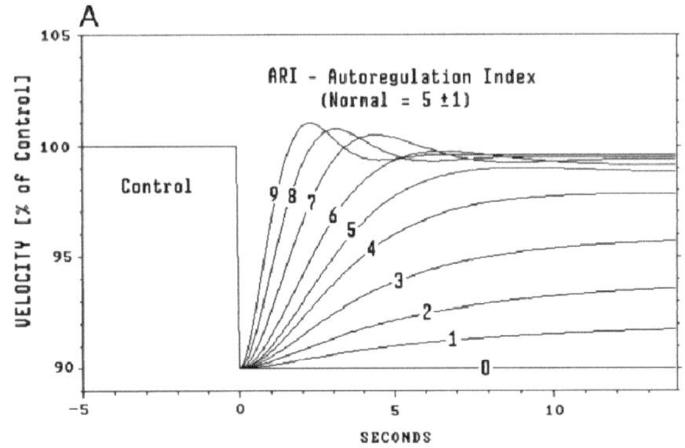

B

T, s	D	K	ARI	dROR, %/s
...	0.00	0	0	0 (No autoregulation)
2.00	1.60	0.20	1	2.5
2.00	1.50	0.40	2	5.0
2.00	1.15	0.60	3	10.0
2.00	0.90	0.80	4	15.0
1.90	0.75	0.90	5	20.0 ("Normal" autoregulation)
1.60	0.65	0.94	6	30.0
1.20	0.55	0.96	7	40.0
0.87	0.52	0.97	8	60.0
0.65	0.50	0.98	9	80.0 (Fastest autoregulation)

Fig. 4. (A) Responses of CA model (ARI) to step changes in blood pressure. The CBFV response curve model with 10 different degrees of dynamic CA is calculated by this method. 9 is the highest degree of dynamic CA. (B) Tabular comparison of ARI, and associated constants, with percentage RoR; T indicates time constant; D, damping factor; K, autoregulatory dynamic gain; ARI, autoregulation index; and dROR, dynamic rate of regulation.

$x1_n$ are state variables (equal to 0 at baseline); mV_n is modeled mean velocity; $MCAv_{base}$ is baseline $MCAv_{mean}$; f is the sampling frequency, and n is the sample number. The mV_n generated from ten predefined combinations of parameters T (time constant), D (dampening factor) and k (autoregulatory gain) that best fit the actual $MCAv_{mean}$ recording is taken as an index of dynamic CA. A value of 0 represents no autoregulation where CBV passively follows perfusion pressure, and a value of 9 represents perfect CA where changes in perfusion pressure produce no alteration to CBV. The autoregulatory index has also been derived from spontaneously occurring blood pressure and cerebral blood vessel velocity fluctuations using transfer function analysis (Panerai *et al.*, 1999a; Panerai *et al.*, 2001). However, the validity of comparison between a linear model and that from a transient hypotensive stimulus may be questionable (see *Transfer function analysis* below).

5.2 Postural alterations

Because of the confounders inherent to both pharmacological and non-physiological methods of BP alteration (e.g., thigh-cuff release) postural maneuvers to alter blood pressure have been utilized for CA assessment. The simple act of standing from a sitting, supine, or squat position is enough to elicit a transient drop in BP of ~35 mmHg and associated drop in CBV (Thomas *et al.*, 2009; Murrell *et al.*, 2009; Murrell *et al.*, 2007). RoR (Sorond *et al.*, 2005), ARI, and transfer function analysis (Claassen *et al.*, 2009) have all been used to quantify the *d*CA response to postural changes in BP.

5.3 Valsalva maneuver

Forced expiration against a closed glottis regularly occurs during normal daily activities such as during defecation and lifting. The Valsalva maneuver has been well described in the literature (Smith *et al.*, 1996; Tiecks *et al.*, 1996) and consists of four phases: (1) increased MAP due to increased intrathoracic pressure; (2a) impaired atrial filling and resultant drop in MAP, followed by; (2b) a baroreceptor mediated tachycardia and increase in MAP; (3) release of strain and drop in intrathoracic pressure which decreases MAP; and (4) baroreceptor mediated sympathetic activity that drives MAP above baseline in the face of transient hypotension. Due to impaired atrial filling, combined with raised intracranial pressure induced by increased intrathoracic pressure during strain, there is a marked decrease in cerebral perfusion pressure during the onset of phase 2a. This drop in perfusion pressure provides an adequate stimulus for measurement of *d*CA (Tiecks *et al.*, 1996; Tiecks *et al.*, 1995b; Zhang *et al.*, 2002). The Valsalva maneuver may, however, be confounded by its inherent physiological complexity. Changes in $PaCO_2$ are likely to occur over the course of the breath-hold, and although it has been suggested that there is sufficient time delay between changes in end-tidal PCO_2 ($PetCO_2$) and subsequent changes in CBF to preclude the breath-hold from effecting measured values of CA, this is not known for certain (Hetzel *et al.*, 2003). Furthermore, changes in intrathoracic pressure likely vary between individuals, and throughout the maneuver there are changes in intracranial pressure, venous outflow pressure and resistance. And though there is a period of relatively stable intracranial pressure, the possibility of these changes confounding measures of CA certainly exist. Nonetheless, Tiecks *et al* (1996) described the Valsalva ARI as the ratio between the relative changes in cerebral blood flow velocities and blood pressure, calculated as:

$$ARI_{Valsalva} = ((CBFV(iv)/CBFV(i)/(BP(iv)/BP(i))$$

where I and IV signify phases one and four of the Valsalva response, respectively. CBF is modified proportionally more than BP, implying that autoregulation is preserved, if the ratio is found to be >1. Because minor variations in expiratory pressure results in changes in the various stages of the maneuver, it is imperative to standardize the technique between and within subjects.

5.4 Transfer function analysis

Transfer function analysis (TFA) for the assessment of dynamic CA is based on analysis of the coherence, frequency and phase components of spontaneous changes in MAP, and the resultant degree to which these changes are reflected in CBV (Zhang *et al.*, 1998). It is thought that CA acts as a high pass-filter, effectively dampening low-frequency oscillations (<0.07Hz) (Panerai *et al.*, 1998; Zhang *et al.*, 1998). An advantage to this method is the ability to complete the measurement in a subject at baseline without the need for any pharmacological or physiological manipulation of BP. However, the corollary is that TFA cannot be used to analyze the CA response to a transient and directional change in BP (i.e., it cannot distinguish between "upward" and "downward" fluctuations in BP). Furthermore, TFA assumes that the dynamic autoregulatory responses to spontaneous fluctuations in BP are linear. This is to say that TFA assumes CA is equally effective in attenuating changes in cerebral perfusion in response to both hyper and hypotensive changes in MAP; however, this may not be the case (Aaslid *et al.*, 2007; Tzeng *et al.*, 2010b). If hysteresis is a natural characteristic of CA (i.e., differential CA depending on directionality of the blood pressure change), than the assumptions of linear techniques such as TFA may not be valid. An extension of TFA is impulse response analysis, whereby spontaneous changes in MAP are inversely transformed back to the time domain (Panerai, 2008). In other words, the impulse response function is an inverse algorithm of the Fast Fourier analysis of frequency shifts of blood velocity, as a time domain function. This allows time-domain models such as the ARI to be applied to spontaneous data (Czosnyka *et al.*, 2009). Again, if the CA response is not linear, comparison of ARI's generated from linear models, to those generated from a transient hypotensive or hypertensive stimulus, may also not be valid. A limitation of CA assessment using spontaneous data is the small magnitude and inconsistency of spontaneous pressure oscillations (Taylor *et al.*, 1998).See Table (appendix).

5.5 The Oxford technique

The Oxford technique is the method of using vasoactive drug injections (most often phenylephrine hydrochloride and sodium nitroprusside; the modified Oxford technique) to provoke baroreflex responses, and has been widely used since (Smyth *et al.*, 1969) utilized bolus angiotensin injected intravenously during wakefulness and sleep; the R-R interval response to changes in arterial BP provides an index of cardiac baroreflex sensitivity. Despite its prevalence in baroreflex research until recently, the technique had not been utilized for assessment of CA, despite providing some distinct advantages in CA quantification. Blood pressure can be raised or lowered, allowing both positive and negative CA gains to be assessed independently - an important consideration given evidence that CA may be more effective at dealing with increases in blood pressure than decreases in blood pressure (Aaslid *et al.*, 2007; Tzeng *et al.*, 2010b). The Oxford technique is also largely painless, reducing the influence of pain induced sympathetic activity. *d*CA is quantified by taking the slope of the linear regression between CBV and MAP - the slope is inversely proportional to the efficacy of cerebral autoregulation in maintaining CBV. This is to say, a slope of zero would imply perfect autoregulation where CBF remains constant across the entire range of MAP, while a gain equal to 1 would reflect the total absence of autoregulation (Tzeng *et al.*, 2010b). The limitations inherent to any pharmacological approach remain manifest with this technique, and although there is supportive evidence (Greenfield & Tindall, 1968) the assumption that there is no direct drug-effect on the cerebral vasculature has been questioned (Brassard *et al.*, 2010). However, direct effects of PE and SNP on cerebral vasculature are considered unlikely given that the blood-brain barrier normally prevents endogenous circulating catecholamine from binding to α_1-adrenoreceptors in small cerebral vessels (Ainslie & Tzeng, 2010; MacKenzie *et al.*, 1976; McCalden *et al.*, 1977).

5.6 Oscillating blood pressure

A criticism of TFA is that it analyses relatively small natural swings in blood pressure. Coherence between pressure and CBF is often low (<0.5) making it difficult to ascertain the statistical and TFA model reliability, as well as the causal relationship between these variables. These difficulties have been partially overcome by inducing large-amplitude blood pressure oscillations through either repeated squat-standing or oscillatory lower body negative pressure at frequencies associated with CA (Claassen *et al.*, 2009; Hamner *et al.*, 2004). See Figure 5 for detailed explication of this technique.

5.7 Cerebrovascular reactivity

Cerebrovascular reactivity gives an index of reactivity of the intracranial vessels in response to a stimulus - typically either pharmaceutical (e.g., acetazolamide) or through ventilatory alterations of $PaCO_2$. There is differential reactivity to CO_2 across the cerebral vasculature. Cerebrovascular CO_2 reactivity assessed by TCD gives a global measure of reactivity compared to more sophisticated techniques such as pulsed arterial spin labeling MRI and positron emission tomography that both allow a specific brain area to be assessed. Typically, a hypercapnic stimulus is utilized to assess reactivity, and using TCD to assess CBV reactivity can be given by:

$$CA = \Delta CBV(\Delta PetCO_2)^{-1}$$

Similarly, volitional hyperventilation can be utilized decrease $PetCO_2$, such that reactivity to hypo and hypercapnia can be assessed. From a clinical perspective, impairment of cerebrovascular reactivity to CO_2 - as assessed by TCD - has been linked to such pathologies as obstructive and central sleep apnea (Burgess *et al.*, 2010; Reichmuth *et al.*, 2009), carotid artery stenosis (Widder *et al.*, 1994), hypertension (Serrador *et al.*, 2005), congestive heart failure (Xie *et al.*, 2005), and cerebral ischemic events (Wijnhoud *et al.*, 2006). It is also an established independent predictor of ischemic stroke (Markus & Cullinane, 2001; Silvestrini *et al.*, 2000; Vernieri *et al.*, 2001).

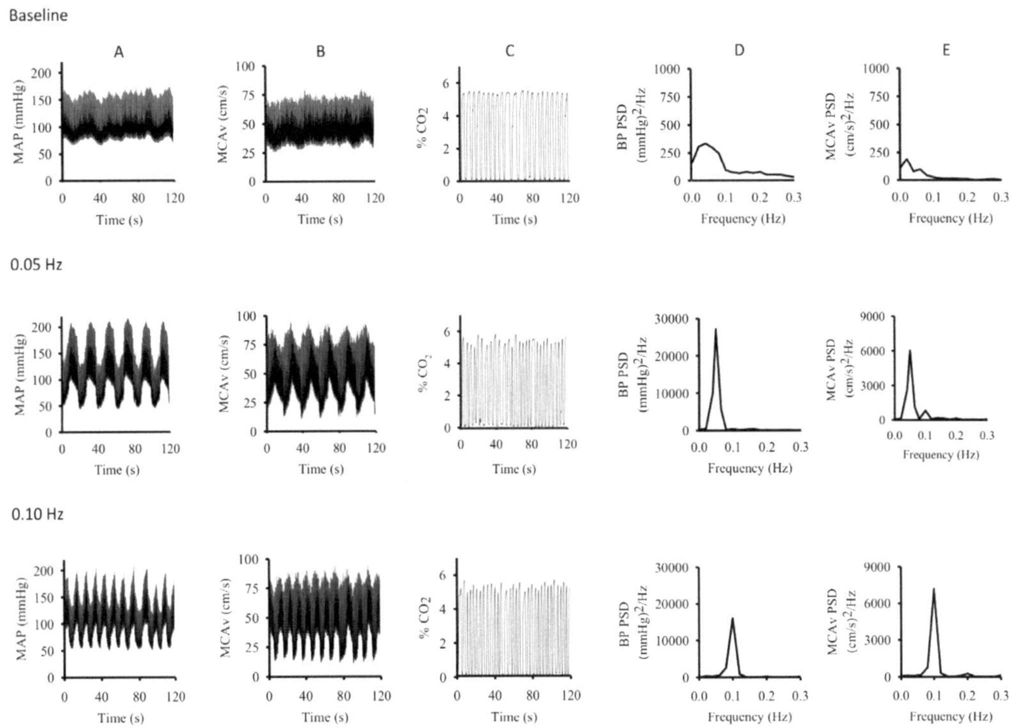

Fig. 5. Effects of repeated squat-stand maneuvers on (**A**) mean arterial blood pressure (Finapres; MAP), (**B**) middle cerebral artery blood velocity (Transcranial Doppler; MCAv), and (**C**) end-tidal CO_2. Raw waveforms are shown from a representative individual at rest (baseline, top row) and during repeated squat-stand maneuvers at 0.05 Hz (5-s squat, 5-s stand; middle row), and 0.1 Hz (10-s squat, 10-s stand; bottom row). A total of 600 s is displayed at rest and at 0.1 and 0.05 Hz; over the 120 s, 6 and 12 full cycles of the 0.05 and 0.1 Hz maneuvers occur, respectively. Note: 1) the large and coherent oscillations in MAP and MCAv during these maneuvers relative to resting conditions; 2) despite the strong hemodynamic effects, there is no distortion of MCAv and MAP waveforms; 3) end-tidal PCO_2 is well maintained; 4) the influence of 'targeting' 0.05Hz and 0.01Hz frequency ranges on blood pressure (BP) and MCAv power spectral densities (panels (**D**) and (**E**) respectfully). For example, the repeated squat-stand maneuvers at 0.05 results in a 40-fold increases in BP spectral power (compared with spontaneous VLF oscillations), while at 0.1 Hz, a 100-fold increase occurs relative to spontaneous LF oscillations. These augmented oscillations in BP led to 20-, and 100-fold increases in MCAv spectral power at 0.05, and 0.1 Hz, respectively. Thus increases in MCAv oscillations are relatively smaller than increases in BP oscillations at 0.05 Hz but not at 0.1 Hz, indicating more effective damping at the lower frequencies. Importantly, the coherence between BP and MCAv is typically much higher for repeated squat-stand maneuvers than for spontaneous oscillations (e.g., range (n=8): 0.6 to 0.99 vs 0.2 to 0.6, respectively). Thus, large oscillations in BP and MCAv induced during repeated squat-stand maneuvers not only provided strong and physiologically relevant hemodynamic perturbations, but also led to improved estimation of transfer function to assess dynamic cerebral autoregulation at the very low and low frequencies.

Acetazolamide can also be used to assess cerebrovascular reactivity. Acetazolamide inhibits carbonic anhydrase, the enzyme responsible for reversible catalyzation of H_2CO_3 formation from CO_2 + H_2O. Consequently it increases tissue PCO_2, leads to metabolic acidosis, and increased CBF. Although the exact mechanisms of acetazolamide-induced increases in CBF are not fully understood they likely involve both metabolic factors and direct as well as indirect vascular effects (Pickkers *et al.*, 2001); and reviewed by Settakis *et al.*, 2003). The use of acetazolamide for cerebrovascular reactivity assessment necessitates intravenous administration. However, in this form the drug can be costly, and depending on the country, difficult to procure. Regardless, confounds associated with cerebrovascular reactivity quantification using acetazolamide are not well understood, but it may directly effect the cerebral vasculature and can indirectly drive increased ventilation, which when combined with the need for intravenous administration and high-cost, makes acetazolamide less utilized than alteration of inspired CO_2. Regardless of the stimulus used, when assessing cerebrovascular reactivity, an absolute measurement of CBV is not as important as resolution of beat-to-beat changes in CBF from a pre-stimulus baseline.

5.8 Neurovascular coupling

Functional hyperemia describes the increased CBF to active areas of the brain where the demand for both nutrient delivery, and clearance of metabolic by-products is increased. The functional anatomy of the brain allows this neurovascular coupling to be easily and reliably examined by measurement of the sensorimotor or cognitive stimulatory effects on CBV – a method termed functional TCD (fTCD; Figure 6). This technique was first utilized by Aaslid *et al* (1987) who showed that blood velocity in the PCA changed with visual stimulation (see Hubel & Wiesel, 2005 for a comprehensive report of visual system physiology), but there are numerous studies in the neuro-cognitive literature that demonstrate consistent CBF changes in response to cognitive, verbal, and motor tasks (Rosengarten *et al.*, 2003; Aaslid, 1987; Deppe *et al.*, 2004; Klingelhöfer *et al.*, 1997; Silvestrini *et al.*, 1993; Stroobant & Vingerhoets, 2000).

Despite the poor spatial resolution inherent to TCD, many studies have examined the relationship between cognitive activation and CBF. For example, chronic hypotension depresses cognitive activity (Jegede *et al.*, 2009; Duschek *et al.*, 2008; Duschek & Schandry, 2007). Conversely, cognitive activity can be improved with pharmacological treatment of hypotension (Duschek *et al.*, 2007). These studies demonstrate that cognitive activity is positively related to neural tissue oxygen delivery, but the scope of fTCD is very broad. Studies have examined the effect of pharmacological agents (Rosengarten *et al.*, 2002a), Type I diabetes (Rosengarten *et al.*, 2002b), Alzheimer's disease (Rosengarten *et al.*, 2007), voluntary movements (Orlandi & Murri, 1996; Sitzer *et al.*, 1994), hemispheric language lateralization (Knecht *et al.*, 1998b; Dorst *et al.*, 2008; Markus & Boland, 1992; Knecht *et al.*, 1998a; Knecht *et al.*, 1998b), emotional processing (Troisi *et al.*, 1999), and attentional processes (Schnittger *et al.*, 1996; Schnittger *et al.*, 1997; Helton *et al.*, 2007; Knecht *et al.*, 1997) on neurovascular coupling. It has also been well characterized in clinical populations (Silvestrini *et al.*, 1993; Silvestrini *et al.*, 1995; Silvestrini *et al.*, 1998; Silvestrini *et al.*, 2000; Thie *et al.*, 1992; Njemanze, 1991; Bruneau *et al.*, 1992), and may be a useful paradigm for the evaluation of cerebrovascular function in certain disease states (Boms *et al.*, 2010).

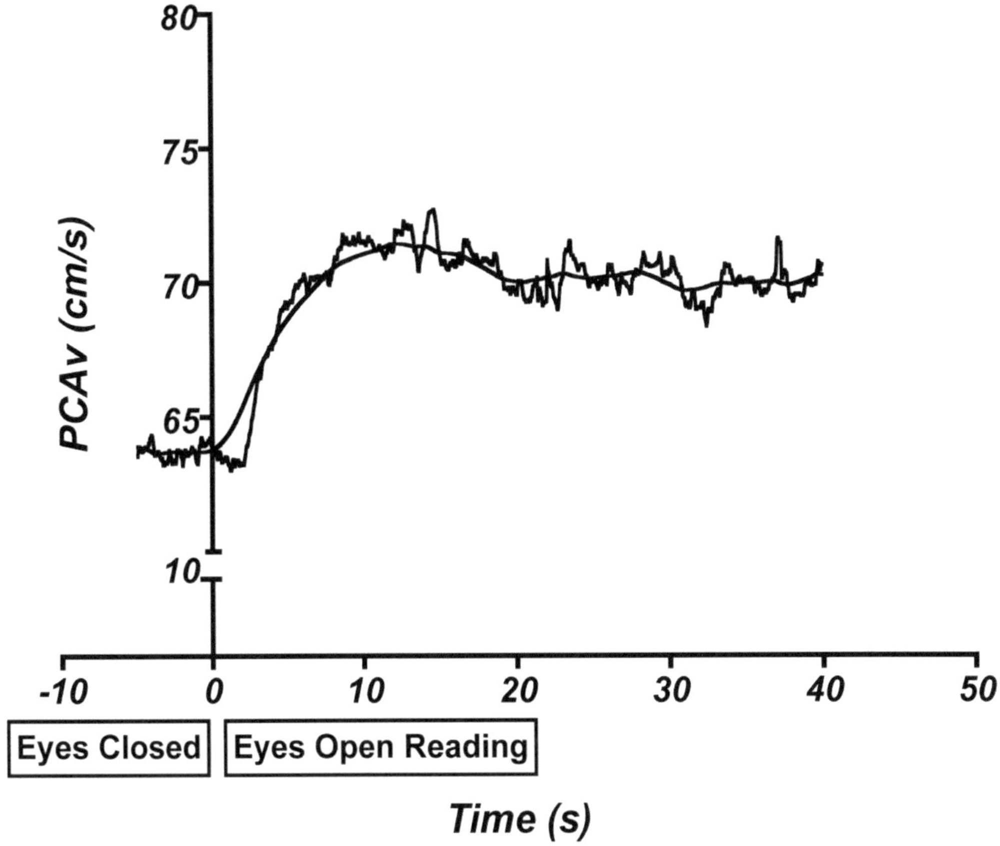

Fig. 6. Mean time course of peak systolic PCAv during visual stimulation (reading) while at upright-seated rest in 10 healthy young volunteers. Smooth line generated by locally weighted polynomial regression.

5.9 Estimation of intracranial and critical closing pressure using TCD

The critical closing pressure is the theoretical pressure at which blood flow within the cerebral vessels drops to zero, due to failure of the transmural pressure across a vessel to counteract the tension created by the vessel's smooth muscle. Measures of cerebrovascular resistance or compliance assume proportional linearity between blood flow and pressure, and that flow through a vessel ceases when the pressure is zero. Aaslid et al. (Aaslid *et al.*, 2003) demonstrated in humans that flow stops due to vessel collapse when perfusion pressure remains positive, making CCP a potentially better measure of cerebrovascular tone. CCP can be estimated by extrapolation of the CBV - blood pressure relationship to the pressure at which zero flow would theoretically occur. However, regardless of whether the entire pressure and velocity waveforms are used (Aaslid *et al.*, 2003), or the systolic and diastolic values only (Ogoh *et al.*, 2010), this technique typically yields an underestimate of CCP. Indeed, in some individuals the estimated CCP may even be negative, which is difficult to interpret physiologically. Furthermore, most studies have used peripheral blood pressure recordings that do not take into account pulse wave amplification in the periphery, which further contaminate CCP estimation. The reader is referred to (Panerai, 2003) for a detailed review of the concept.

6. Clinical applicability of TCD

The low cost, excellent temporal resolution, and bedside availability of TCD make it an ideal tool for clinical diagnosis of acute and chronic cerebrovascular diseases. The principle area of clinical application of TCD is the assessment of pathologies that alter blood velocity within the intracranial arteries or veins. We particularly focus on vasospasm, stenosis, intracranial occlusions, thrombosis, critical closing pressure, brain death, and patent foramen ovale.

6.1 Vasospasm

Vasospasm is observed as a complication of subarachnoid hemorrhage with an incidence ranging between 30% and 70% depending if the vasospasm is symptomatic or angiographic, respectively. Because blood velocity within a vessel is inversely proportional to its cross-sectional area, the primary pathological condition that affects flow-velocity is vasospasm, which is therefore detectable with TCD (Aaslid *et al.*, 1982). Vasospasm can remain asymptomatic, but the factors leading to symptom presentation are largely unknown. Although diagnosis of vasospasm requires the presence of hyperaemia in addition to increased blood flow velocities (see the Lindegaard index, below), at least within the MCA, threshold values of MCAv are fairly well accepted. Velocities between 120 and 200 cm/s are indicative of a reduction in lumen diameter between 25% and 50%, and serious vasospasm and lumen diameter reduction greater than 50% is indicated with velocities above 200 cm/s (Tsivgoulis *et al.*, 2009). Hyperaemia must also be present to diagnose vasospasm; the Lindegaard Index is a ratio between the mean flow velocity in the MCA and that in the ICA, where values greater than 6 indicate severe vasospasm, between 3 and 6 indicate moderate vasospasm, and less than 3, hyperaemia (Rasulo *et al.*, 2008). The disadvantage of using the Lindegaard ratio is that it assumes a dichotomous condition - where there is either vasospasm or not - which may be misleading in certain patients. A promising diagnostic criterion is the use of a daily increase in the systolic pressure of more than 50 cm/sec; this avoids dichotomous classification of vasospasm, informs about the physiopathological trend towards vasospasm, thereby allowing the early identification of patients at risk. To further increase the accuracy of transcranial Doppler in the identification of cerebral vasospasm, thresholds in mean velocities of more than 160 cm/sec have accurately diagnosed cerebral vasospasm (Mascia *et al.*, 2003).

6.2 Stenosis

Typically TCD does not provide sufficient data for accurate identification of stenosis of a cerebral vessel, particularly in the posterior vessels that are more tortuous and have greater anatomic variability. Diagnosis of stenosis using TCD requires: (1) acceleration of flow velocity through the stenotic segment, 2) decrease in velocity below the stenotic segment, (3) bilateral asymmetry in flow, and (4) disturbances in flow (i.e., turbulence and murmurs) (Rasulo *et al.*, 2008). Diagnosis of stenosis using TCD has greater sensitivity and specificity in the anterior than in the posterior circulation due to the lower anatomic variability and relative ease of insonation of the anterior vessels.

6.3 Intracranial occlusion

TCD has excellent utility in diagnosis of occlusion within the cerebral vessels with sensitivity and specificity over 90% - particularly in patients where cerebral ischemia is present (Camerlingo *et al.*, 1993). Diagnosis is through absence or a profound reduction of flow at the normal position and depth, and/or consequent lack of signal for the vessels in the immediate vicinity of the occluded region. Furthermore, due to its non-invasiveness, TCD can easily be used to track the progression of an occlusion both before and after treatment (Rasulo *et al.*, 2008). Furthermore, recent data suggest an independent effect of the ultrasound in augmenting the thrombolysis of the occlusion in patients with acute MCA thrombosis (Eggers *et al.*, 2003; Eggers *et al.*, 2009). The Clotbust trial (Alexandrov *et al.*, 2004) demonstrated that the presence of residual flow signal, dampened waveform, and microembolic signals prior to thrombolysis was associated with increased likelihood of complete recanalisation after thrombolysis. Furthermore, in patients with acute ischemic stroke, continuous TCD significantly increased tissue plasminogen activator-induced arterial recanalization (Alexandrov, 2009). See (Alexandrov, 2006) for a review of the use of TCD in thrombolytic treatment of stroke.

6.4 Sickle cell disease and risk of arterial thrombosis

Sickle cell disease is associated with an increased risk of stroke in children (Adams *et al.*, 1998). Level I evidence has been established for the use of TCD in the diagnostic screening of patients with sickle cell anemia. A MCAv threshold of 170 cm/sec was identified as indicative for the need of blood transfusion, such that a 30% reduction in circulating hemoglobin-s was achieved (Adams *et al.*, 1997). A randomized trial subsequently demonstrated that application of the above Doppler criteria yielded a 92% absolute reduction in the risk of stroke in children (Adams *et al.*, 1998). Additionally, reference CBV values were recently outlined for the purpose of screening for intracranial vessel narrowing in children with sickle cell disease (Krejza *et al.*, 2000).

6.5 Brain death

Electroencephalography or angiography can be utilized for clinical diagnosis of brain death. Angiography is typically preferred because EEG gives little information regarding brainstem function and signals can be difficult to attain within the intensive care unit. However, angiography requires injectable contrast media, and cannot be completed bedside at all. Typically, increased intracranial pressure concomitant with brain death reduces diastolic blood flow velocity in the intracerebral vessels. Further increases in intracranial pressure produce reversed flow during diastole in the circle of Willis, and finally, spiked and reverberating flow is considered indicative of brain death (de Freitas & André, 2006; Ropper *et al.*, 1987; Tsivgoulis *et al.*, 2009).

6.6 Shunt and emboli detection

In the presence of right-to-left cardiac shunt microbubbles injected into the venous circulation - that are largely filtered out in the lungs - will appear in the cerebral circulation within 5-15 seconds. There are reports of up to 100% sensitivity in right-to-left shunt detection (Droste *et al.*, 2002); however, it seems unlikely that the TCD technique can differentiate between various forms of shunt. For example, that microbubbles appear in the systemic circulation could be indicative of a patent foramen ovale, pulmonary arteriovenous malformation, or an atrial septal defect. But given that up to 60% of the normal population may present with right-to-left shunt of either intracardiac or pulmonary arteriovenous malformations (Woods *et al.*, 2010), an inexpensive means of screening such as TCD, as part of a diagnostic battery, may be very useful.

Both gaseous and solid microemboli can be detected using TCD through recognition of irregularities within the Doppler signal (Padayachee *et al.*, 1987; Deverall *et al.*, 1988; Ringelstein *et al.*, 1998). Although these microemboli are often clinically silent, their detection may be of prognostic value in assessing risk of stroke, and of use during cardiac or vascular surgeries where gaseous emboli may originate from the oxygenator. The detection of emboli using TCD is complicated and relies on 10 technical parameters and Ringelstein *et al.* provide a detailed description of the technique (Ringelstein *et al.*, 1998). There is some difficulty in distinguishing between gaseous and solid emboli. This is of clinical importance as each has distinct clinical relevance, particularly in cases where both types of emboli may be present (e.g., mechanical heart valve patients, patients with carotid stenosis (reviewed in: (Rodriguez *et al.*, 2009; Markus & Punter, 2005).

7. Utility of assessment of neck artery blood flow

Measurement of CBF by quantification of inflowing blood through the neck is not a new technique, but has not seen the prolific utilization of TCD or MRI, for example. Nonetheless, the technique has recently seen a resurgent popularity because it facilitates estimation of both flow proper (as opposed to blood velocity), and regional distribution of CBF during a variety of conditions (exercise, standing, environmental stress, etc.) not possible with MRI. The technique is nonetheless especially prone to measurement error, both for technical reasons and because of the apparent ease with which an untrained individual can pick up a vascular ultrasound probe, image a carotid artery, and believe the resulting measurement is accurate.

The aim of this section is to outline the virtues and caveats of the measurement of CBF via quantification of neck artery blood flow using high-resolution vascular ultrasound. First, we will discuss the vascular anatomy providing blood to the head. Then, we will address principals of linear vascular ultrasound, methods of analysis, sources of measurement error and our perspective on the appropriate use of the technique. Finally, the utility of the technique will be discussed in conjunction with an overview of the current literature.

7.1 The arteries of the neck

Early Greek physicians termed the principal arteries of the neck Karatides, after the adjective for stupefying, because their compression yielded unconsciousness. Such were these vessels' importance recognized early, even before the physiological function of blood was understood. Indeed, the carotid arteries are the principle conduit for blood transport to the brain, carrying approximately 70% of global CBF.

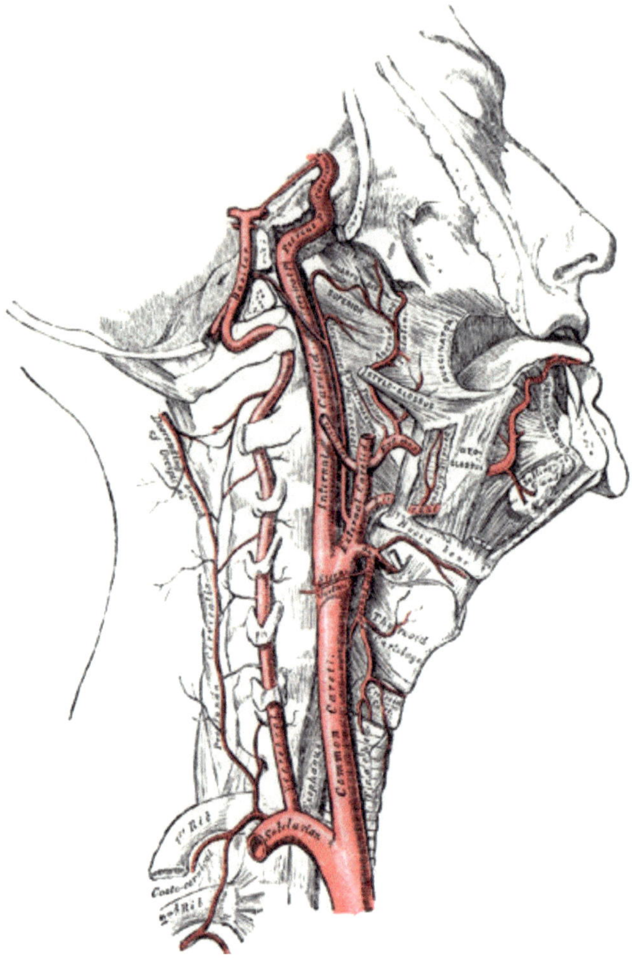

Fig. 7. Diagram of the right carotid arteries and vertebral artery.

The carotid system originates with the common carotid arteries (CCA), that branch from the aortic arch and brachiocephalic trunk on the left and right sides, respectively. The CCA bifurcates into the external (ECA) and internal (ICA) carotid arteries. The position and morphology of the carotid bifurcation exhibits some variation, lying somewhere between the level of the thyroid cartilage and hyoid bone in the majority of individuals. The ECA is most often positioned either anteromedial or medial to the ICA (Al-Rafiah *et al.*, 2011), giving off the superior thyroid artery and ascending pharangeal artery within the first two centimeters distal from the bifurcation. There is, however, variation in the loci of these arteries origins, occasionally branching from the CCA or ICA, and more often from the bifurcation itself. The ICA normally does not give off any branches until after entering the base of the skull through the foramen lacerum. The ophthalmic artery and a number of smaller arteries branch prior to the circle of Willis, where the ICA terminates to form the middle, anterior, and posterior communicating arteries. Because in the majority of individuals there are no branches off of the ICA prior to entering the skull, ICA blood flow is an accurate metric of CBF.

The vertebral arteries (VA) arise as the most proximal branches off the subclavian arteries, then course through the foremen of the transverse processes of C6-C2, into the spinal canal and skull to join bilaterally forming the basilar artery. The vessel can be imaged proximal to entering C6, and between each of the vertebra until entering the skull. There are numerous anastomoses with the VA both extra- and intracranially. The VA communicates with branches of the deep cervical artery, and inferior thyroid artery extracranially, and upon entering the skull gives off branches to the cerebellum before joining to form the basilar artery (BA). A number of arteries project from the BA to supply the cerebellum and pons before the BA bifurcates to form the poster circle of Willis as the posterior communicating arteries. The figure 8 below provide typical ultrasound example of the different waveforms commonly observed in the ICA, ECA and VA.

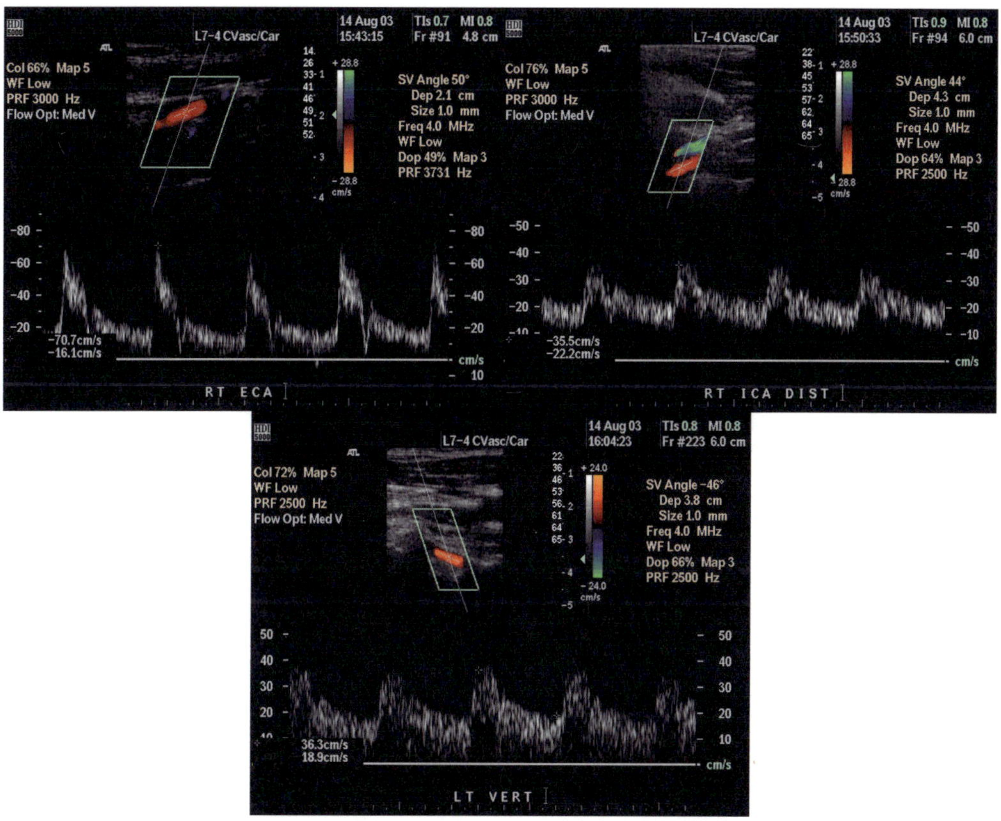

Fig. 8. From left to right, ultrasound examples of the ECA (left), ICA (middle) and VA (right). Note: 1) The ECA waveform should have a sharp upstroke and a low end-diastolic velocity, as it supplies a high resistance vascular bed. ECA may have a flow reversal component (flow below the baseline) in late systole or early diastole; 2) ICA waveform should have a more gradual upstroke (slower acceleration) in systole, and an elevated end-diastolic velocity. This is because it supplies a low resistance vascular bed (i.e., the brain). Thus flow should be above the baseline for the entire cardiac cycle; and 3) The VA waveform should have a gradual upstroke and relatively high end-diastolic velocity as it also supplies a low resistance vascular bed.

7.2 Technical aspects of vascular ultrasound

Neck artery ultrasound accurately quantifies global and regional CBF non-invasively and with high spatial and temporal resolution; indeed, it is the only known method of CBF measurement possessing these attributes. The principal limitation is consequently that of the operator, not the technique *per se.* But in fact the technique is so easily confounded by user error that this limitation obviates flippant dismissal. For example, a one degree error in the angle of insonation; a 0.1mm error in diameter measurement; and, one cm/s error in mean blood velocity each yield a 3, 4, and 4% error in the measurement of flow. It is obvious that very minor operator errors during insonation and during subsequent analysis quickly compound and can easily produce significant inaccuracies (Schoning *et al.*, 1994). For every 1-degree error in the insonation angle an approximate 3% error in velocity, and therefore in flow, results. But, whereas the velocity and flow error are linearly related, inaccuracies in the measurement of diameter have an exponentially larger effect (because the diameter is squared to calculate luminal area). The appropriate measurement of diameter is a topic of extensive debate within other fields reliant on ultrasonic measure of blood flow (Black *et al.*, 2008; Green *et al.*, 2011). It is unfortunate, then, that the accurate measurement of luminal diameter presents a number of problems that have largely been unaddressed since the invention of the technique. The majority of investigators utilize calipers typically part of the ultrasound software to manually measure from one luminal surface to the other. Some authors have accounted for the pulsatile nature of most arteries by measuring both systolic and diastolic diameters, and calculate a mean diameter based on a third to two-thirds systolic-diastolic ratio (Sato *et al.*, 2011; Sato & Sadamoto, 2010). Other authors have discordantly reported the ICA, ECA, and VA to be without pulsatile changes throughout the cardiac cycle (Scheel *et al.*, 2000a; Scheel *et al.*, 2000b; Schoning & Hartig, 1996; Schoning *et al.*, 2005a; Schoning *et al.*, 1994). Proprietary and commercially available software that automatically tracks the vessel internal walls on the B-mode image with high temporal resolution facilitates calculation of other metrics such as pulsatility and shear stress, and moreover dramatically increases the precision of the diameter measurement. Manual measurement of vessel lumen is also likely to prevent observation of any change in diameter, as arterial response to changes in shear or blood gases involves a temporal latency with stimulus related and inter -individual variability impossible to observe when only a few measures are taken.

8. Integrative assessment and future directions

Cerebrovascular function is clearly regulated by an array of functionally integrated processes. Measurement of only one process will provide an inadequate representation of this complex physiology. We therefore suggest that in both the research and clinical setting, assessment of cerebrovascular function with TCD should ideally include measures of four principle factors: (1) baseline CBV; (2) cerebrovascular reactivity; (3) cerebral autoregulation; and (4) neurovascular coupling. Furthermore, there is evidence that CBF and CA varies with time of day, exercise, body position, caffeine, food intake, and menstrual cycle; as such, these variables should be carefully standardized for each of the following metrics both between and within subjects or patients.

8.1 Baseline cerebral blood flow and velocities in arteries of interest

Because normative data for blood flow velocities is well known within the literature for the MCA (Aaslid *et al.*, 1984; Ringelstein *et al.*, 1990) and related neck arteries (Scheel *et al.*, 2000b; Schoning *et al.*, 1994); thus, baseline blood flow and CBFv should always be collected for all arteries of interest. Indeed, diagnosis of atypical flow patterns within the cerebral circulation is indicative of a number of conditions such as intracerebral stenosis or occlusion (Aaslid, 1986b; Aaslid, 2006). Because in a normal population cerebrovascular function is largely determined by its ability to adjust to changes in perfusion pressure, it is largely the change from baseline following a stimulus that is of greatest importance in assessing autoregulation.

8.2 Cerebrovascular reactivity

Cerebrovascular reactivity is an accepted independent predictor of ischemic stroke (Markus & Cullinane, 2001). That it has been linked with a spectrum of vascular pathologies justifies its inclusion when assessing cerebrovascular function. Arterial CO_2 can be increased through inhalation of a hypercapnic gas or simple re-breathing paradigm. Ainslie & Duffin (2009) have recently detailed the assessment and related interpretation of cerebrovascular reactivity. Furthermore, $PetCO_2$ should always be measured because of its direct effects on cerebrovascular calibre. Moreover, spontaneous measures of *d*CA are affected differentially by hypercapnia and hypocapnia (Panerai *et al.*, 1999b).

8.3 Cerebral autoregulation

Quantification of cerebral autoregulation (CA) is clearly an important factor in any study assessing cerebrovascular function. Despite caveats inherent to each methods of CA quantification most studies to date have applied only one measure of CA, and generally in the hypotensive range. Moreover, recent studies have largely focused on spontaneous CA analysis using TFA. However, we recommend that it is critical to 'force' the BP challenge in order to reliably engage CA. Driving BP oscillations using either squat-stand, or oscillating lower body negative pressure at the frequency of interest will enhance the reliability and validity of TFA measures (Claassen *et al.*, 2009; Hamner *et al.*, 2004). Like the Oxford method, this approach also permits the assessment and separation of the cerebral responses to both hypotension and hypertension. Given the apparent difference in efficacy of CA to managing falling or rising perfusion pressures, and the distinct consequences to dysregulation (i.e., ischemia versus hemorrhage, respectively), this is an important consideration.

8.4 Neurovascular coupling

Neurovascular coupling (NVC) is likely involved in maintenance of adequate nutrient and oxygen supply to specific regions of the brain. It is a relatively simple addition to any experimental design, and should be measured if time permits. The regional task specificity within the brain allows coupling to be easily assessed; simple sensory stimuli (e.g., turning on a light) provides adequate stimulus to assess neurovascular coupling in the cortex by measurement of CBV in the PCA (Aaslid, 1987). Coupling between neural activity is decreased in a number of pathologies, including hypertension, Alzheimer's disease, ischemic stroke (reviewed by Girouard & Iadecola, 2006), and in long-term smokers (Woods *et al.*, 2010).

9. TCD and neck blood flow utility

It is clear that there is tremendous utility in the assessment of cerebrovascular function with TCD. Surprisingly, integrative assessment of cerebrovascular function is currently lacking and no studies to date have combined the assessment of these four fundamental measurements. Given that regulation of cerebrovascular function involves the complex integration of each of the above factors, only experimental designs that incorporate holistic assessment of multiple mechanisms can hope to clarify the complex physiology responsible for maintaining brain O_2 and nutrient delivery in such narrow margins.

In the clinical setting, depending on the key measurement question, the implementation of a simplified protocol that encompasses each of these metrics is prudent. Measurement of MCAv, PCAv, ECG, beat-to-beat BP, and end-tidal gases should be recorded throughout. The following protocol would likely be adequate: 5 minutes supine baseline; 2 minutes eyes closed; 2 minutes of reading followed by 5-10 cycles of 20 seconds eyes closed followed by 40 seconds reading to assess NVC; 2 minutes of either rebreathing or breathing of a 5% CO2 gas mixture to assess cerebrovascular reactivity; and finally one BP stimulus - either using the Oxford technique, thigh cuffs, Valsalva maneuver, or squat-stand cycles. Such a protocol, with one or two skilled experimenters, can be completed within 45-60 minutes on both healthy subjects and a variety of patient groups (Figure 9).

The prototype for the assessment of both blood velocity and vessel diameter was introduced in 1974 (Barber *et al.*, 1974). Several years later pulsed-Doppler ultrasound was utilized for the quantification of blood velocity in the internal carotid and vertebral arteries during changes in inspired CO_2 (Hauge *et al.*, 1980). This early technology lacked B-mode functionality to allow visualization of the vessel, and measurement of diameter. Consequently, the diameter of the vessel had to be assumed constant for the velocity to be indicative of flow, a problem overcome several years later following diagnostic utilization of combined B-mode and Doppler (Duplex) scanning for identification of artherosclerotic pathology (Blackshear *et al.*, 1979; Strandness, 1985). The "logical progression" came soon after when Leopold et al (1987) applied Duplex scanning to the internal carotid artery to quantify CBF and CO_2 reactivity. The method's principal use has since been for the evaluation of neck artery pathology, however a handful of studies have utilized the technique for the quantification of CBF decline through aging (Schoning & Hartig, 1996; Schoning *et al.*, 1994) and to assess cerebrovascular reactivity to CO_2 and O_2 (Fortune *et al.*, 1992; Hauge *et al.*, 1980; Leopold *et al.*, 1987; Schoning *et al.*, 1994). The results of these studies are broadly consistent with studies assessing cerebrovascular reactivity and global brain blood flow using indicator dilution techniques (Ainslie & Duffin, 2009; Battisti *et al.*, 2010; Fan *et al.*, 2008) (Ackerman *et al.*, 1973; Grubb *et al.*, 1974; Harper & Glass, 1965), and TCD.

Use of ICA blood flow has been extended to the bedside diagnostic assessment of myriad cerebrovascular pathologies. There is a small body of literature describing insonation of the ICA for the assessment of periventricular leukomlacia (Kehrer & Schoning, 2009), cerebral vasculitis (Kamm *et al.*, 2008; Kuker *et al.*, 2008), evaluation of cerebral circulatory arrest (Schoning *et al.*, 2005b), and for establishing normative values for CBF during natal development (Kehrer *et al.*, 2005; Kehrer & Schoning, 2009). Ultrasonic study of the vertebral arteries has also received attention with respect to risk identification involved with chiropractic cervical spine manipulation (Bowler *et al.*, 2011; Mitchell, 2005), though many of the conclusions herein remain speculative.

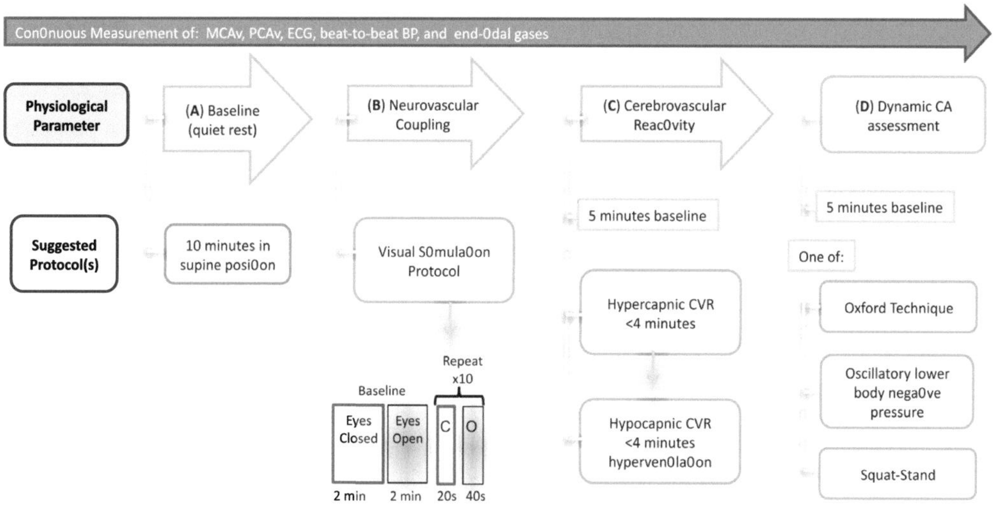

Fig. 9. (A) A complete resting assessment of intracranial blood flow using TCD should include blood velocities of middle cerebral artery (MCA), posterior cerebral artery (PCA), anterior cerebral artery (ACA) and basilar artery. The probe(s) can then be fixed on the arteries of interest for the remainder of the protocol. Electrocardiogram, end-tidal gases, and beat-to-beat blood pressure should be measured concomitantly with cerebral blood velocity metrics throughout the experiment. (B) The neurovascular coupling protocol should consist of 2 minutes each of resting with eyes open and closed, followed by 5-10 cycles of 20 seconds eyes closed and 40 seconds of reading with concurrent measurement of MCA and PCA velocities. (C) Assessment of cerebrovascular reactivity in both hypercapnic and hypocapnic ranges can be carried out in <4 minutes of rebreathing or inhalation of 5% CO_2, or, hyperventilation, respectively. (D) Dynamic cerebral autoregulation can be assessed using any of: supra-systolic thigh-cuff release (Section 5.1), the Valsalva maneuver (Section 5.3), the Oxford technique, or oscillatory blood pressure perturbations. The Oxford technique (Section 5.5) or transfer function analysis using either squat-stand cycles or oscillating lower body negative pressure at 0.05 and 0.1 Hz are recommended for reasons detailed in Section 5.6 and Figure 5.

More recently neck artery blood flow quantification has seen a resurgent application in physiology research. Sato et al conducted two studies (Bowler *et al.*, 2011; Mitchell, 2005; Sato *et al.*, 2011; Sato & Sadamoto, 2010) utilizing the technique to quantify changes in regional head perfusion during varying degrees of semi-recumbent cycling exercise. They measured blood flow in the external, internal, and common carotid arteries, as well as in the vertebral artery to show that the well-documented increase-plateau-decrease with progressive exercise to intensities above the ventilator threshold was only evident in the anterior circulation. Their data indicate, and support previous suggestions, that the poster and anterior cerebral circulations possess disparate blood flow regulation and CO_2

sensitivities. In this respect the possibility that the arteries of the neck were directly involved in the regulation of CBF was raised by their data (Hellström *et al.*, 1996).

From an integrative systems approach, numerous factors independently, synergistically, and sometimes antagonistically participate in the regulation of CBF. In addition to the traditional mechanisms describing CBF regulation (e.g. autoregulation, partial pressure of arterial carbon dioxide), a variety of other factors, such as cardiac output, the arterial baroreflex and chemoreflex control, are very likely involved in this complex regulatory physiology. Research exploring these complex interactions, especially in relation to neurovascular coupling, is currently lacking. Future studies with particular focus on these integrative physiological mechanisms are clearly warranted in both health and disease states.

10. Conclusions

Many methods are available for the assessment of CBF, but the high temporal resolution, non-invasiveness, and relative low-cost of TCD make it functional in both clinical and research settings. The ability to assess cerebral reactivity, CA, and neurovascular coupling, makes TCD extremely useful for the assessment of integrative cerebrovascular function. Four principle components of cerebrovascular regulation can, and should, be assessed using TCD, as collectively these provide insight into a complex physiology. Measurement of (1) velocities within the major cerebral vessels; (2) measurement of ICA, ECA and VA blood flow, (3) assessments of autoregulation, (4) cerebrovascular reactivity and (5) neurovascular coupling together facilitate holistic appraisal of cerebrovascular function.

11. Appendix

	Methodology			Blood Flow Parameters								
Study	**Intervention**	**Imaging Technique**	**Analysis Method**	**Vessel**	**PSV (cm/s)**	**EDV (cm/s)**	**Vmean (cm/s)**	**Diameter (mm)**	**Blood Flow (ml/min)**	**Other**		
	Resting Studies											
Yazici *et al.*, 2005	Rest	Duplex ultrasound	CCA measurements taken 2 cm proximal to the bifurcation; ICA and ECA measurements taken 1-2 cm distal to the bifurcation; VA measurements taken bilaterally between the 4th and 5th cervical vertebral transverse processes in the sagittal plane. B-mode images. Age is presented in parentheses. (*n*=96)	CCA (21-50)	98 ± 20	26 ± 6		6.2 ± 0.6	427 ± 106			
				CCA (51-80)	74 ± 15	20 ± 5		6.8 ± 0.8	408 ± 95			
				ECA (21-50)	71 ± 15	16 ± 5		4.1 ± 0.5	128 ± 45			
				ECA (51-80)	73 ± 19	14 ± 5		4.1 ± 0.7	139 ± 57			
				ICA (21-50)	76 ± 14	30 ± 7		4.5 ± 0.5	238 ± 57			
				ICA (51-80	65 ± 14	25 ± 6		4.6 ± 0.7	225 ± 60			
				VA (21-50)	53 ± 10	18 ± 5		3.5 ± 0.4	86 ± 34			
				VA (51-80)	48 ± 12	15 ± 17		3.6 ± 0.5	77 ± 41			
										CBF volume (ml/min)		
										Combined	**Male**	**Female**
Scheel *et al.*, 2000	Rest	Duplex ultrasound	Flow volume measurements were in the C4-C5 inter-transverse segment of the VA, 1.5-2 cm below the carotid bulb in the ECA and ICA. Luminal diameter determined on the enlarged B-mode. Angle of insonation = ~60°. 3-5 cardiac cycles. Age is presented in parentheses. (*n*=78).	VA (20-85)					158 ± 48	657 ±120	670 ± 117	644 ± 123
				VA (20-39)					173 ± 41	727 ± 102	725 ± 87	730 ± 87
				VA (40-59)					147 ± 36	656 ± 121	663 ± 126	648 ± 120
				VA (60-85)					155 ± 58	603 ± 106	648 ± 120	572 ± 99
				ICA (20-85)					499 ± 108			
				ICA (20-39)					554 ± 99			
				ICA (40-59)					508 ± 114			
				ICA (60-85)					448 ± 85			
				ECA (20-85)					328 ± 111			
				ECA (20-39)					290 ± 63			
				ECA (40-59)					350 ± 146			
				ECA (60-85)					340 ± 103			
				CCA (20-85)					816 ± 198			
				CCA (20-39)					853 ± 197			
				CCA (40-59)					868 ± 223			
				CCA (60-85)					745 ± 160			

Scheel *et al.*, 2000	Rest	Colour duplex sonography	Flow volume measurements were most frequently taken in the C4-C5 intertransverse segment of the VA, 1.5 -2 cm below the carotid bulb in the CCA, and 1-2 cm above the carotid bulb in ECA and ICA. D = B-mode; measure diameter of CCA in end-diastolic phase. Angle of insonation = 60°. Age is presented in parentheses. (*n*=78).	CCA (20-39)	101 ± 22	25 ± 5	25 ± 5	6.0 ± 0.7	426 ± 99	
				CCA (40-59)	89 ± 17	26 ± 5	25 ± 5	6.1 ± 0.8	434 ± 111	
				CCA (60-85)	81 ± 21	20 ± 7	21 ± 6	6.2 ± 0.9	373 ± 80	
				ECA (20-39)	86 ± 14	16 ± 4	19 ± 3	4.0 ± 0.4	145 ± 32	
				ECA (40-59)	85 ± 18	19 ± 3	22 ± 5	4.1 ± 0.7	175 ± 73	
				ECA (60-85)	81 ± 30	15 ± 6	20 ± 7	4.3 ± 0.7	170 ± 73	
				ICA (20-39)	72 ± 18	26 ± 5	26 ± 5	4.8 ± 0.5	277 ± 49	
				ICA (40-59)	65 ± 10	26 ± 5	25 ± 5	4.7 ± 0.6	254 ± 57	
				ICA (60-85)	58 ± 11	20 ± 5	21 ± 6	4.9 ± 0.8	224 ± 43	
				VA (20-39)	52 ± 6	17 ± 3	17 ± 3	3.3 ± 0.3	87 ± 20	
				VA (40-59)	47 ± 8	15 ± 3	14 ± 2	3.2 ± 0.4	74 ± 18	
				VA (60-85)	45 ± 11	12 ± 3	12 ± 4	3.6 ± 0.4	78 ± 29	
Schoning & Hartig, 1996	Rest	Duplex ultrasound	CCA measurements taken 1.5-2 cm proximal to bifurcation . ICA and ECA measurements taken 1.5-2 cm distal to bifurcation. VA measurements taken between C4-C5 vertebral transverse process. B-mode imaging. Age is presented in parentheses. (*n*=94).	CCA (3-9.9)					775 ± 117	
				CCA (10-18)					750 ± 119	
				ECA (3-9.9)					113 ± 43	
				ECA (10-18)					189 ± 64	
				ICA (3-9.9)					585 ± 90	
				ICA (10-18)					543 ± 90	
				VA (3-9.9)					236 ± 51	
				VA (10-18)					184 ± 36	
				CBFV (3-9.9)					821 ± 116	
				CBFV (10-18)					727 ± 106	
									Blood Flow (ml/min)	
									Observer A	**Observer B**
Schoning & Scheel, 1996	Rest	Doppler flowmetry and colour duplex sonography	ECA and ICA measurements taken 1.5-2 cm above the bifurcation. B-mode to take luminal diameter. (*n*=32).	LICA Day 1					276 ± 68	266 ± 63
				RICA Day 1					268 ± 54	260 ± 57
				LICA Day 2					269 ± 65	257 ± 52
				RICA Day 2					254 ± 60	249 ± 44
				LVA Day 1					99 ± 44	97 ± 44
				RVA Day 1					74 ± 38	79 ± 41
				LVA Day 2					94 ± 41	92 ± 38
				RVA Day 2					75 ± 38	74 ± 36
				CBFV Exam 1					723 ± 153	699 ± 155
				CBFV Exam 2					709 ± 146	694 ± 146
				CBFV Exam 3					693 ± 136	672 ± 110
Schoning *et al.*, 1994	Rest	Duplex ultrasonography	Measurements taken 1.5 cm below carotid bulb in the CCA and 1.0 to 1.5 cm away from the bifurcation in ICA and ECA. VA was measured at the C4-C5 intertransverse area. D = B-mode ICA, ECA and VA; M-mode for CCA. (*n*=48).	CCA	96 ± 25	26 ± 6	25.4 ± 5.4	6.3 ± 0.9	470 ± 120	
				ICA	66 ± 16	26 ± 6	24.9 ± 5.2	4.8 ± 0.7	265 ± 62	
				ECA	83 ± 17	17 ± 5	19.6 ± 4.1	4.1 ± 0.6	160 ± 66	
				VA	48 ± 10	16 ± 4	15.6 ± 3.6	3.4 ± 0.6	85 ± 33	
	Exercise Studies									
Sato *et al.*, 2011	Rest	Duplex ultrasound	Measurements for the ICA were taken 1.0-1.5 cm distal to bifurcation on the left ICA, chin slightly elevated; VA measured between the transverse process of the C3 and subclavian artery. Left ECA and right CCA measured 1.0-1.5 cm above the carotid. Mean diameter = [(systolic diameter x 1/3)] + [(diastolic diameter x 2/3)]. (*n*=10).	CCA			28.5 ± 1.0	5.2 ± 0.1	363 ± 18	
				ICA			28.4 ± 1.3	4.2 ± 0.1	239 ± 14	
				ECA			19.6 ± 1.6	3.8 ± 0.1	129 ± 12	
				VA			20.1 ± 1.0	3.1 ± 0.2	90 ± 12	
	40% VO_2 Peak			CCA			31.3 ± 0.7	5.3 ± 0.1	420 ± 14	
				ICA			33.7 ± 1.3	4.2 ± 0.1	280 ± 14	
				ECA			24.2 ± 1.9	3.9 ± 0.1	163 ± 10	
				VA			25.2 ± 2.5	3.1 ± 0.2	117 ± 13	
	60% VO_2 Peak			CCA			34.2 ± 1.0	5.4 ± 0.1	463 ± 20	
				ICA			34.4 ± 1.6	4.2 ± 0.1	291 ± 16	
				ECA			25.6 ± 2.2	4.0 ± 0.1	183 ± 12	
				VA			27.8 ± 1.9	3.1 ± 0.2	129 ± 12	
	80% VO_2 Peak			CCA			35.9 ± 1.2	5.4 ± 0.1	500 ± 31	
				ICA			30.4 ± 1.0	4.2 ±0.1	258 ± 13	
				ECA			31.8 ± 2.2	4.0 ± 0.1	238 ± 13	
				VA			30.3 ± 2.0	3.2 ± 0.2	144 ± 14	

Sato *et al.*, 2009	Voluntary elbow flexion/ extension (no load; 2 min)	Duplex ultrasound	Motor-driven lever arm rotated at constant velocity. Measured vessel diameter and blood flow velocity at 2-3 cm proximal to the carotid bifurcation using an insonation angle as low as possible <60° (*n*=11).	CCA		23.9 ± 2.6	378 ± 41	
	Passive mechanoreflex activating elbow extension			CCA		24.2 ± 3.2	370 ± 43	
Hellstrom *et al.*, 1996	Rest	Duplex ultrasonography	5- to 10-MHz-wide band linear-array transducer. Vessel diameter measured in B mode. M-mode for use in flow calculations. Increase exercise workload every 6 min. Ergometer cycle. (*n*=11).	CCA			591 ± 200	
	20-22% VO_2 max			CCA			610 ± 200	
	40-44%VO_2 max			CCA			698 ± 399	
	60-67% VO_2 max			CCA			784 ± 300	
	80-90% VO_2 max			CCA			839 ± 300	
	Rest			CCA			752 ± 200	
	Rest			ICA			332 ± 50	
	20-22% VO_2 max			ICA			366 ± 60	
	40-44%VO_2 max			ICA			367 ± 60	
	60-67% VO_2 max			ICA			387 ± 70	
	80-90% VO_2 max			ICA			360 ± 70	
	Rest			ICA			340 ± 70	
	Postitional Studies							
Bowler *et al.*, 2011	Neutral	Duplex ultrasound	Doppler angle = 56°. Measurements ICA 1-2 cm above the carotid bulb (C2/3); VA measured at C2/3. Vmean = [(PSV - EDV)/3] + EDV. (*n*=14).	LICA	92.4 ± 22.4	33.6 ± 6.8	53.2 ± 11.4	
				RICA	98.8 ± 21.7	38.2 ± 7.0	58.4 ± 10.5	
				LVA	55.0 ± 9.5	18.5 ± 3.0	30.7 ± 4.6	
				RVA	54.1 ± 18.7	18.0 ± 5.7	30.0 ± 9.8	
	SMP (LR,RSF)			LICA	95.2 ±19.2	39.7 ± 9.2	58.2 ± 11.5	
				RICA	96.4 ± 19.7	36.3 ± 7.1	56.3 ± 10.1	
				LVA	50.6 ± 11.7	18.3 ± 3.9	29.1 ± 6.3	
				RVA	45.9 ± 8.6	17.5 ± 4.4	26.9 ± 5.3	
	Neutral			LICA	95.7 ± 20.1	36.0 ± 7.7	55.9 ± 10.5	
				RICA	96.7 ± 17.1	35.9 ± 6.3	56.1 ± 7.3	
				LVA	57.1 ± 13.7	20.2 ± 4.4	32.5 ± 6.7	
				RVA	53.2 ± 16.3	19.3 ± 7.0	30.6 ±9.9	
	SMP (RR, LSF)			LICA	91.2 ± 22.5	32.7 ± 7.6	52. 2 ± 11.2	
				RICA	100.6 ± 23.4	37.3 ± 11.3	58.4 ± 13.4	
				LVA	54.5 ± 14.0	19.0 ± 4.2	30.8 ± 7.0	
				RVA	50.3 ± 15.8	19.5 ± 7.5	29.8 ± 10.1	
	Pharmaceutical Studies							
Bokker *et al.*, 2011	Pre-acetazolamide	Arterial spin labelling; 3T MRI scanner.	For positioning at low-resolution T1-weighted spin-echo sequence was obtained in the sagittal plane. Perfusion images consisted of 17 7 mm slices aligned parallel to the orbitomeatal angle, acquired in ascending fashion with an in-plance resolution 3x3 mm 9 true acquisition resolution. (*n*=16).	ICA				51.8 ± 8.1
	Post-acetazolamide			ICA				78.6 ± 12.4
	Pathological Studies							
Albayrak *et al.*, 2006	Healthy	Duplex ultrasound	Measurements for ICA 1.5 cm distal to the carotid bifurcation. VA examined between the transverse processes of the vertebrae C4 and C5. TAV = integral of the mean flow velocities of all moving particles passing the sample volume over 3-5 complete cardiac cycles. (*n*=29).	LICA	51.8 ±14.9	18.1 ± 6.6		
				RICA	54.4 ± 14.4	18.1 ± 5.2		
				LVA	37.7 ± 12.1	11.3 ± 5.6		
				RVA	36.6 ± 11.3	10.3 ± 4.5		
	COPD			LICA	62.1 ± 18.9	18.9 ± 6.7		
				RICA	54.5 ± 18.3	16.9 ± 5.4		
				LVA	40.9 ± 12.5	11.7 ± 4.8		
				RVA	38.4 ± 13.9	9.9 ± 4.3		

Abbreviations: CBFV; cerebral blood flow volume. CCA; common carotid artery. COPD; chronic obstrutive pulmonary disease. ECA; external carotid artery. EDV; end-diastolic velocity. ICA; internal carotid artery. LICA; left internal carotid artery. LVA; left vertebral artery. PSV; peak systolic velocity. RICA; right intrnal carotid artery. RVA; right vertrbral artery. SMP; simulated manipulation position [LR, RSF; left rotation, right side flexion or RR, LSF; right rotation, left side flexion]. TAV; time averaged maximum blood flow velocity, VA; vertebral artery. Vmean; mean velocity

12. References

Aaslid R (1986a). The Doppler principle applied to measurement of blood flow velocity in cerebral arteries. In *Transcranial Doppler sonography* ed. Aaslid R, Springer-Verlag, New York.

Aaslid R (1986b). Transcranial Doppler Examination Techniques. In *Transcranial Doppler Sonography* ed. Aaslid R, pp. 39–59. Springer-Verlag, New York.

Aaslid R (1987). Visually evoked dynamic blood flow response of the human cerebral circulation. *Stroke* 18, 771–775.

Aaslid R (2006). Cerebral autoregulation and vasomotor reactivity. *Frontiers of neurology and neuroscience* 21, 216–228.

Aaslid R, Blaha M, Sviri G, Douville CM & Newell DW (2007). Asymmetric dynamic cerebral autoregulatory response to cyclic stimuli. *Stroke* 38, 1465–1469.

Aaslid R, Huber P & Nornes H (1984). Evaluation of cerebrovascular spasm with transcranial Doppler ultrasound. *J Neurosurg* 60, 37–41.

Aaslid R, Lash SR, Bardy GH, Gild WH & Newell DW (2003). Dynamic pressure--flow velocity relationships in the human cerebral circulation. *Stroke* 34, 1645–1649.

Aaslid R, Lindegaard KF, Sorteberg W & Nornes H (1989). Cerebral autoregulation dynamics in humans. *Stroke* 20, 45–52.

Aaslid R, Markwalder TM & Nornes H (1982). Noninvasive transcranial Doppler ultrasound recording of flow velocity in basal cerebral arteries. *J Neurosurg* 57, 769–774.

Ackerman RH, Zilkha E, Bull JW, Du Boulay GH, Marshall J, Russell RW & Symon L (1973). The relationship of the CO 2 reactivity of cerebral vessels to blood pressure and mean resting blood flow. *Neurology* 23, 21–26.

Adams RJ, McKie VC, Carl EM, Nichols FT, Perry R, Brock K, McKie K, Figueroa R, Litaker M, Weiner S & Brambilla D (1997). Long-term stroke risk in children with sickle cell disease screened with transcranial Doppler. *Ann Neurol* 42, 699–704.

Adams RJ, McKie VC, Hsu L, Files B, Vichinsky E, Pegelow C, Abboud M, Gallagher D, Kutlar A, Nichols FT, Bonds DR & Brambilla D (1998). Prevention of a first stroke by transfusions in children with sickle cell anemia and abnormal results on transcranial Doppler ultrasonography. *N Engl J Med* 339, 5–11.

Ainslie P & Duffin J (2009). Integration of cerebrovascular CO2 reactivity and chemoreflex control of breathing: mechanisms of regulation, measurement, and interpretation. *AJP: Regulatory, Integrative and Comparative Physiology* 296, R1473–R1495.

Ainslie P & Tzeng Y (2010). On the regulation of the blood supply to the brain: old age concepts and new age ideas. *Journal of Applied Physiology* 108, 1447–1449.

Ainslie PN & Ogoh S (2010). Regulation of cerebral blood flow in mammals during chronic hypoxia: a matter of balance. *Exp Physiol* 95, 251–262.

Al-Rafiah A, EL-Haggagy AA, Aal IH & Zaki AI (2011). Anatomical study of the carotid bifurcation and origin variations of the ascending pharyngeal and superior thyroid arteries. *Folia Morphol (Warsz)* 70, 47–55.

Alexandrov AV (2006). Ultrasound enhanced thrombolysis for stroke. *International journal of stroke : official journal of the International Stroke Society* 1, 26–29.

Alexandrov AV (2009). Ultrasound enhancement of fibrinolysis. *Stroke* 40, S107–10.

Alexandrov AV, Molina CA, Grotta JC, Garami Z, Ford SR, Alvarez-Sabin J, Montaner J, Saqqur M, Demchuk AM, Moyé LA, Hill MD, Wojner AW & Investigators

CLOTBUST (2004). Ultrasound-enhanced systemic thrombolysis for acute ischemic stroke. *N Engl J Med* 351, 2170–2178.

Barber FE, Baker DW, Nation AW, Strandness DEJ & Reid JM (1974). Ultrasonic duplex echo-Doppler scanner. *IEEE Trans Biomed Eng* 21, 109–113.

Battisti A, Fisher JA & Duffin J (2010). Measuring the hypoxic ventilatory response. *Advances in experimental medicine and biology* 669, 221–224.

Bishop CC, Powell S, Rutt D & Browse NL (1986). Transcranial Doppler measurement of middle cerebral artery blood flow velocity: a validation study. *Stroke* 17, 913–915.

Black MA, Cable NT, Thijssen DH & Green DJ (2008). Importance of measuring the time course of flow-mediated dilatation in humans. *Hypertension* 51, 203–210.

Blackshear WMJ, Phillips DJ, Thiele BL, Hirsch JH, Chikos PM, Marinelli MR, Ward KJ & Strandness DEJ (1979). Detection of carotid occlusive disease by ultrasonic imaging and pulsed Doppler spectrum analysis. *Surgery* 86, 698–706.

Boms N, Yonai Y, Molnar S, Rosengarten B, Bornstein NM, Csiba L & Olah L (2010). Effect of smoking cessation on visually evoked cerebral blood flow response in healthy volunteers. *J Vasc Res* 47, 214–220.

Bowler N, Shamley D & Davies R (2011). The effect of a simulated manipulation position on internal carotid and vertebral artery blood flow in healthy individuals. *Man Ther* 16, 87–93.

Brassard P, Seifert T, Wissenberg M, Jensen P, Hansen C & Secher N (2010). Phenylephrine decreases frontal lobe oxygenation at rest but not during moderately intense exercise. *Journal of Applied Physiology* 108, 1472–1478.

Bruneau N, Dourneau MC, Garreau B, Pourcelot L & Lelord G (1992). Blood flow response to auditory stimulations in normal, mentally retarded, and autistic children: a preliminary transcranial Doppler ultrasonographic study of the middle cerebral arteries. *Biol Psychiatry* 32, 691–699.

Burgess KR, Fan JL, Peebles K, Thomas K, Lucas S, Lucas R, Dawson A, Swart M, Shepherd K & Ainslie P (2010). Exacerbation of obstructive sleep apnea by oral indomethacin. *Chest* 137, 707–710.

Camerlingo M, Casto L, Censori B, Ferraro B, Gazzaniga GC & Mamoli A (1993). Transcranial Doppler in acute ischemic stroke of the middle cerebral artery territories. *Acta Neurol Scand* 88, 108–111.

Cassaglia P, Griffiths R & Walker A (2009). Cerebral sympathetic nerve activity has a major regulatory role in the cerebral circulation in REM sleep. *Journal of Applied Physiology* 106, 1050–1056.

Cassaglia PA, Griffiths RI & Walker AM (2008). Sympathetic withdrawal augments cerebral blood flow during acute hypercapnia in sleeping lambs. *Sleep* 31, 1729–1734.

Chapman RW, Santiago TV & Edelman NH (1979). Effects of graded reduction of brain blood flow on chemical control of breathing. *Journal of applied physiology: respiratory, environmental and exercise physiology* 47, 1289–1294.

Claassen JA, Levine BD & Zhang R (2009). Dynamic cerebral autoregulation during repeated squat-stand maneuvers. *J Appl Physiol* 106, 153–160.

Czosnyka M, Brady K, Reinhard M, Smielewski P & Steiner LA (2009). Monitoring of cerebrovascular autoregulation: facts, myths, and missing links. *Neurocritical care* 10, 373-386.

de Freitas GR & André C (2006). Sensitivity of transcranial Doppler for confirming brain death: a prospective study of 270 cases. *Acta Neurol Scand* 113, 426–432.

Deegan BM, Devine ER, Geraghty MC, Jones E, Olaighin G & Serrador JM (2010). The relationship between cardiac output and dynamic cerebral autoregulation in humans. *J Appl Physiol* 109, 1424–1431.

Deppe M, Ringelstein EB & Knecht S (2004). The investigation of functional brain lateralization by transcranial Doppler sonography. *Neuroimage* 21, 1124–1146.

Deverall PB, Padayachee TS, Parsons S, Theobold R & Battistessa SA (1988). Ultrasound detection of micro-emboli in the middle cerebral artery during cardiopulmonary bypass surgery. *Eur J Cardiothorac Surg* 2, 256–260.

DeWitt LD & Wechsler LR (1988). Transcranial Doppler. *Stroke* 19, 915-921.

Dorst J, Haag A, H. OW, Hamer HM & Rosenow F (2008). Functional transcranial Doppler sonography and a spatial orientation paradigm identify the non-dominant hemisphere. *Brain and cognition* 68, 53–58.

Droste DW, Lakemeier S, Wichter T, Stypmann J, Dittrich R, Ritter M, Moeller M, Freund M & Ringelstein EB (2002). Optimizing the technique of contrast transcranial Doppler ultrasound in the detection of right-to-left shunts. *Stroke* 33, 2211-2216.

Duschek S, Hadjamu M & Schandry R (2007). Enhancement of cerebral blood flow and cognitive performance following pharmacological blodd pressure elevation in chronic hypotension. *Psychophysiology* 44, 145–153.

Duschek S, Heiss H, Werner N & Reyes del Paso GA (2009). Modulations of autonomic cardiovascular control following acute alpha-adrenergic treatment in chronic hypotension. *Hypertens Res* 32, 938–943.

Duschek S & Schandry R (2007). Reduced brain perfusion and cognitive performance due to constitutional hypotension. *Clin Auton Res* 17, 69–76.

Duschek S, Werner N, Kapan N & Reyes del Paso GA (2008). Patterns of cerebral blood flow and systemic hemodynamics during arithmetic processing. *Journal of Psychophysiology* 22, 81–90.

Eckberg DL (1980). Nonlinearities of the human carotid baroreceptor-cardiac reflex. *Circ Res* 47, 208–216.

Edvinsson L & Krause DN (2002). Lippincott, Williams & Wilkins, Philadelphia.

Eggers J, Koch B, Meyer K, König I & Seidel G (2003). Effect of ultrasound on thrombolysis of middle cerebral artery occlusion. *Ann Neurol* 53, 797–800.

Eggers J, Ossadnik S & Seidel G (2009). Enhanced clot dissolution in vitro by 1.8-MHz pulsed ultrasound. *Ultrasound in medicine & biology* 35, 523–526.

Fadel PJ, Stromstad M, Hansen J, Sander M, Horn K, Ogoh S, Smith ML, Secher NH & Raven PB (2001). Arterial baroreflex control of sympathetic nerve activity during acute hypotension: effect of fitness. *Am J Physiol Heart Circ Physiol* 280, H2524–32.

Fan J, Burgess K, Basnyat R, Thomas K, Peebles K, Lucas S, Lucas R, Donnelly J, Cotter J & Ainslie P (2010a). Influence of high altitude on cerebrovascular and ventilatory responsiveness to CO2. *J Physiol (Lond)* 588, 539–549.

Fan JL, Burgess KR, Thomas KN, Peebles KC, Lucas SJ, Lucas RA, Cotter JD & Ainslie PN (2010b). Influence of indomethacin on ventilatory and cerebrovascular responsiveness to CO2 and breathing stability: the influence of PCO2 gradients. *Am J Physiol Regul Integr Comp Physiol* 298, R1648–58.

Fan J-L, Cotter JD, Lucas RAI, Thomas K, Wilson L & Ainslie PN (2008). Human cardiorespiratory and cerebrovascular function during severe passive hyperthermia: effects of mild hypohydration. *Journal of applied physiology (Bethesda, Md : 1985)* 105, 433–445.

Fortune JB, Bock D, Kupinski AM, Stratton HH, Shah DM & Feustel PJ (1992). Human cerebrovascular response to oxygen and carbon dioxide as determined by internal carotid artery duplex scanning. *J Trauma* 32, 618–27; discussion 627-8.

Galvin SD, Celi LA, Thomas KN, Clendon TR, Galvin IE, Bunton RW & Ainslie PN (2010). Effects of age and coronary artery disease on cerebrovascular reactivity to carbon dioxide in humans. *Anaesth Intensive Care* 38, 710–717.

Gerriets T, Postert T, Goertler M, Stolz E, Schlachetzki F, Sliwka U, Seidel G, Weber S & Kaps M (2000). DIAS I: duplex-sonographic assessment of the cerebrovascular status in acute stroke. A useful tool for future stroke trials. *Stroke* 31, 2342–2345.

Girouard H & Iadecola C (2006). Neurovascular coupling in the normal brain and in hypertension, stroke, and Alzheimer disease. *J Appl Physiol* 100, 328–335.

Green DJ, Jones H, Thijssen D, Cable NT & Atkinson G (2011). Flow-mediated dilation and cardiovascular event prediction: does nitric oxide matter? *Hypertension* 57, 363–369.

Greenfield JC & Tindall GT (1968). Effect of norepinephrine, epinephrine, and angiotensin on blood flow in the internal carotid artery of man. *J Clin Invest* 47, 1672–1684.

Grubb RLJ, Raichle ME, Eichling JO & Ter-Pogossian MM (1974). The effects of changes in PaCO2 on cerebral blood volume, blood flow, and vascular mean transit time. *Stroke* 5, 630–639.

Hamner JW, Cohen MA, Mukai S, Lipsitz LA & Taylor JA (2004). Spectral indices of human cerebral blood flow control: responses to augmented blood pressure oscillations. *The Journal of Physiology* 559, 965–973.

Harper AM & Glass HI (1965). Effect of alterations in the arterial carbon dioxide tension on the blood flow through the cerebral cortex at normal and low arterial blood pressures. *J Neurol Neurosurg Psychiatr* 28, 449–452.

Hauge A, Thoresen M & Walloe L (1980). Changes in cerebral blood flow during hyperventilation and CO2-breathing measured transcutaneously in humans by a bidirectional, pulsed, ultrasound Doppler blood velocitymeter. *Acta Physiol Scand* 110, 167–173.

Hellström G, Fischer-Colbrie W, Wahlgren NG & Jogestrand T (1996). Carotid artery blood flow and middle cerebral artery blood flow velocity during physical exercise. *Journal of applied physiology (Bethesda, Md : 1985)* 81, 413–418.

Helton WS, Hollander TD, Warm JS, Tripp LD, Parsons K, Matthews G, Dember WN, Parasuraman R & Hancock PA (2007). The abbreviated vigilance task and cerebral hemodynamics. *Jounral of Clinical and Experimental Neurophysiology* 29, 545–552.

Hendrikse J, van der Grond J, Lu H, van Zijl PC & Golay X (2004). Flow territory mapping of the cerebral arteries with regional perfusion MRI. *Stroke* 35, 882–887.

Hetzel A, Reinhard M, Guschlbauer B & Braune S (2003). Challenging cerebral autoregulation in patients with preganglionic autonomic failure. *Clin Auton Res* 13, 27–35.

Hoksbergen AW, Fulesdi B, Legemate DA & Csiba L (2000). Collateral configuration of the circle of Willis: transcranial color-coded duplex ultrasonography and comparison with postmortem anatomy. *Stroke* 31, 1346–1351.

Hossmann KA (1994). Viability thresholds and the penumbra of focal ischemia. *Ann Neurol* 36, 557–565.

Hubel DH & Wiesel TN (2005). Oxford University Press, New York.

Iadecola C & Nedergaard M (2007). Glial regulation of the cerebral microvasculature. *Nat Neurosci* 10, 1369–1376.

Immink R, Van Den Born B, Van Montfrans G, Kim Y, Hollmann M & Van Lieshout J (2008). Cerebral Hemodynamics During Treatment With Sodium Nitroprusside Versus Labetalol in Malignant Hypertension. *Hypertension* 52, 236–240.

Ito S, Mardimae A, Han J, Duffin J, Wells G, Fedorko L, Minkovich L, Katznelson R, Meineri M, Arenovich T, Kessler C & Fisher JA (2008). Non-invasive prospective targeting of arterial P(CO2) in subjects at rest. *J Physiol (Lond)* 586, 3675–3682.

Jakovcevic D & Harder DR (2007). Role of astrocytes in matching blood flow to neuronal activity. *Curr Top Dev Biol* 79, 75–97.

Jegede AB, Rosado-Rivera D, Bauman WA, Cardozo CP, Sano M, Moyer JM, Brooks M & Wecht JM (2009). Cognitive performance in hypotensive persons with spinal cord injury. *Clin Auton Res* .

Kamm C, Nagele T, Mittelbronn M, Schoning M, Melms A, Gasser T & Schols L (2008). Primary central nervous system vasculitis in a child mimicking parasitosis. *J Neurol* 255, 130–132.

Kehrer M, Blumenstock G, Ehehalt S, Goelz R, Poets C & Schoning M (2005). Development of cerebral blood flow volume in preterm neonates during the first two weeks of life. *Pediatr Res* 58, 927–930.

Kehrer M & Schoning M (2009). Quantitative sonographic measurement of cerebral blood flow volume in infants with periventricular leukomalacia. *Brain Dev* 31, 473.

Kety S & Schmidt C (1945). The determination of cerebral blood flow in man by the use of nitrous oxide in low concentrations. *Americal Journal of Physiology* 33–52.

Kety SS (1999). Mental illness and the sciences of brain and behavior. *Nat Med* 5, 1113–1116.

Kety SS & Schmidt CF (1948). The nitrous oxide method for the quantitative determination of cerebral blood flow in man; theory, procedure and normal values. *J Clin Invest* 27, 476–483.

Klingelhöfer J, Matzander G, Sander D, Schwarze J, Boecker H & Bischoff C (1997). Assessment of functional hemispheric asymmetry by bilateral simultaneous cerebral blood flow velocity monitoring. *J Cereb Blood Flow Metab* 17, 577–585.

Knecht S, Deppe M, Bäcker M, Ringelstein EB & Henningsen H (1997). Regional cerebral blood flow increases during preparation for and processing of sensory stimuli. *Experimental brain research Experimentelle Hirnforschung Expérimentation cérébrale* 116, 309–314.

Knecht S, Deppe M, Ebner A, Henningsen H, Huber T, Jokeit H & Ringelstein EB (1998a). Noninvasive determination of language lateralization by functional transcranial Doppler sonography: a comparison with the Wada test. *Stroke* 29, 82–86.

Knecht S, Deppe M, Ringelstein EB, Wirtz M, Lohmann H, Dräger B, Huber T & Henningsen H (1998b). Reproducibility of functional transcranial Doppler sonography in determining hemispheric language lateralization. *Stroke* 29, 1155–1159.

Kolb JC, Ainslie PN, Ide K & Poulin MJ (2004). Protocol to measure acute cerebrovascular and ventilatory responses to isocapnic hypoxia in humans. *Respiratory physiology & neurobiology* 141, 191–199.

Krejza J, Mariak Z, Melhem ER & Bert RJ (2000). A guide to the identification of major cerebral arteries with transcranial color Doppler sonography. *AJR Am J Roentgenol* 174, 1297-1303.

Kuker W, Gaertner S, Nagele T, Dopfer C, Schoning M, Fiehler J, Rothwell PM & Herrlinger U (2008). Vessel wall contrast enhancement: a diagnostic sign of cerebral vasculitis. *Cerebrovasc Dis* 26, 23-29.

Lassen NA (1959). Cerebral blood flow and oxygen consumption in man. *Physiol Rev* 39, 183-238.

Lassen NA, HOEDT-RASMUSSEN K, SORENSEN SC, SKINHOJ E, CRONQUIST S, BODFORSS B & INGVAR DH (1963). REGIONAL CEREBRAL BLOOD FLOW IN MAN DETERMINED BY KRYPTON. *Neurology* 13, 719-727.

Leopold PW, Shandall AA, Feustel P, Corson JD, Shah DM, Popp AJ, Fortune JB, Leather RP & Karmody AM (1987). Duplex scanning of the internal carotid artery: an assessment of cerebral blood flow. *Br J Surg* 74, 630-633.

Lohmann H, Ringelstein EB & Knecht S (2006). Functional transcranial Doppler sonography. *Frontiers of neurology and neuroscience* 21, 251-260.

Lucas SJ, Tzeng YC, Galvin SD, Thomas KN, Ogoh S & Ainslie PN (2010a). Influence of changes in blood pressure on cerebral perfusion and oxygenation. *Hypertension* 55, 698-705.

Lucas SJ, Burgess KR, Thomas KN, Donnelly J, Peebles KC, Lucas RA, Fan JL, Basnyat R, Cotter JD & Ainslie PN (2010b). Alterations in cerebral blood flow and cerebrovascular reactivity during 14 days at 5050 m. *J Physiol*

MacKenzie ET, McCulloch J, O'Kean M, Pickard JD & Harper AM (1976). Cerebral circulation and norepinephrine: relevance of the blood-brain barrier. *Am J Physiol* 231, 483-488.

Mahony PJ, Panerai RB, Deverson ST, Hayes PD & Evans DH (2000). Assessment of the thigh cuff technique for measurement of dynamic cerebral autoregulation. *Stroke* 31, 476-480.

Mandell DM, Han JS, Poublanc J, Crawley AP, Kassner A, Fisher JA & Mikulis DJ (2008). Selective reduction of blood flow to white matter during hypercapnia corresponds with leukoaraiosis. *Stroke* 39, 1993-1998.

Markus H & Cullinane M (2001). Severely impaired cerebrovascular reactivity predicts stroke and TIA risk in patients with carotid artery stenosis and occlusion. *Brain* 124, 457-467.

Markus HS & Boland M (1992). "Cognitive activity" monitored by non-invasive measurement of cerebral blood flow velocity and its application to the investigation of cerebral dominance. *Cortex* 28, 575-581.

Markus HS & Punter M (2005). Can transcranial Doppler discriminate between solid and gaseous microemboli? Assessment of a dual-frequency transducer system. *Stroke* 36, 1731-1734.

Martin PJ, Evans DH & Naylor AR (1995). Measurement of blood flow velocity in the basal cerebral circulation: advantages of transcranial color-coded sonography over conventional transcranial Doppler. *J Clin Ultrasound* 23, 21-26.

Mascia L, Fedorko L, terBrugge K, Filippini C, Pizzio M, Ranieri VM & Wallace MC (2003). The accuracy of transcranial Doppler to detect vasospasm in patients with aneurysmal subarachnoid hemorrhage. *Intensive Care Med* 29, 1088-1094.

McCalden TA, Eidelman BH & Mendelow AD (1977). Barrier and uptake mechanisms in the cerebrovascular response to noradrenaline. *Am J Physiol* 233, H458–65.

Mitchell J (2005). The vertebral artery: a review of anatomical, histopathological and functional factors influencing blood flow to the hindbrain. *Physiother Theory Pract* 21, 23–36.

Miyazaki M & Kato K (1965). Measurement of cerebral blood flow by ultrasonic Doppler technique; hemodynamic comparison of right and left carotid artery in patients with hemiplegia. *Jpn Circ J* 29, 383–386.

Mosso A (1880). Sulla circolazione del cervello dell'uomo. *Att R Accad Lincei* 5, 237–358.

Murrell C, Cotter J, George K, Shave R, Wilson L, Thomas K, Williams M, Lowe T & Ainslie P (2009). Influence of age on syncope following prolonged exercise; differential responses but similar orthostatic intolerance. *J Physiol (Lond)* 1-11.

Murrell C, Wilson L, Cotter JD, Lucas S, Ogoh S, George K & Ainslie PN (2007). Alterations in autonomic function and cerebral hemodynamics to orthostatic challenge following a mountain marathon. *J Appl Physiol* 103, 88–96.

Nabavi DG, Droste DW, Schulte-Altedorneburg G, Kemeny V, Panzica M, Weber S & Ringelstein EB (1999). Diagnostic benefit of echocontrast enhancement for the insufficient transtemporal bone window. *J Neuroimaging* 9, 102–107.

Njemanze PC (1991). Cerebral lateralization in linguistic and nonlinguistic perception: analysis of cognitive styles in the auditory modality. *Brain and language* 41, 367–380.

Nöth U, Kotajima F, Deichmann R, Turner R & Corfield DR (2008). Mapping of the cerebral vascular response to hypoxia and hypercapnia using quantitative perfusion MRI at 3 T. *NMR in biomedicine* 21, 464–472.

Nuttall GA, Cook DJ, Fulgham JR, Oliver WC & Proper JA (1996). The relationship between cerebral blood flow and transcranial Doppler blood flow velocity during hypothermic cardiopulmonary bypass in adults. *Anesth Analg* 82, 1146–1151.

Ogoh S & Ainslie PN (2009a). Regulatory mechanisms of cerebral blood flow during exercise: new concepts. *Exercise and sport sciences reviews* 37, 123–129.

Ogoh S & Ainslie PN (2009b). Cerebral blood flow during exercise: mechanisms of regulation. *J Appl Physiol* 107, 1370–1380.

Ogoh S, Brothers R, Jeschke M, Secher N & Raven P (2010). Estimation of cerebral vascular tone during exercise; evaluation by critical closing pressure in humans. *Exp Physiol* 95, 678–685.

Ogoh S, Fadel PJ, Nissen P, Jans Ø, Selmer C, Secher NH & Raven PB (2003). Baroreflex-mediated changes in cardiac output and vascular conductance in response to alterations in carotid sinus pressure during exercise in humans. *J Physiol (Lond)* 550, 317–324.

Ogoh S, Fisher JP, Fadel PJ & Raven PB (2007). Increases in central blood volume modulate carotid baroreflex resetting during dynamic exercise in humans. *J Physiol (Lond)* 581, 405–418.

Ogoh S, Tzeng YC, Lucas SJ, Galvin SD & Ainslie PN (2009). Influence of baroreflex-mediated tachycardia on the regulation of dynamic cerebral perfusion during acute hypotension in humans. *J Physiol (Lond)* .

Orlandi G & Murri L (1996). Transcranial Doppler assessment of cerebral flow velocity at rest and during voluntary movements in young and elderly healthy subjects. *Int J Neurosci* 84, 45–53.

Padayachee TS, Parsons S, Theobold R, Linley J, Gosling RG & Deverall PB (1987). The detection of microemboli in the middle cerebral artery during cardiopulmonary bypass: a transcranial Doppler ultrasound investigation using membrane and bubble oxygenators. *Ann Thorac Surg* 44, 298-302.

Panerai R (2009). Complexity of the human cerebral circulation. *Philosophical Transactions of the Royal Society A: Mathematical, Physical and Engineering Sciences* 367, 1319-1336.

Panerai RB (2003). The critical closing pressure of the cerebral circulation. *Medical engineering & physics* 25, 621-632.

Panerai RB (2008). Cerebral autoregulation: from models to clinical applications. *Cardiovascular engineering (Dordrecht, Netherlands)* 8, 42-59.

Panerai RB, Dawson SL, Eames PJ & Potter JF (2001). Cerebral blood flow velocity response to induced and spontaneous sudden changes in arterial blood pressure. *Am J Physiol Heart Circ Physiol* 280, H2162-74.

Panerai RB, Dawson SL & Potter JF (1999a). Linear and nonlinear analysis of human dynamic cerebral autoregulation. *Am J Physiol* 277, H1089-99.

Panerai RB, Deverson ST, Mahony P, Hayes P & Evans DH (1999b). Effects of CO2 on dynamic cerebral autoregulation measurement. *Physiological measurement* 20, 265-275.

Panerai RB, Rennie JM, Kelsall AW & Evans DH (1998). Frequency-domain analysis of cerebral autoregulation from spontaneous fluctuations in arterial blood pressure. *Medical & biological engineering & computing* 36, 315-322.

Peebles KC, Richards AM, Celi L, McGrattan K, Murrell CJ & Ainslie PN (2008). Human cerebral arteriovenous vasoactive exchange during alterations in arterial blood gases. *J Appl Physiol* 105, 1060-1068.

Pickkers P, Hughes AD, Russel FG, Thien T & Smits P (2001). In vivo evidence for K(Ca) channel opening properties of acetazolamide in the human vasculature. *Br J Pharmacol* 132, 443-450.

Piechnik SK, Chiarelli PA & Jezzard P (2008). Modelling vascular reactivity to investigate the basis of the relationship between cerebral blood volume and flow under CO2 manipulation. *Neuroimage* 39, 107-118.

Postert T, Federlein J, Przuntek H & Buttner T (1997). Insufficient and absent acoustic temporal bone window: potential and limitations of transcranial contrast-enhanced color-coded sonography and contrast-enhanced power-based sonography. *Ultrasound Med Biol* 23, 857-862.

Powers J, Averkiou M & Bruce M (2009). Principles of cerebral ultrasound contrast imaging. *Cerebrovasc Dis* 27 Suppl 2, 14-24.

Querido JS & Sheel AW (2007). Regulation of cerebral blood flow during exercise. *Sports medicine (Auckland, NZ)* 37, 765-782.

Rasulo FA, De Peri E & Lavinio A (2008). Transcranial Doppler ultrasonography in intensive care. *European journal of anaesthesiology Supplement* 42, 167-173.

Reichmuth K, Dopp JM, Barczi SR, Skatrud JB, Wojdyla P, Hayes Jr D & Morgan BJ (2009). Impaired Vascular Regulation in Patients with Obstructive Sleep Apnea: Effects of CPAP Treatment. *Am J Respir Crit Care Med* .

Ringelstein EB, Droste DW, Babikian VL, Evans DH, Grosset DG, Kaps M, Markus HS, Russell D & Siebler M (1998). Consensus on microembolus detection by TCD. International Consensus Group on Microembolus Detection. *Stroke* 29, 725-729.

Ringelstein EB, Kahlscheuer B, Niggemeyer E & Otis SM (1990). Transcranial Doppler sonography: anatomical landmarks and normal velocity values. *UMB* 16, 745-761.
Robbins PA, Swanson GD & Howson MG (1982). A prediction-correction scheme for forcing alveolar gases along certain time courses. *Journal of applied physiology: respiratory, environmental and exercise physiology* 52, 1353-1357.
Rodriguez RA, Nathan HJ, Ruel M, Rubens F, Dafoe D & Mesana T (2009). A method to distinguish between gaseous and solid cerebral emboli in patients with prosthetic heart valves. *European journal of cardio-thoracic surgery : official journal of the European Association for Cardio-thoracic Surgery* 35, 89-95.
Ropper AH, Kehne SM & Wechsler L (1987). Transcranial Doppler in brain death. *Neurology* 37, 1733-1735.
Rosengarten B, Aldinger C, Kaufmann A & Kaps M (2002a). Neurovascular coupling remains unaffected by glyceryl trinitrate. *Cerebrovasc Dis* 14, 58-60.
Rosengarten B, Dost A, Kaufmann A, Gortner L & Kaps M (2002b). Impaired cerebrovascular reactivity in type 1 diabetic children. *Diabetes Care* 25, 408-410.
Rosengarten B, Paulsen S, Molnar S, Kaschel R, Gallhofer B & Kaps M (2007). Activation-flow coupling differentiates between vascular and Alzheimer type of dementia. *J Neurol Sci* 257, 149-154.
Rosengarten B, Spiller A, Aldinger C & Kaps M (2003). Control system analysis of visually evoked blood flow regulation in humans under normocapnia and hypercapnia. *European journal of ultrasound : official journal of the European Federation of Societies for Ultrasound in Medicine and Biology* 16, 169-175.
Sato K, Ogoh S, Hirasawa A, Oue A & Sadamoto T (2011). The distribution of blood flow in the carotid and vertebral arteries during dynamic exercise in humans. *J Physiol (Lond)* .
Sato K & Sadamoto T (2010). Different blood flow responses to dynamic exercise between internal carotid and vertebral arteries in women. *J Appl Physiol* 109, 864-869.
Scheel P, Ruge C, Petruch UR & Schoning M (2000a). Color duplex measurement of cerebral blood flow volume in healthy adults. *Stroke* 31, 147-150.
Scheel P, Ruge C & Schoning M (2000b). Flow velocity and flow volume measurements in the extracranial carotid and vertebral arteries in healthy adults: reference data and the effects of age. *Ultrasound Med Biol* 26, 1261-1266.
Schnittger C, Johannes S, Arnavaz A & Münte TF (1997). Blood flow velocity changes in the middle cerebral artery induced by processing of hierarchical visual stimuli. *Neuropsychologia* 35, 1181-1184.
Schnittger C, Johannes S & Münte TF (1996). Transcranial Doppler assessment of cerebral blood flow velocity during visual spatial selective attention in humans. *Neuroscience Letters* 214, 41-44.
Schoning M & Hartig B (1996). Age dependence of total cerebral blood flow volume from childhood to adulthood. *J Cereb Blood Flow Metab* 16, 827-833.
Schoning M, Scheel P, Holzer M, Fretschner R & Will BE (2005a). Volume measurement of cerebral blood flow: assessment of cerebral circulatory arrest. *Transplantation* 80, 326-331.
Schoning M, Scheel P, Holzer M, Fretschner R & Will BE (2005b). Volume measurement of cerebral blood flow: assessment of cerebral circulatory arrest. *Transplantation* 80, 326-331.

Schoning M, Walter J & Scheel P (1994). Estimation of cerebral blood flow through color duplex sonography of the carotid and vertebral arteries in healthy adults. *Stroke* 25, 17–22.

Serrador JM, Picot PA, Rutt BK, Shoemaker JK & Bondar RL (2000). MRI measures of middle cerebral artery diameter in conscious humans during simulated orthostasis. *Stroke* 31, 1672-1678.

Serrador JM, Sorond FA, Vyas M, Gagnon M, Iloputaife ID & Lipsitz LA (2005). Cerebral pressure-flow relations in hypertensive elderly humans: transfer gain in different frequency domains. *J Appl Physiol* 98, 151–159.

Settakis G, Molnár C, Kerényi L, Kollár J, Legemate D, Csiba L & Fülesdi B (2003). Acetazolamide as a vasodilatory stimulus in cerebrovascular diseases and in conditions affecting the cerebral vasculature. *Eur J Neurol* 10, 609–620.

Silvestrini M, Caltagirone C, Cupini LM, Matteis M, Troisi E & Bernardi G (1993). Activation of healthy hemisphere in poststroke recovery. A transcranial Doppler study. *Stroke* 24, 1673–1677.

Silvestrini M, Troisi E, Matteis M, Cupini LM & Caltagirone C (1995). Involvement of the healthy hemisphere in recovery from aphasia and motor deficit in patients with cortical ischemic infarction: a transcranial Doppler study. *Neurology* 45, 1815–1820.

Silvestrini M, Troisi E, Matteis M, Razzano C & Caltagirone C (1998). Correlations of flow velocity changes during mental activity and recovery from aphasia in ischemic stroke. *Neurology* 50, 191–195.

Silvestrini M, Vernieri F, Pasqualetti P, Matteis M, Passarelli F, Troisi E & Caltagirone C (2000). Impaired cerebral vasoreactivity and risk of stroke in patients with asymptomatic carotid artery stenosis. *JAMA* 283, 2122–2127.

Sitzer M, Knorr U & Seitz RD (1994). cerebral hemodynamics during sensorimotor activation in humans. *Journal of Applied Physiology* 77, 2804–2811.

Slessarev M, Han J, Mardimae A, Prisman E, Preiss D, Volgyesi G, Ansel C, Duffin J & Fisher J (2007). Prospective targeting and control of end-tidal CO2 and O2 concentrations. *The Journal of Physiology* 581, 1207–1219.

Sloan MA, Alexandrov AV, Tegeler CH, Spencer MP, Caplan LR, Feldmann E, Wechsler LR, Newell DW, Gomez CR, Babikian VL, Lefkowitz D, Goldman RS, Armon C, Hsu CY & Goodin DS (2004). Assessment: transcranial Doppler ultrasonography: report of the Therapeutics and Technology Assessment Subcommittee of the American Academy of Neurology. *Neurology* 62, 1468–1481.

Smith ML, Beightol LA, Fritsch-Yelle JM, Ellenbogen KA, Porter TR & Eckberg DL (1996). Valsalva's maneuver revisited: a quantitative method yielding insights into human autonomic control. *Am J Physiol* 271, H1240–9.

Smyth HS, Sleight P & Pickering GW (1969). Reflex regulation of arterial pressure during sleep in man. A quantitative method of assessing baroreflex sensitivity. *Circ Res* 24, 109–121.

Sorond FA, Khavari R, Serrador JM & Lipsitz LA (2005). Regional cerebral autoregulation during orthostatic stress: age-related differences. *J Gerontol A Biol Sci Med Sci* 60, 1484–1487.

Strandness DEJ (1985). Echo-Doppler (duplex) ultrasonic scanning. *J Vasc Surg* 2, 341–344.

Stroobant N & Vingerhoets G (2000). Transcranial Doppler ultrasonography monitoring of cerebral hemodynamics during performance of cognitive tasks: a review. *Neuropsychology review* 10, 213–231.

Taylor JA, Carr DL, Myers CW & Eckberg DL (1998). Mechanisms underlying very-low-frequency RR-interval oscillations in humans. *Circulation* 98, 547–555.

ter Minassian A, Melon E, Leguerinel C, Lodi CA, Bonnet F & Beydon L (1998). Changes in cerebral blood flow during PaCO2 variations in patients with severe closed head injury: comparison between the Fick and transcranial Doppler methods. *J Neurosurg* 88, 996–1001.

Thie A, Carvajal-Lizano M, Schlichting U, Spitzer K & Kunze K (1992). Multimodal tests of cerebrovascular reactivity in migraine: a transcranial Doppler study. *J Neurol* 239, 338–342.

Thomas KN, Cotter JD, Galvin SD, Williams MJ, Willie CK & Ainslie PN (2009). Initial orthostatic hypotension is unrelated to orthostatic tolerance in healthy young subjects. *J Appl Physiol* 107, 506–517.

Tiecks FP, Douville C, Byrd S, Lam AM & Newell DW (1996). Evaluation of impaired cerebral autoregulation by the Valsalva maneuver. *Stroke* 27, 1177–1182.

Tiecks FP, Lam AM, Aaslid R & Newell DW (1995a). Comparison of static and dynamic cerebral autoregulation measurements. *Stroke* 26, 1014–1019.

Tiecks FP, Lam AM, Matta BF, Strebel S, Douville C & Newell DW (1995b). Effects of the Valsalva Maneuver on Cerebral Circulation in Healthy Adults : A Transcranial Doppler Study. *Stroke* 26, 1386–1392.

Troisi E, Silvestrini M, Matteis M, Monaldo BC, Vernieri F & Caltagirone C (1999). Emotion-related cerebral asymmetry: hemodynamics measured by functional ultrasound. *J Neurol* 246, 1172–1176.

Tsivgoulis G, Alexandrov AV & Sloan MA (2009). Advances in transcranial Doppler ultrasonography. *Current neurology and neuroscience reports* 9, 46–54.

Tzeng YC, Lucas SJ, Atkinson G, Willie CK & Ainslie PN (2010a). Fundamental relationships between arterial baroreflex sensitivity and dynamic cerebral autoregulation in humans. *J Appl Physiol* 108, 1162–1168.

Tzeng YC, Willie CK, Atkinson G, Lucas SJ, Wong A & Ainslie PN (2010b). Cerebrovascular regulation during transient hypotension and hypertension in humans. *Hypertension* 56, 268–273.

Tzeng YC, Willie CK & Ainslie PN (2010c). Baroreflex, cerebral perfusion, and stroke: integrative physiology at its best. *Stroke* 41, e429.

Valdueza JM, Balzer JO, Villringer A, Vogl TJ, Kutter R & Einhäupl KM (1997). Changes in blood flow velocity and diameter of the middle cerebral artery during hyperventilation: assessment with MR and transcranial Doppler sonography. *AJNR American journal of neuroradiology* 18, 1929–1934.

Vernieri F, Pasqualetti P, Matteis M, Passarelli F, Troisi E, Rossini PM, Caltagirone C & Silvestrini M (2001). Effect of collateral blood flow and cerebral vasomotor reactivity on the outcome of carotid artery occlusion. *Stroke* 32, 1552–1558.

Widder B, Kleiser B & Krapf H (1994). Course of cerebrovascular reactivity in patients with carotid artery occlusions. *Stroke* 25, 1963–1967.

Wijnhoud AD, Koudstaal PJ & Dippel DW (2006). Relationships of transcranial blood flow Doppler parameters with major vascular risk factors: TCD study in patients with a recent TIA or nondisabling ischemic stroke. *Journal of clinical ultrasound : JCU* 34, 70–76.

Willie CK, Cowan EC, Ainslie PN, Taylor CE, Smith KJ, Sin PYW & Tzeng YC (2011a). Neurovascular coupling and distribution of cerebral blood flow during exercise. *Journal of Neuroscience Methods* 198, 270–273.

Willie CK, Colino FL, Bailey DM, Tzeng YC, Binsted G, Jones LW, Haykowsky MJ, Bellapart J, Ogoh S, Smith KJ, Smirl JD, Day TA, Lucas SJ, Eller LK & Ainslie PN (2011b). Utility of transcranial Doppler ultrasound for the integrative assessment of cerebrovascular function. *Journal of Neuroscience Methods* 196, 221–237.

Wilson LC, Cotter JD, Fan JL, Lucas RA, Thomas KN & Ainslie PN (2010). Cerebrovascular reactivity and dynamic autoregulation in tetraplegia. *Am J Physiol Regul Integr Comp Physiol* 298, R1035–42.

Wintermark M, Sesay M, Barbier E, Borbély K, Dillon WP, Eastwood JD, Glenn TC, Grandin CB, Pedraza S, Soustiel JF, Nariai T, Zaharchuk G, Caillé JM, Dousset V & Yonas H (2005). Comparative overview of brain perfusion imaging techniques. *Stroke* 36, e83–99.

Woods T, Harmann L, Purath T, Ramamurthy S, Subramanian S, Jackson S & Tarima S (2010). Small- and Moderate-Size Right-to-Left Shunts Identified by Saline Contrast Echocardiography Are Normal and Unrelated to Migraine Headache. *Chest* 138, 264–269.

Xie A, Skatrud JB, Khayat R, Dempsey JA, Morgan B & Russell D (2005). Cerebrovascular response to carbon dioxide in patients with congestive heart failure. *Am J Respir Crit Care Med* 172, 371–378.

Zagorac D, Yamaura K, Zhang C, Roman RJ & Harder DR (2005). The effect of superoxide anion on autoregulation of cerebral blood flow. *Stroke* 36, 2589–2594.

Zhang R, Zuckerman JH, Giller CA & Levine BD (1998). Transfer function analysis of dynamic cerebral autoregulation in humans. *Am J Physiol* 274, H233–41.

Zhang R, Zuckerman JH, Iwasaki K, Wilson TE, Crandall CG & Levine BD (2002). Autonomic neural control of dynamic cerebral autoregulation in humans. *Circulation* 106, 1814–1820.

2

Theory and Practice of MRA-Guided Transcranial Doppler Sonography

Francisco L. Colino and Gordon Binsted
Department of Human Kinetics, Faculty of Health and Social Development, The University of British Columbia, Kelowna, BC, Canada

1. Introduction

Despite consisting of 2 - 3% of total body mass, the brain accounts for ~20% of the body's oxygen consumption and therefore must receive significant blood supply to maintain homeostasis (Ainslie & Duffin, 2009). This profound dependency on blood supply belies the brain's apparent ability to regulate blood supply so tightly. Hence, the brain's ability to regulate its blood supply has been, and still is, the subject of considerable research (e.g., Kety & Schmidt, 1948; Panerai et al., 2009; Willie & Smith, 2011; Willie et al., 2011; also see Ainslie & Duffin, 2009 for a recent review). However, the dense cortical bone of the skull does not lend itself easily to normal ultrasound techniques.

The most common tool for assessing cerebral blood flow regulation is transcranial Doppler sonography (TCD) as it operates at lower frequencies (usually 1 - 2 MHz), relative to conventional ultrasound frequencies (≥ 5 MHz), to penetrate the skull. Traditionally, researchers rely solely on an M-mode display[1] for information regarding depth, blood flow velocity, pulsatility index, etc. (Aaslid et al., 1986). Based on historical indicators they infer which vessel is insonated; for example, the user can perform simple stimulus-response tests to confirm that the identity of the vessel. A reduction in blood flow velocity following the vibration/compression of the external carotid would confirm middle cerebral artery (MCA) insonation. In a similar fashion, flow variation accompanying the opening/closing of the eyes is a simple confirmatory test for the posterior cerebral artery (PCA).

Despite these well-established procedures to determine vessel identity, there are several notable problems with the current approach. First, TCD measures blood flow velocity, which is a relative measure; absolute flow cannot be estimated without knowing the vessel diameter. Specifically, according to Poiseuille's Law, flow (Q) is determined by the vessel length (L), pressure difference (P), viscosity (η) and, most notably, vessel radius (α).

$$Q = \frac{pa^4 P}{8Lh} \qquad (1)$$

---

[1] M-mode stands for 'motion mode'. This modality returns echoes over time for one line of the B-mode image. Thus, movement of structures positioned in that line can be visualized in a time-varying fashion. Often M-mode and B-mode are displayed together on the ultrasound monitor.

While each factor is relevant to an accurate estimate of flow, vessel radius has the most profound influence as it is raised to the fourth power. For example, if an occlusion (e.g., due to thrombus etc.) decreases vessel radius by 1/2 then blood flow decreases 16-fold. Thus, it is critical to know the *veridical* radius when estimating absolute volumetric flow - even if the other factors are known.

However, it is also important to note that intracranial arteries are distensible (Monson et al. 2008) and therefore the reliance on Poiseuille's Law is inappropriate. Notably, a recent computer simulation of the cerebral circulation has identified vascular compliance as an important determinant of dynamic cerebral pressure-flow relationships characterized in the frequency domain (Zhang et al. 2009). Based on a Windkessel model, they reported that increases in steady state cerebrovascular resistance and or decreases in compliance could alter dynamic pressure-flow velocity relations within the cerebral circulation. This finding suggests added complexity to the study of cerebrovascular physiology because the current characteristics, derived largely from transfer function analysis (TFA), are commonly ascribed to active vascular control mechanisms without acknowledging the dynamic mechanical properties of the cerebral vasculature. Specifically, vascular compliance necessitates the consideration of the rate of pressure change driving the volume expansion in compliant vessels (i.e. capacitive blood flow) in addition to the instantaneous blood pressure that drives blood flow directly through small resistive vessels (Chan et al. 2011).

When estimating blood flow velocity using TCD, insonation angle can also profoundly impact measure accuracy. The accuracy of the flow-measure estimate increases as the insonation angle decreases (i.e. becomes closer to parallel). An oblique angle results in underestimation (see Aaslid, 1986). Problematically however, information regarding insonation angle is rarely available. Indeed, blood velocity data garnered from TCD are often compared to control conditions using percent change metric as an attempt to control for this shortcoming. Such an approach makes comparison between individuals and/or groups problematic at best. Information regarding vessels course, depth and diameter would reasonably aid estimation of absolute blood flow, while confirmation of insonation location (e.g., segment of vessel) and insonation angle will aid replication and reliability. Thus, with this knowledge, researchers would be able to employ more varied designs, enabling consideration of absolute, multi-day measures and between-subject comparisons. While we certainly acknowledge that the majority of TCD users adopt attenuation methods as opposed to absolute velocities (for the reasons highlight above), it is nonetheless important to recognize the limitations of stimulus-response relationships (e.g., for reactivity or autoregulation testing. read: Ainslie & Duffin; and Willie et al) and present more comprehensive alternatives.

There are limited number of examples in the literature exist that attempted to address the problem of TCD guidance (Auer et al., 1999; Kantelhardt et al., 2011). A recent study looked at neurological patients with various forms of head trauma using computerized tomography of the basal cerebral arterial architecture (Kantelhardt et al., 2011). These authors demonstrated that CT-guided TCD is a viable and efficient means to re-examine neurology patients. Specifically, this group was able to reduce initial examinations to approximately 8 minutes of all measured vessels (i.e., internal carotid artery, MCA, MCA bifurcation, PCA, anterior cerebral artery (ACA), and posterior communicating arteries). Kantelhardt and colleagues concluded that navigated TCD provides faster and more reliable insonation of all basal cerebral vessels given visualized anatomical references. Incredibly, subsequent examination times on the same patient were reduced by approximately 50%. The development of a standardized protocol for image-guided TCD, to establish spatial coordinates of vascular structures, should aid multi-day investigations by improving inter-session precision, reducing inter- and intra-investigator variability, and accommodating cases of atypical vascular architecture.

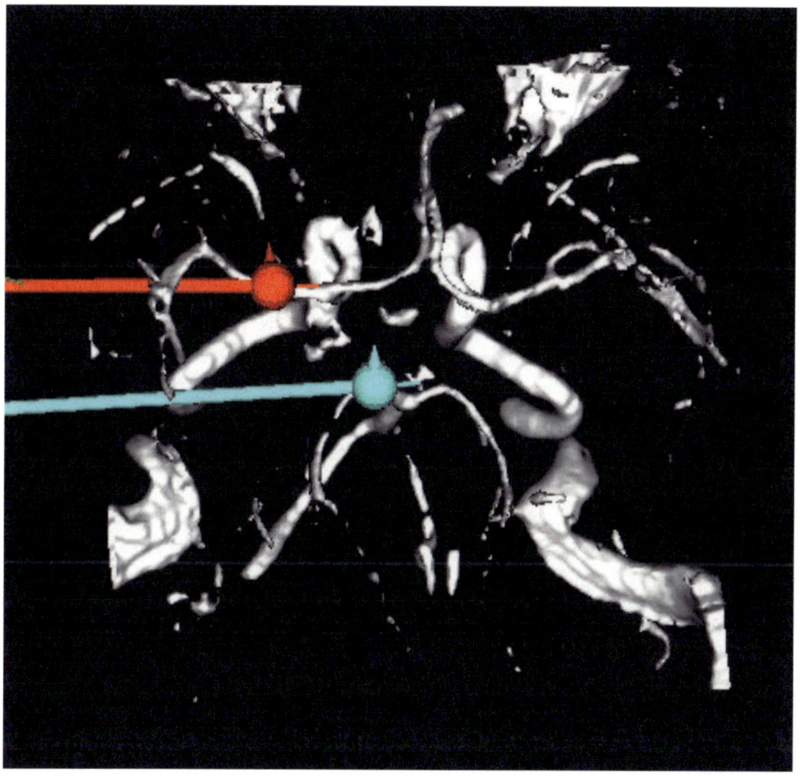

Fig. 1. Example of targets on MCA (red trajectory) and PCA (light blue trajectory) for TCD guidance. The experimenter is guided to the target vessel relative to the targets set by the experimenter. The angle of the probe relative to the these target gives insonation angle as well as target depth. However, it is important to note that target selection is entirely based on experimenter judgment. Therefore, it is recommended that the target is set as parallel as possible to the blood vessel's longitudinal axis. Indeed, a tortuously coursed vessel complicates the procedure.

The limitations presented for TCD stem largely from its inability, due to low ultrasonic frequency, to resolve a useful 2D image. Higher ultrasound frequencies cannot adequately penetrate the bones of the skull. B-mode duplex ultrasonography used in neurosurgical settings (e.g., Mathiesen et al., 2007; Mercier et al., 2010; Weiss et al., 2008) is only possible due to the availability of an open window free of boney obstruction. In most physiological experiments the researcher does not have this luxury and are limited to relying on "windows" (i.e., areas of thin bone) to interrogate the vessels of interest (Grolimund, 1986). A way to overcome this physical barrier is achieved by magnetic resonance angiography

(MRA) which, when coupled with existing neuronavigation systems (Gronningsaeter et al., 2000; Mathiesen et al., 2007), can provide an effective means to help direct the TCD probe. While there are other imaging modalities in available (e.g., CT), MRA is a non-invasive method that does not emit ionizing radiation nor does it require contrast agents (Kantelhardt et al., 2011).

2. Magnetic Resonance Angiography: Basic principles

Magnetic resonance angiography (MRA) uses a combination of static magnetic fields and radiofrequency pulses to generate images that can readily be used to assess the cerebral arteries and veins (Wedeen et al., 1985). Tissues have inherent magnetic relaxation times (e.g., T_1, T_2) that principally determine how they appear in an image. Blood has a long T_1 relaxation time (~1.2 secs), which is exploited to generate MR angiograms. A typical MRA image acquisition utilizes the "time-of-flight" (TOF) imaging method whereby (in one variant) the flow of blood from one position to the next will change the returned signal, thus differentiating blood from stationary tissues. Conventional spin-echo and fast spin-echo images result in "dark blood" (i.e., flowing blood returns no signal and, therefore, appears dark), however researchers interested in the arteries themselves often seek images via a gradient-echo pulse sequence. Unlike spin-echo or fast spin-echo sequence, only one radiofrequency pulse is emitted during each repetition cycle to negate the image wash-out (Edelman & Meyer, 2003). The resulting angiograms are referred to as "bright blood" images because the blood in the cerebral vessels returns much more signal than the surrounding tissue. In general, three-dimensional TOF MRA is best for high anatomical resolution, whereas two-dimensional TOF MRA is best to image slow or turbulent blood flow (Baumgartner et al., 1995). Thus, three-dimensional TOF MRA is most appropriate for TCD navigation.

MRA-guided duplex ultrasound has been used in neurosurgical settings (Akdemir et al., 2007; Mathiesen et al., 2007), but transcranial examinations are of limited use because of the acoustic windows of the skull (Baumgartner et al., 1995; Gerriets et al., 1999; Grolimund, 1986). Similarly then, MRA-guided TCD can reduce search times dramatically and improve examiner anatomical orientation (Kantelhardt et al., 2011) with several examples commercially packages available[2]: Kolibri navigation system (Softouch, Brainlab AG), Brainsight 2 (Rogue Research). Once the images are collected and downloaded into the guidance software, a threshold-based segmentation of the arteries from the surrounding tissue and three-dimensional reconstruction must be performed (Figure 1). A 3D reconstruction of the vascular architecture that is spatially matched with a subject's anatomical MRI image provides a virtual representation for easy vessel identification and ultrasound interrogation. Further, based on this abstraction, the experimenter can calculate vessel diameter and insonation angle (discussed below).

The above guidance systems use frameless image guidance. The use of passive infrared tracking systems in combination with a relative guidance coordinate system permits subjects to move freely (see Figure 2). In general, the registration process begins with the

[2] These systems are employable with some modification. No system is natively able to physically accommodate a TCD probe nor optimally configured to target Doppler signal.

acquired MRA image and identifying anatomical landmarks in the guidance software (e.g., tip of the nose, nasion, left and right inter-tragal notch) and the registration of these fiducial landmarks. Rigid bodies are fixed to the subject and the TCD probe and co-registered (Figure 2). While this approach to image guidance for TCD has shown to dramatically improved acquisition of circle of Willis arteries (Auer et al., 1999; Kantelhardt et al., 2011), this data does not speak to the accuracy of tracking the subject and tool.

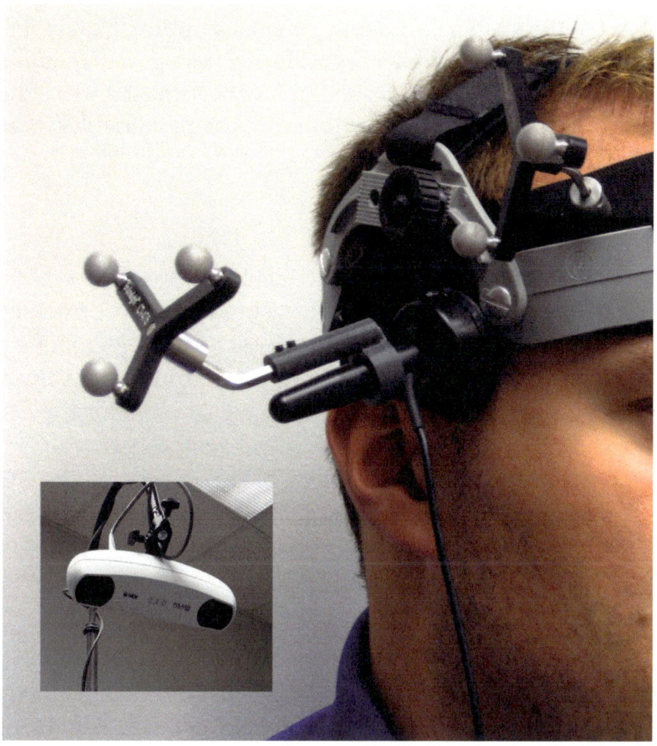

Fig. 2. Rigid bodies attached to example participant's head to track the three-dimensional position of the TCD probe relative to the participant's head. The rigid bodies are tracked by an infrared-emitting camera (inset; Polaris Vicra IR camera, Northern Digital Inc., Waterloo, ON, Canada) that emits IR light that reflects back to the camera by the passive IR markers fixed to each rigid body. Pictured is a TCD probe, a MARC 600 head mount (Spencer Technologies, Seattle, WA, USA) and rigid bodies (Brainsight, Rogue Research, Montreal, QC, Canada).

3. Measurement errors and insonation angle

Despite image guidance's utility, using rigid body reconstructions to track tools (i.e., markers attached to the TCD probe and the subject in this case) has inherent uncertainty. This is particularly concerning when an experimenter attempts to acquire a deep vessel (e.g., middle cerebral artery). Most motion capture manufacturers claim sub-millimeter precision performance of their products, however the published errors assume measurements are taken at the rigid body (see Figure 2). For the purposes of TCD it is useful to consider the minimum tracking uncertainty as expressed as per unit insonation depth. As exemplar, consider a camera system with a volume accuracy of 0.25 mm with a 0.5 mm confidence interval. That is, the tool being tracked can be tracked to the nearest 0.25 mm with an uncertainty of 0.5 mm (*N.B.* these numbers describe the Polaris Vicra, Northern Digital Inc. To view these specifications, see http://www.ndigital.com/medical/polarisfamily-techspecs.php). Further, the rigid body tracking the TCD probe is 8 cm long and the skin-to-skull distance is 0.25 cm. Thus, we can calculate the "tracking uncertainty" using simple trigonometry; the result of which gives $x \approx 0.63$ mm of error for every 10 mm of insonation depth. Thus, with a 50 mm insonation depth generates approximately 5.8 mm of tracking uncertainty. Therefore every researcher considering using image-guiding systems for experiments must keep in mind when designing an experiment and taking measurements. Let us review the calculations and point out important variables that affect tracking uncertainty.

3.1 Estimating insonation angle

Classically, the insonation angle is unknown in TCD-based vascular experiments. This leads to uncertainty as to how much velocity measurements are underestimated during measurement. Also, we already know from the physics of Doppler shifts (see Aaslid, 1986 for a complete review of the physics behind Doppler shift in blood velocity measurement) that the higher the degree of perpendicularity to the signal of interest, the higher the degree of underestimation. Indeed, when insonating a vessel an observer who is not aware of this potential issue can mistakenly take the observed blood velocity as the true blood velocity when, in fact, observed blood velocity may be much lower than that observed (Aaslid, 1986). Specifically,

$$v = |v'| \cos\sigma \tag{2}$$

where v is observed blood velocity, v' is the true blood flow velocity, and σ is the angle of the ultrasonic beam relative to the flow vector (i.e., insonation angle). However, it is unlikely that insonation angle is zero for any given TCD measurement. Almost more importantly however, the experimenter does not know the insonation angle and, therefore, does not know by how much blood velocity is underestimated. For example, we have observed insonation angles as great as 30° while interrogating the posterior cerebral artery (PCA) while observing an average blood velocity of 55 cm/sec (unpublished observations). The observed blood velocity is therefore underestimated by approximately 14% and the absolute blood velocity is approximately 64 cm/sec. However, researchers must keep in mind that a relatively perpendicular insonation angle may be the only approach to insonate an artery given the limitations imposed by the temporal acoustic window.

4. Measuring temporal bone thickness

The cranial bones are made up of three layers; each influences the ultrasound beam in a different way (White et al., 1978). In most cases however, ultrasonic power is markedly reduced by transmission through the temporal bone. Power loss is primarily a function of bone thickness as long as the bone is structurally homogeneous (i.e., no thickness variation). If the temporal bone thickness varies, the bone acts as an acoustic lens by scattering the acoustic energy across space (Grolimund, 1986). Nontheless, researchers should be aware that increased bone thickness impedes TCD measurements. Insonating at an angle that is normal (i.e., 90 degrees) to the bone diminishes boney impediment to the ultrasound beam (Ammi et al., 2008). Furthermore, possessing a library of anatomical MRI images that can be acquired with an MRA, from subjects opens the possibility for screening subjects for adequately thin acoustic windows.

Bone thickness, for the purpose of TCD, can be estimated at the temporal bone rostral to the ear and dorsal to the zygomatic arch using any standard MRI imaging software (e.g., Osirix). The experimenter can therefore judge variations in the temporal acoustic window by measuring thickness of the cortical bone in sequential order from the point where the zygomatic arch meets the ear dorsally and rostrally. Grolimund (1986) observed that cortical bone in the temporal acoustic window as thin as 2.5 mm resulted in 99% energy loss in the ultrasound beam, as well as significant scattering of the beam (Ammi et al., 2008; Grolimund et al., 1986). Measuring the borders of the temporal acoustic window can assist experimenters to visualize it appropriately. Thus, they can determine the best approach to the cerebral vessels given the acoustic constraints provided by a subject's anatomy. Also, knowing the window boundaries can help reduce experiment time by eliminating the need to reposition the TCD probe during vessel acquisition.

Having a defined acoustic window can inform experimenters how to optimally approach a blood vessel by maximizing signal and reducing insonation angle. Unfortunately, for some subjects the available acoustic window may not afford a good approach to underlying vessels. In other words, the approach that optimizes insonation angle may not be optimal for good signal acquisition. Indeed, in our laboratory we observed maximum signal from the PCA was reached with an insonation angle > thirty degrees. However, when the probe was adjusted for optimal insonation angle ($<5^{\circ}$) the signal quality suffered severely due to bone occlusion. That is, the image guiding system confirmed that the probe was pointed at the PCA but there was insufficient signal from the PCA for any useful analysis (unpublished observations).

Certainly, these observations demonstrate the inherent drawback of insonating through bone - signal will always be lost and in some cases, completely. Indeed, in a recent study Ammi et al. (2008) conducted a study of ultrasound beam penetration through human skull specimens. They found that all ultrasonic pulses sent from various ultrasonic emitters of differing frequencies (i.e., 1.03 and 2.0 MHz) were attenuated as a function of bone thickness. Furthermore, sound pressure level of a 2.0 MHz probe, measured by a hydrophone, was diminished by more than 75% at the location they calculated the MCA would be *in vivo* (for details on this hydrophone alignment procedure see Ammi et al., 2008, *pp.* 1581-2). Thus, despite the informative benefits of using an imaging system for experimental optimization, these results highlight the fact that no guidance system can overcome the physical barrier of the temporal bone.

5. MRA and TCD vessel diameter measurement: Method agreement

We mentioned in the introduction that the brain requires an adequate supply of oxygen to maintain normal functions (Ainslie & Duffin, 2009), and the methods by which the brain does this is difficult to determine without a reliable estimate of absolute blood flow, and therefore vessel diameter. Due to obvious physical and ethical limitations, indirect measures must be employed leaving the true value of a physiological quantity unknown. Generally, new measures are compared against a "gold standard" method to assess the newer measure's reliability, or, in other words, quantify measurement error (Atkinson & Nevill, 2006). Atkinson & Nevill (1998) defined reliability as "the amount of measurement error that has been deemed *acceptable for the effective practical use* of a measurement tool" (emphasis added). It is important to note that it is inevitable that different measures will have a degree of disagreement but it is important to measure *how much* disagreement exists between two measures (Bland & Altman, 1999) the impact of this difference. In the context of this review, the methods of interest are TCD and MRA and the practical impact on flow estimates was considered.

In a recently published study, Wilson et al. (2011) compared vessel diameter measurements from transcranial color Doppler ultrasound (TCCD) and MRA. In brief, they correlated transcranial Doppler and MRA vessel diameter estimates and found them to correlate (Pearson's $r = 0.82$, $r^2 = 0.67$). The robustness of this correlation superficially suggests a degree of confidence can be had in TCD estimates, as they appear to correspond well to MR values. However, the Wilson et al. (2011) study only included 7 subjects in their comparison between TCCD and MRA diameter comparisons (although it must be noted that this was *not* the primary research question of Wilson et al., 2011). Atkinson and Nevill (2006) suggest that 40 participants is the minimum number required to perform a measurement comparison study. As such, this correlation should be interpreted with caution, due to insufficient power, however it would similarly be inappropriate to discount it, as the data appear externally valid.

Despite a strong correlation, the presence of systematic bias between the TCD and MRA methods was not addressed by Wilson et al (2011). What is immediately apparent is from their data (see Table 1) is that TCCD vessel diameters generally larger than the MRA-derived diameters. Plotting these differences using a Bland-Altman approach (Figure 3) reveals clear systematic bias in which the ultrasound-derived vessel diameters are nearly twice those measured from MRA. Proportional bias is also evident whereby systematic differences between method sensitivities across the measurement range (Atkinson & Nevill, 2006). We can further assess measurement differences by determining their limits of agreement (LOA). The LOA expresses maximum deviation between any two repeated observations with a 95% certainty. Notably, a sizeable proportion of the data lies above the upper limit of agreement ($LOA_{upper} = 3.23$; $LOA_{lower} = 2.04$), indicating poor agreement between MRA and TCCD. However, in the present case of due to the proportional bias present in this data LOA should be interpreted with caution for determination of agreement between TCCD and MRA vessel measurements (Bland & Altman, 1999). A similar caution should be taken when considering intraclass correlation coefficients for the same purpose, as they too assume no relationship between error and magnitude of a measured value.

Fortunately, the proportional biases in TCCD/MRA reliability can be corrected using a logarithm transformation of the raw data (see Table 2). The log-transformed differences can be plotted (Figure 4) and thus permit the LOA to be determined for this bias-free data (see Table 2). LOA for the log-transformed data show that the two methods appear to agree fairly well; data points fall within the limits of agreement ($LOA_{upper} = 0.71$; $LOA_{lower} = 0.50$). However, once again, given that these results are derived from a sample of seven participants they must be interpreted with reservation (for a summary of results from other studies, see Table 3).

Participant	TCCD	MRA	Mean	Difference	Calculated LOA
Normoxia					3.23 (upper limit)
1	6.03	3.34	4.69	2.69	2.04 (lower limit)
2	5.77	3.36	4.57	2.41	
3	5.55	3.07	4.31	2.48	
4	5.29	3.16	4.23	2.13	
5	5.25	2.76	4.01	2.49	
6	5.14	2.60	3.87	2.54	
7	5.01	2.93	3.97	2.08	
Hypoxia					
1	6.67	3.52	5.10	3.15	
2	6.40	3.62	5.01	2.78	
3	6.35	3.34	4.85	3.01	
4	6.11	3.04	4.58	3.07	
5	5.93	3.24	4.59	2.69	
6	5.86	3.16	4.51	2.70	
7	5.58	2.84	4.21	2.74	
			SD	0.31	

Table 1. MCA vessel diameters measured by TCCD and MRA, as well as the calculated mean of the two measures along with the difference scores and standard deviation of the difference scores. Also, see the calculated LOA for the raw diameter scores. SD is the standard deviation of all the difference scores used to calculate LOA. Thus, despite the initially stated concern regarding sample size and lack of consideration of both random and systematic error, the original assertion made by Wilson et al. (2011) appears well founded. A good degree of agreement does appear to exist between MRA and TCCD vessel diameter measurements, suggesting that (in the absence of MR) TCD can generate reliable values.

Participants	Log TCD	Log MRA	Mean	Difference	Calculated Log LOA
Normoxia					0.72 (upper limit)
1	1.80	1.21	1.50	0.59	0.50 (lower limit)
2	1.75	1.21	1.48	0.54	
3	1.71	1.12	1.42	0.59	
4	1.67	1.15	1.41	0.52	
5	1.66	1.02	1.34	0.64	
6	1.64	0.96	1.30	0.68	
7	1.61	1.08	1.34	0.54	
Hypoxia					
1	1.90	1.26	1.58	0.64	
2	1.86	1.29	1.57	0.57	
3	1.85	1.21	1.53	0.64	
4	1.81	1.11	1.46	0.70	
5	1.78	1.18	1.48	0.60	
6	1.77	1.15	1.46	0.62	
7	1.72	1.04	1.38	0.68	
			SD	0.05	

Table 2. Log transformed scores from Table 1. The mean of each trial and the difference between each measure for every subject was calculated. This was done to eliminate the proportional bias that was present in difference data from the raw numbers. SD is the standard deviation of all the difference scores used to calculate LOA.

Measurement Tool	Mean MCA diameter (mm)	Study	No. participants	Notes
Cadaver	2.5 -- 4 (mean = 3.35)	Pai et al., 2005	5	
MRA (1.5T)	2.9	Serrador et al., 2000	12	
	2.73	Schreiber et al., 2000	8	
	2.23	Tarasow et a., 2007	36	
	2.95	Hansen et al., 2007	12	
	3.4	Valdueza et al., 1997	6	
	3.04 (Normoxia) 3.27 (Hypoxia)	Wilson et al., 2011	7	
Angiography	2.38	Tarasow et al., 2007	36	
Power Doppler				
Proximal MCA	5.2	Muller et al., 2000	17	Participants suspected of having vasospasm
Distal MCA	4.3	Muller et al., 2000		
TCCD				
Proximal MCA	5.9	Muller et al., 2000	17	Participants suspected of having vasospasm
Distal MCA	4.9	Muller et al., 2000		
	5.44 (Normoxia) 6.23 (90-min Hypoxia) 6.28 (180-min Hypoxia)	Wilson et al., 2011	7	

Table 3. Summary of results from several studues measureing MCA diameter using various measurement tools. MCA, middle cerebral artery; MRA, magnetic resonance angiography; TCCD, transcranial color-coded Doppler sonography. Please note the fairly constant relationship in the diameter measurements from MRA and TCCD (Wilson et al., 2011). Adapted from Wilson et al. (2011).

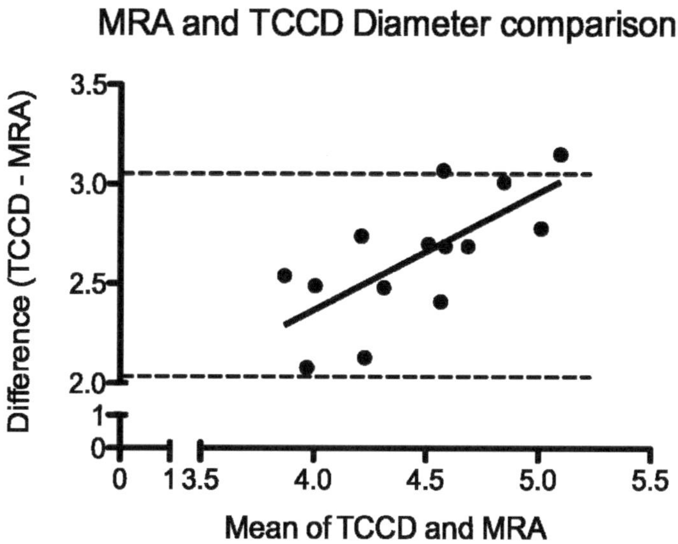

Fig. 3. MRA and TCCD MCA vessel diameter comparison. The abscissa depicts the mean of TCCD and MRA diameter measurement in a participant-wise manner. The ordinate depicts the difference of TCCD and MRA within each subject. Clearly, there is a proportional bias in the sample measured by the regression line ($y = 0.59x + 0.01$). The LOA (depicted by two dashed lines) cannot be used to measure agreement because it assumes there is no relationship between error and the magnitude of the measured value (Bland & Altman, 1999; Atkinson & Nevill, 2006). Therefore, this data needs to be transformed to eliminate the proportional bias (see Figure 4).

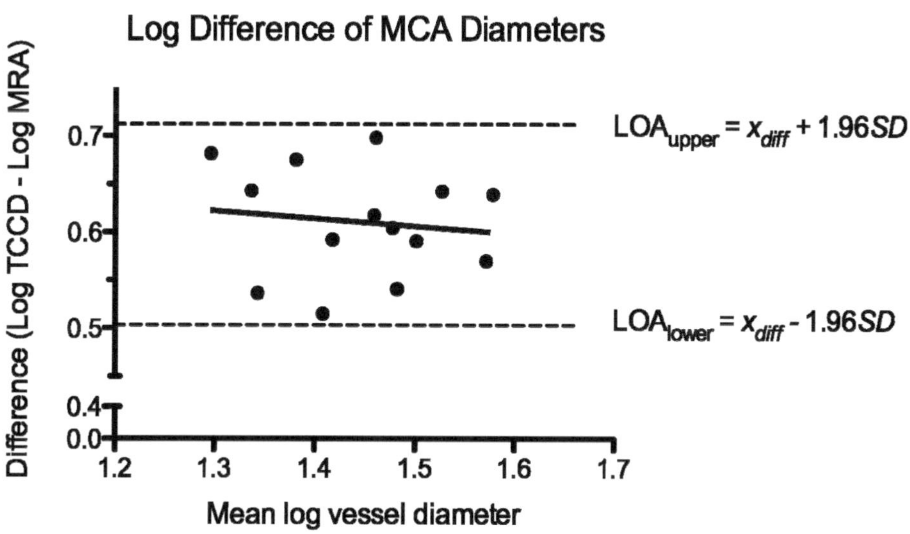

Fig. 4. MRA and TCCD log MCA vessel diameter comparison. The abscissa depicts the mean log TCCD and MRA diameter measurement in a participant-wise manner.

The ordinate depicts the difference of the log TCCD and log MRA within each subject. Logarithmic transformation of the data virtually eliminated the proportional bias in the sample (regression line: -0.08x + 0.72). The LOA (depicted by two dashed lines) is better suited to this transformed data (Bland & Altman, 1999; Atkinson & Nevill, 2006). From a sample of 14 data points, we can see that there is good agreement between TCCD and MRA vessel diameter measurements, despite a systematic bias. Therefore, a correction factor need only be applied to the data to correct the bias.

Another variable to consider is the random error. In the present example, we can see that the data points in Figure 4 are homoscedastic (uniform over a measurement range, parametrically confirmable via Levene's test), thus random error can be estimated using the standard error of measurement (SEM), coefficient of variation (CV) and SD_{diff}. CV from the log-transformed data is uniform across the measurement range (Atkinson & Nevill, 2006; Bland & Altman, 1999) and maintains value of ~4.1%.[3] This indicates that the measurement tools are well calibrated.

6. Conclusions

In this chapter we explored the use of MRA as means of optimizing TCD use and as a way of confirming TCD measures. While the utility of MRA as a tool for estimating insonation properties cannot be understated, there can be no replacement for experimenter skill in determining probe placement in clinical and research settings. Specifically, there is no fixed solution to determining the optimal insonation vector, on a subject-to-subject basis, given variations in cranial thickness and vascular peculiarities. However, despite this caveat, MRA as a guidance tool does generate some clear benefits: multi-day experimental methods may be considered due to accurate repositioning of the TCD probe; estimates of blood flow velocity can be corrected in order to account for subject-required sacrifices in insonation angle; subjects may be screened for significant variation on vascular architecture. MRA is also a useful supplementary tool for determining estimated signal loss due to bone-related degradation. Finally, although MR methods are indisputably the clinical standard for estimates of vessel diameter, TCD is surprisingly functional, however owing to significant proportional bias TCD derived diameter measurements need to be examined in a more exhaustive fashion to establish appropriate norms and corrections.

7. References

Aaslid, R. (1986). Transcranial Doppler Examination Techniques. In *Transcranial Doppler Sonography*, R. Aaslid, (Ed.), 39-59, Springer-Verlag, ISBN 321-181-935-5, Vienna, Austria.

[3] For non-parametric methods to calculate complex relationships between error magnitude and measured values see Bland and Altman (1999).

Aaslid, R., Markwalder, T. M., & Nornes, H. (1982). Non-invasive transcranial Doppler ultrasound recording of flow velocity in basal cerebral arteries. *Journal of Neurosurgery*, Vol. 57, No. 2, (January 1984), 769-774, ISSN 0022-3050.

Ainslie, P. N., & Duffin, J. (2009). Integration of cerebrovascular CO2 reactivity and chemoreflex control of breathing: mechanisms of regulation, measurement and interpretation. *American Journal of Physiology- Regulatory, Integrative and Comparative Physiology*, Vol. 296, No. 5, (February 2009), R1473-95, ISSN 0363-6119.

Akdemir, H., Oktem, I. S., Menku, A., Tucer, B., Tugcu, B., & Gunaldi, O. (2007). Image-guided microneurosurgical management of small arteriovenous malformation: role of neuronavigation and intraoperative Doppler sonography. *Minimally Invasive Neurosurgery*, Vol. 50, No. 3, (June 2007), 163-169, ISSN 0946-7211.

Alexandrov, A. V., Sloan, M. A., Wong, L. K. S., Douville, C., Razumovsky, A. Y., Koroshetz, W. J. et al. (2007). Practice standards for transcranial Doppler ultrasound: part I -- test performance. *Journal of Neuroimaging*, Vol. 17, No. 1, (January 2007), 11-18, ISSN 1552-6569.

Ammi, A. Y., Mast, T. D., Huang, I.-H., Abruzzo, T. A., Coussios, C.-C., Shaw, G. J. et al. (2008). Characterization of ultrasound propagation through ex-vivo human temporal bone. *Ultrasound in Medicine & Biology*, Vol. 34, No. 10, (October 2008), 1578-1589, ISSN 0301-5629.

Atkinson, G. (2003). What is this thing called measurement error? In *Kinanthropometry VIII: Proceedings of the 8th International Conference of the International Society for the Advancement of Kinathropometry (ISAK)*, T. Reilly & M. Marfell-Jones (Eds.), 3-14, Routledge, ISBN 041-528-969-6, London, England.

Atkinson, G., & Nevill, A. (1998). Statistical methods for Assessing Measurement Error (Reliability) in Variables Relevant to Sports Medicine. *Sports Medicine*, Vol. 26, No. 4, (October 1998), 217-238, ISSN 0112-1642.

Atkinson, G., & Nevill, A. (2006). Method agreement and measurement error in the physiology of exercise. In *Sport and Exercise Physiology Testing Guidelines*, E. M. Winter, T. Mercer, P. D. Bromley, A. M. Davison, & A. M. Jones (Eds.), 41-48, Routledge, ISBN 041-537-966-0, London, England.

Auer, A., Felber, S., Lutz, W., Kremser, C., Schmidauer, C., Hochmair, E. et al. (1999). Transcranial Doppler sonography guided by magnetic resonance angiography for improved monitoring of intracranial arteries. *Journal of Neuroimaging*, Vol. 9, No. 1, (January 1999), 34-38, ISSN 1552-6569.

Baumgartner, R. W., Mattle, H. P., & Aaslid, R. (1995). Transcranial color-coded duplex sonography, magnetic resonance angiography, and computed tomography angiography: methods, applications, advantages, and limitations. *Journal of Clinical Ultrasound*, Vol. 23, No. 2, (February 1995), 89-111, ISSN 1097-0096.

Bland, J. M., & Altman, D. G. (1999). Measuring agreement in methods comparison studies. *Statistical Methods in Medical Research*, Vol. 8, No. 2, (April 1999), 135-160, ISSN 0962-2802.

Edelman, R. R., & Meyer, J. (2003). MR angiography of the head and neck: basic principles and clinical applications. In *Magnetic Resonance Imaging in Stroke,* S. Davis, M. Fisher, & S. Warach (Eds.), 85-101, Cambridge University Press, ISBN 052-180-683-6, Cambridge.

Gerriets, T., Seidel, G., Fiss, I., Modrau, B., & Kaps, M. (1999). Contrast-enhanced transcranial color-coded duplex sonography: efficiency and validity. *Neurology,* Vol. 52, No. 6, 1133-1137, ISSN 0028-3878.

Grolimund, O. (1985). Transmission of Ultrasound Through the Temporal Bone. In *Transcranial Doppler Sonography,* R. Aaslid (Ed.), 10-21, Springer-Verlag, ISBN 321-181-935-5, Vienna, Austria.

Gronninsaeter, A., Kleven, A., Omnedal, S., Aarseth, T. E., Lie, T., Lindseth, F. et al. (2000). SonoWand, an ultrasound-based neuronavigation system. *Neurosurgery,* Vol. 47, No. 6, (June 2000), 1373-1379, ISSN 0148-396X.

Hansen, J. M., Pedersen, D., Larsen, V. A., Sanchez-del-Rio, M., Alvarez Linera, J. R., Olesen, J. et al. (2007). Magnetic resonance angiography shows dilatation of the middle cerebral artery after infusion of glyceryl trinitrate in healthy volunteers. *Cephalalgia,* Vol. 27, No. 2, (February 2007), 118-127, ISSN 1468-2982.

Kantelhardt, S. R., Greke, C., Keric, N., Vollmer, F., Thiemann, I., & Giese, A. (2011). Image-guidance for trancranial Doppler ultrasonography. *Neurosurgery,* doi: 10.1227/NEU.0b013e31821553b2, ISSN 0148-396X.

Kety, S. S., & Schmidt, C. F. (1948). The effects of altered arterial tensions of carbon dioxide and oxygen on cerebral blood flow and cerebral oxygen consumption of normal young men. *The Journal of Clinical Investigation,* Vol. 27, No. 4, (July 1948), 484-492, ISSN 1558-8238.

Mathiesen, T., Peredo, I., Edner, G., Kihlstrom, L., Svensson, M., Ulfarsson, E. et al. (2007). Neuronavigation for arteriovenous malformation surgery by intraoperative three-dimensional ultrasound angiography. *Neurosurgery,* Vol. 60, No. 4 (Supp 2), (April 2007), 345-350, ISSN 1524-4040.

Mercier, L., Del Maestro, R. F., Petrecca, K., Kochanowska, A., Drouin, S., Yan, C. X. B. et al. (2011). New prototype neuronavigation system based on preoperative imaning and intraoperative freehand ultrasound: system description and validation. *International Journal of Computer Assisted Radiology & Surgery,* Vol. 6, No. 4, (July 2011), 507-522, ISSN 1861-6410.

Muller, M., Schwerdtfeger, K., & Zieroth, S. (2000). Asessment of middle cerebral artery diameter after aneurysmal subarachnoid hemorrhage by transcranial color-coded duplex sonography. *European Journal of Ultrasound,* Vol. 11, No. 1, (January 2000), 15-19 ISSN 0929-8266.

Northern Digital Inc. Polaris Spectra and Polaris Vicra Technical Specifications. Retrieved Wednesday June 15, 2011, Available from http://www.ndigital.com/medical/polarisfamily-techspecs.php.

Pai, S. B., Varma, R. G., & Kulkarni, R. N. (2005). Microsurgical anatomy of the middle cerebral artery. *Neurol India,* Vol. 53, No. 2, (April – June 2005) 186-190, ISSN 0028-3886.

Panerai, R. B. (2009). Transcranial Doppler for evaluation of cerebral autoregulation. *Clinical Autonomic Research*, Vol. 19, No. 4, (August 2009) 1977-1211, ISSN 1619-1560.

Schreiber, S.J., S., Gottschalk, S., Weih, M., Villringer, A., & Valdueza, J. M. (2000). Assessment of blood flow velocity and diameter of the middle cerebral artery during the acetazolamide provocation test by use of transcranial Doppler sonography and MR imaging. *American Journal of Neuroradiology*, Vol. 21, No. 7, (August 2000), 1207-1211, ISSN 0195-6108.

Serrador, J.M., S., Picot, P. A., Rutt, B. K., Shoemaker, J. K., & Bondar, R. L. (2000). MRI measures of middle cerebral artery diameter in conscious humans during simulated orthostasis. *Stroke*, Vol. 31, No. 7, (July 2000), 1672-1678, ISSN 0039-2499.

Tarasow, E., Abdulwahed Saleh Ali, A., Lewszuk, A., & Walecki, J. (2007). Measurements of the middle cerebral artery in digital subtraction angiography and MR angiography. *Medical Science Monitor*, Vol. 13, No. 1(Supp), (May 2007), 65-72, ISSN 1234-1010.

Tsivgoulis, G., Alexandrov, A. V., & Sloan, M. A. (2009). Advances in transcranial Doppler ultrasonography. *Current Neurology & Neuroscience Reports*, Vol. 9, No. 1, (January 2009), 46-54, ISSN 1528-4042.

Valdueza, J. M., Belzer, J. O., Villringer, A., Vogl, T. J., Kutter, R., & Einhaupl, K. M. (1997). Changes in blood flow velocity and diameter of the middle cerebral artery during hyperventilation: assessment with MR and transcranial Doppler sonography. *American Journal of Neuroradiology*, Vol. 18, No. 10, (October 1997), 1929-1934, ISSN 0195-6108.

Wedeen, V. J., Meuli, R. A., Edelman, R. R., Geller, S. C., Frank, L. R., Brady, T. J. et al. (1985). Projective imaging of pulsatile flow with magnetic resonance. *Science*, Vol. 230, No. 4728, (November 1985), 946-948, ISSN 1095-9203.

Weiss, C. R., Nour, S. G., & Lewin, J. S. (2008). MR-guided biopsy: a review of current techniques and applications. *Journal of Magnetic Resonance Imaging*, Vol. 27, No. 2, (February 2008), 311-325, ISSN 1522-2586.

White, D. N., Curry, G. R., & Stevenson, R. J. (1978). The acoustic characteristics of the skull. *Ultrasound in Medicine & Biology*, Vol. 4, No. 3, (November 1978), 225-252, ISSN 0301-5629.

Willie, C. K., Ainslie, P. N., Taylor, C. E., Jones, H., Sin, P. Y. W., & Tzeng, Y. C. (2011). Neuromechanical features of the cardiac baroreflex after exercise. *Hypertension*, Vol. 57, No. 5, (May 2011), 927-933, ISSN 0194-911X.

Willie, C. K., Colino, F. L., Bailey, D. M., Tzeng, Y. C., Binsted, G., Jones, L. W. et al. (2011). Utility of transcranial Doppler ultrasound for the Integrative assessement of Cerebrovascular Function. *Journal of Neuroscience Methods*, Vol. 196, No. 2, (March 2011), 221-237, ISSN 0165-0270.

Willie, C. K., & Smith, K. J. (2011). Fuelling the exercising brain: a regulatory quagmire for lactate metabolism. *Journal of Physiology (London)*, Vol. 589, No. 4, (February 2011), 779-780, ISSN 0022-3751

Wilson, M. H., Edsell, M. E. G., Davagnanam, I., Hirani, S. H., Martin, D. S., Levett, D. Z. H. et al. (2011). Cerebral artery dilatation maintains cerebral oxygenation at extreme altitude and in acute hypoxia -- an ultrasound and MRI study. *Journal of Cerebral Blood Flow & Metabolism*, Vol. 31, *doi: 10.1038/jcbfm.2011.81*, Published online June 2011.

3

Transcranial Color-Coded Sonography

Akke Bakker[1] and Philip N. Ainslie[2]
[1]MIRA Institute, University of Twente
[2]University of British Columbia Okanagan
[1]The Netherlands
[2]Canada

1. Introduction

Transcranial color-coded sonography (TCCS) was first described in 1988 (Berland et al., 1988); it combines blood flow velocity measurements with non-invasive imaging of intracranial vessels and parenchymal structures at a high spatial resolution (Zipper & Stolz, 2002). TCCS is a combination of B-mode and pulsed wave (PW) Doppler sonography; therefore, it is possible to give a color-coded demonstration of the frequency shift or the reflected energy. Because of the addition of a B mode image to the PW Doppler function (Zipper et al., 2001), TCCD also offers a number of advantages and extensions compared to its precursor transcranial Doppler (TCD). The color-coded flow-velocity map serves as an examination tool for the presence of stenoses, occlusions, and collateral flow through the circle of Willis. This chapter reviews the role of TCCS in cerebrovascular disease and describes the principles, the use of ultrasound agents, the examination procedure and related typical pathological findings. The limitations of TCCS are also considered.

2. Principles of TCCS

TCCS combines gray scale imaging of intracranial parenchymal structures with imaging of intracranial vessels. Due to the presence of narrow ultrasound windows in the skull, transducers with transmission frequencies between 1.8 and 3.6 MHz are most commonly used for insonation (Baumgartner, 2003). The advantage over conventional TCD is that intracranial vascular structures can be displayed in the correct anatomical relationships to parenchymal structures, allowing angle corrected flow velocity measurements (Zipper & Stolz, 2002).

Either the frequency shift (fTCCS) or the energy of the Doppler signal (pTCCS) can be shown from the color-coding: fTCCS is dependent on the Doppler shift resulting from moving erythrocytes, providing information on flow direction and velocity; pTCCS is dependent on the integrated power of the back-scattered signal (Griewing et al., 1998). Both color-coded Doppler modes image the anatomical course of cerebral vessels, allowing estimates of insonation angles and measurement of angle-corrected velocities in defined depths and sample volumes using spectral Doppler sonography. fTCCS can be used to identify flow direction and velocity, which allows the visual estimation of basal cerebral hemodynamics; this process facilitates the positioning of the Doppler sample volume and produces less tissue motion artifacts than pTCCS (Baumgartner et al., 1997a). Compared to fTCCS, pTCCS has a better signal-to-noise ratio, is not dependent on the angle of insonation and is not subject to aliasing (Bude et al., 1994).

3. Ultrasound contrast agents

Adequate bone windows need to be present in order to insonate the cerebral arteries. The temporal bone window becomes smaller and may disappear with advancing age and especially in postmenopausal women. To allow the investigation of patients with insufficient bone windows, ultrasound contrast agents (UCAs) that enhance the backscatter from blood and increase the signal-to-noise ratios can be administered to the patient. For example, the intrasound contrast agent 'Levovist' consists of transpulmonary stable microbubbles formed in a galactose suspension. This causes a signal increase of approximately 25 dB and therefore an improved signal-to-noise ratio (Riet et al., 1997). In general, current UCA are spheric particles, commonly known as microbubbles; microbubbles are typically reflective and can thus be separated from tissue. The microbubble concept comprises a gaseous component trapped by a shell structure. Currently, perfluorocarbon derivates are the gaseous component of choice, whereas phospholipids, human albumin or polymers are mainly used as shell material (Sauerbruch et al., 2009).

UCA are optimized ultrasound- scatters because of their oscillating behavior and their high reflectivity, which is about 1000fold higher in comparison to erythrocytes. The UCA mean diameter of approximately 2-4μm accounts for the strong oscillatory response at ultrasound wavelengths between 1-3.5 MHz (Sauerbruch et al., 2009). Measured flow velocities may therefore be higher when using UCA; therefore, to allow comparisons, follow-up examinations should also be performed with UCA. Although there is varying availability of UCA in different countries and a lack in studies with direct comparison of the different UCA, application of multiple small boli (e.g. in the case of Riet et al. (1997) Levovist was given in the following concentrations: 16 mL of 200 mg/mL; 10 mL of 300 mg/mL; and 8 mL of 400 mg/mL) or continuous intravenous infusion increases the length of the diagnostically useful time window (Nedelmann et al., 2009). Future research on the reliability and validity of different UCA is needed.

4. Examination procedure

For assessment of the cerebral arteries several acoustic windows are described: the transtemporal, transforaminal, transoccipital and transorbital windows. These examination procedures have been descrived in depth elsewhere (Baumgartner, 2003, Sauerbruch et al., 2009; Zipper et al., 2001; Zipper & Stolz, 2002) and will only be briefly overviewed here. The most common plane - to allow depiction of the circle of Willis - for the cerebrovascular exam is via the axial mesencephalic insonation plane through the temporal bone window (Nedelmann et al., 2009). The examination procedure for the temporal bone window is therefore described in this section.

Transtemporal insonation starts in B mode with an axial projection in the orbito-meatal line through the transtemporal window (Fig. 1 & 2). This projection shows the temporal axial mesencephalic or orbitomeatal scanning plane. These planes are essentially characterized in B mode by the butterfly shaped mesencephalon brain stem surrounded by an echogenic border, corresponding to the basal systems at a depth of about 5-9 cm. After identifying the mesencephalon the assessment is continued in color-coded B mode to investigate the cerebral vessels. Slight up- or downwards tilts of the transducer are necessary to follow the course of the vessel segments of the circle of Willis. Using this approach, the distal intracranial part of the internal cerebral artery (ICA) and - in most cases - the carotid siphon, the main stem (M1) and insular (M2) segments of the middle cerebral artery (MCA), the precommunicating (A1) segment of the anterior cerebral artery (ACA), and the precommunicating (P1) and postcommunicating (P2) segments of the posterior cerebral artery (PCA) can be reliably recognized and allocated in the color-coded B mode image (Baumgartner, 2003; Zipper et al., 2001; Zipper & Stolz, 2002). By convention, in fTCCS, a system setting can be chosen that codes a flow towards the probe red and away from the transducer blue; thus the ICA, M1 MCA, and P1 PCA are coded red; and parts of the carotid siphon, the A1 ACA, and the P2 PCA are coded blue (Zipper & Stolz, 2002).

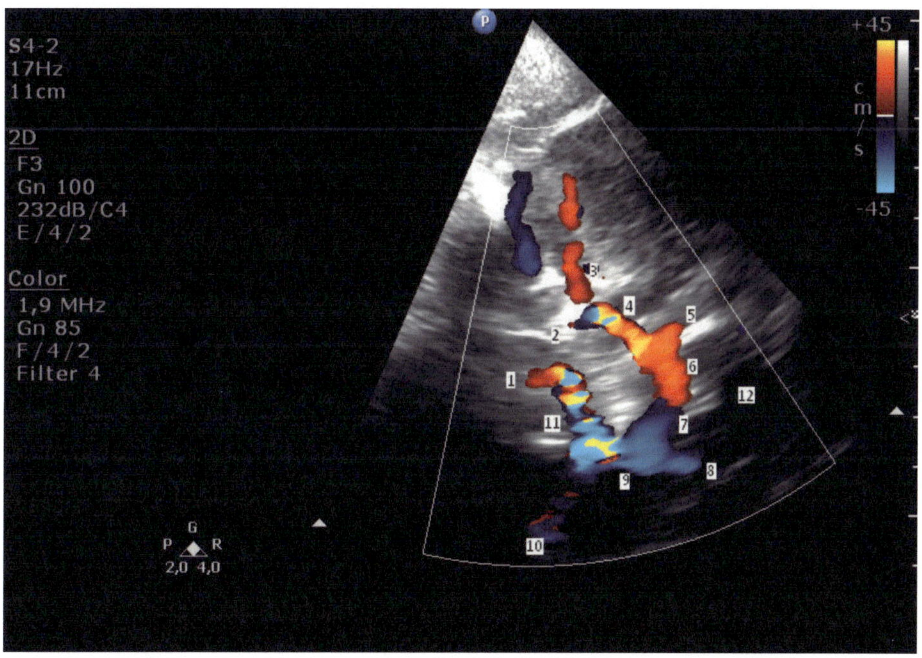

Fig. 1. Transtemporal insonation with fTCCS. Flow towards the probe is red and away from the transducer blue: (1) ipsilateral and contralateral A2 ACA, (2) ipsilateral A1 ACA, (3) ipsilateral M1 MCA, (4) ipsilateral posterior communicating artery, (5) ipsilateral P2 PCA, (6) ipsilateral P1 PCA, (7) contralateral P1 PCA (8) contralateral P2 PCA, (9) contralateral posterior communicating artery, (10) contralateral M1 MCA, (11) contralateral A1 ACA, (12) mesencephalon surrounded by both PCAs.

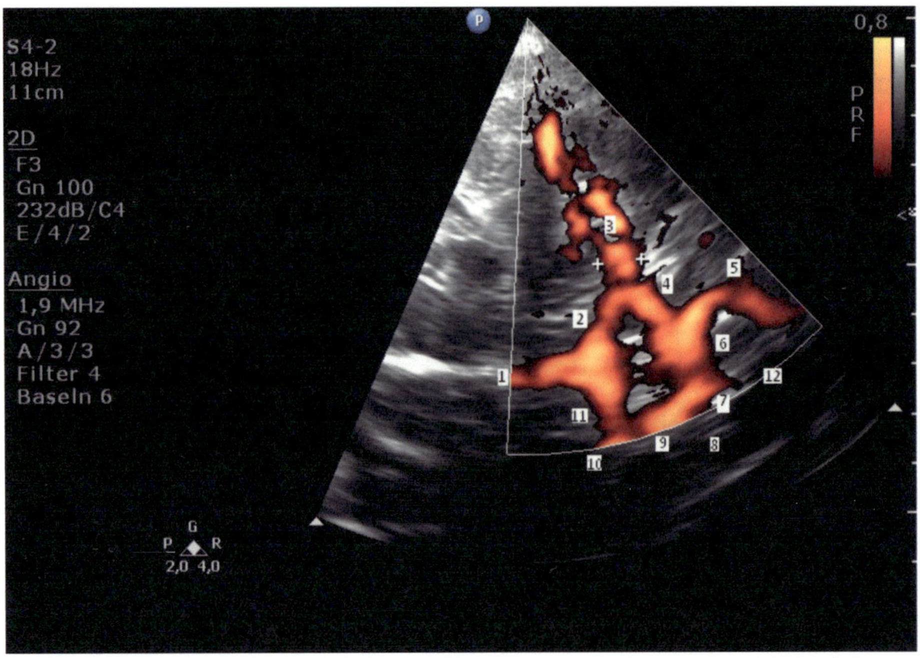

Fig. 2. Transtemporal insonation with pTCCS. (1) ipsilateral and contralateral A2 ACA, (2) ipsilateral A1 ACA, (3) ipsilateral M1 MCA, (4) ipsilateral posterior communicating artery, (5) ipsilateral P2 PCA, (6) ipsilateral P1 PCA, (7) contralateral P1 PCA (8) contralateral P2 PCA, (9) contralateral posterior communicating artery, (10) contralateral M1 MCA, (11) contralateral A1 ACA, (12) mesencephalon surrounded by both PCAs.

4.1 Settings

With TCCS the scale, gain and angle correction settings are of most importance (Hou et al., 2009). For measurements of vessel diameter the scaling of the color-coded B mode image is essential (i.e., a low scale causes more errors). The amount of movement detected by the TCCS can be set by changing the gain. A high gain increases the amount of detected movement and the color-coded B mode image is colorful, while a low gain decreases the amount of detected movement and results in a black and white image.

To determine the angle of insonation, a linear marker can be placed by the sonographer on the color-coded B mode image of the vessel segment being insonated. The direction of the marker should be oriented along the long axis of the segment. The angle between the linear marker and the sonographic beam is displayed automatically; this is considered a two-dimensional approximation of the angle of insonation. The determination of the angle of insonation allows for angle-corrected blood flow velocity measurement (Swiat et al., 2009). Angle-corrected velocity measurements are one of the advantages of TCCS over TCD. The angle between the transtemporally transmitted ultrasound beam and the major intracranial arteries varies considerable due to anatomic variations. For example, variations between different arterial segments, between similar segments of different individuals, and interhemispherically within the same person (Eicke et al., 1994).

5. Utility of TCCS

TCCS is widely used to evaluate the intracranial arterial system in patients with acute stroke. It enables detection of the position of the third ventricle and a potential midline shift in ischemic stroke. Although intracerebral hemorrhage, aneurysms, and arteriovenous malformations may be detected by TCCS, it is not the first-line imaging method in these situations (Nedelmann et al., 2009). Several advantages of TCCS in the diagnosis of cerebrovascular disease are highlighted below.

It has been reported that TCCS used in the diagnosis of cerebral artery stenosis or occlusion has a higher sensitivity, specificity and accuracy compared to digital substraction angiography, though the false-positive and false-negative rate still exists (Hou et al. (2009). It was concluded that TCCS can be used for screening of cerebral artery stenosis or occlusion. However, the degree of stenosis could not be precisely evaluated. Stolz et al. (2008) concluded that transcranial ultrasound provides important information on prognosis in patients with acute stroke. Diagnosis of MCA M1 or branch occlusion by TCD or TCCS on admission without thrombolytic treatment is affected with a significantly increased chance to take a fatal course according to their meta-analysis. Stolz et al. also conclude that these patients also have a more than 10-times higher chance not to clinically improve within the first days after stroke compared to patients with primary patent intracranial vessels.

It is also established that TCCS is useful to identify the presence and extent of intracranial hemorrhage within 3 hours of stroke onset (Pérez et al. (2009). In this study, arly hematoma enlargement within the first hours can be monitored using TCCS showing an excellent correlation with CT scan. However, it was found that the accuracy of TCCS is limited to the initial phase. Monitoring vasospasm in patients after subarachnoid hemorrhage is commonly done using TCD. Swiat et al. (2009) compared TCD with TCCS for the detection of vasospasm; the accuracy of TCCS and TCD was similar, but TCCS was more sensitive than TCD in the detection of MCA spasm. Collectively, these studies highlight the utility of TCCS in a number of clinical settings.

6. Limitations of TCCS

As is the case with all ultrasound procedures, it the quality of TCCS results critically depends on the skills and experience of the examiner. All ultrasound procedures should be performed by sufficiently trained and experienced sonographers (Nedelmann et al., 2009). The main limitation of TCCS, however, arises from poor acoustic insonation conditions. Because of an insufficient temporal bone window, insonation of the basal cerebral arteries is incomplete in approximately 10% of patients with cerebrovascular diseases (Kenton et al., 1997; Krejza et al., 2007; Seidel et al., 1995). Application of an UCA increases the number of conclusive ultrasound studies and allows adequate diagnosis in approximately 80 to 90% of those patients with insufficient temporal bone windows (Baumgartner et al., 1997b; Gerriets et al., 1999; Nedelmann et al., 2009). Another limitation of TCCD when compared to TCD is that the probe cannot be fixed; thus, measurements are limited in each artery of interest. Information about the utility of TCCD for the assessment of cerebrovascular reactivity, autoregulation or neurovascular coupling is not yet available. Future research on the reliability and validity of TCCD with and without different UCA is needed.

7. References

Baumgartner, R., Nirkko, A., Müri, R., & Gönner, F. (1997a). Transoccipital power-based colour-coded duplex sonography of cerebral sinuses and veins. *Stroke,* 28 (January 1997), pp. (1319-1323), ISSN 0039-2499

Baumgartner, R.W., Arnold M., Gonner F., Staikow I., Herrmann C., Rivoir A., & Muri R.M. (1997b). Contrast-enhanced transcranial color-coded duplex sonography in ischemic cerebrovascular disease. *Stroke,* 28 (Dec 1997), pp. (2473-2478), ISSN 0039-2499

Baumgartner, R.W. (2003). Transcranial color duplex sonography in cerebrovascular disease: a systemic review. *Cerebrovasc Dis,* 16, pp. (4-13), ISSN 1276-6355

Berland, L., Bryan, C., & Sekar, B. (1988). Sonographic examination of the adult brain. *Journal of Clinical Ultrasound,* 16 (June 1988), pp. (337-345)

Bude, R.O., Rubin, J.M., & Adler, R.S. (1994). Power versus conventional color Doppler sonography: comparison in the depiction of normal intrarenal vasculature. *Radiology,* 192 (September 1994), pp. (777-780), ISSN 0033-8419

Eicke B.M., Tegeler C.H., Dalley G., & Myers L.G. (1994). Angle correction in transcranial Doppler sonography. *J Neuroimaging,* 4 (January 1994), pp. (29-33), ISSN 1051-2284

Gerriets T., Seidel G., Fiss I., Modrau B., & Kaps M. (1999). Contrast-enhanced transcranial color-doded duplex sonography: efficiency and validity. *Neurology*, 52 (April 1999), pp. (1133-1137), ISSN 0028-3878

Griewing, B., Schminke, U., Motsch, L., Brassel, F., & Kessler, C. (1998). Transcranial duplex sonography of the middle cerebral artery stenosis: a comparison of colour-coding techniques ± frequency or power-based Doppler and contrast enhancement. *Journal of Neuroimaging*, 40 (August 1998), pp. (490-495), ISSN 0028-3940

Hou, W.H., Liu, X., Duan, Y.Y., Wang, J., Sun, S.G., Deng, J.P., Qin, H.Z., & Cao, T.S. (2009). Evaluation of Transcranial Color-Coded Duplex Sonography for Cerebral Artery Stenosis or Occlusion. *Cerebrovascular Diseases*, 27 (March 2009), pp. (479-484), ISSN 1015-9770

Kenton A.R., Martin P.J., Abbott R.J., & Moody A.R. (1997). Comparison of transcranial color-coded sonography and magnetic resonance angiography in acute stroke. *Stroke*, 28 (August 1997), pp. (1601-1606), ISSN 0039-2499

Krejza J., Swiat M., Pawlak M.A., Oszkinis G., Weigele J., Hurst R.W., & Kaser S. (2007). Suitability of temporal bone acoustic window: conventional tcd versus transcranial color-coded duplex sonography. *J Neuroimaging*, 17 (October 2007), pp (311-314), ISSN 1552-4628

Nedelmann, M., Stolz, E., Gerriets, T., Baumgartner, R.W., Malferrari, G., Seidel, G., & Kaps, M. (2009) Consensus recommendations for transcranial color-coded duplex sonography for the assessment of intracranial arteries in cliniacl trials on acute stroke. *Stroke*, 40 (October 2009), pp. (3238-3244), ISSN 1524-4628

Pérez, E.S., Delgado-Mederos, R., Rubiera, M., Delgado, P., Ribó, M., Maisterra, O., Ortega, G., Álvarez-Sabin, J., & Molina, C.A. (2009). Transcranial duplex sonography for monitoring hyperacute intracerebral hemorrhage. *Stroke*, 40 (January 2009), pp. (987-990), ISSN 0039-2499

Sauerbruch, S., Schlachetzki, F., Bogdahn, U., Valaikiene, J.,Hölscher, T. & Harrer, J., (2009). Application of Transcranial Color-Coded Duplex Sonography. *Stroke*, 5, 1 (February 2009), pp. (39-54)

Seidel, G., Kaps, M., & Gerriets, T. (1995). Potential and limitations of transcranial color-coded duplex sonography. *Stroke*, 26 (November 1995), pp. (2061-2066), ISSN 0039-2499

Stolz, E., Cioli, F., Allendoerfer, J., Gerriets, T., Del Sette, M., & Kaps, M. (2008). Can early neurosonology predict outcome in acute stroke? A metaanalysis of prognostic clinical effect sizes related to the vascular status. *Stroke*, 39 (October 2008), pp. (3255-3261), ISSN 0039-2499

Swiat, M., Weigele, J., Hurst, R.W., Kasner, S.E., Pawlak, M. Arkuszewski, M., Al-Okaili, R.N., Swiercz, M. Ustymowicz, A. Opala, G., Melhem, E.R., & Krejza, J. (2009). Middle cerebral artery vasospasm: Transcranial color-coded suplex sonography versus conventional nonimaging transcranial Doppler sonography. *Critical Care Medicine*, 37 (March 2009), 3, pp. (963-968), ISSN 0090-2493

Ries, S., Steinke, W., Neff, K.W. & Hennerici, M. (1997). Echocontrast-Enhanced Transcranial Color-Coded Sonography for the Diagnosis of Transverse Sinus Venous Thrombosis. *Stroke*, 28 (April 1997), pp. (696-700)

Zipper, S.G., Saposnik, G.D., & Weber, S. (2001). Transcranial Color-coded Sonography (TCCS): A Helpful Tool In Clinical Neurology. *The Internet Journal of Neurology*, 1, 1, ISSN 1531-295X

Zipper, S.G., & Stolz, E. (2002). Clinical application of transcranial colour-coded duplex sonography - a review. *European Journal of Neurology*, 9, (January 2002), pp. (1-8), ISSN 1468-1331

4

Near-Infrared Spectroscopy

Akke Bakker[1,2], Brianne Smith[2], Philip Ainslie[2] and Kurt Smith[2]
[1]*University of Twente*
[2]*University of British Columbia Okanagan*
[1]*The Netherlands*
[2]*Canada*

1. Introduction

Near infrared spectroscopy (NIRS) is an imaging technique used in both clinical and emergency medicine, as well as in research laboratories to quantify and measure the oxygenation status of human tissue non-invasively. This is done by monitoring in vivo changes of the oxygen saturation of hemoglobin molecules in the body, based on the absorbance of near-infrared light by hemoglobin. With regards to NIRS in human tissue, this chapter will primarily be concerned with discerning the oxygenation status of cerebral tissue. The importance of such a measure, especially in cerebral physiology, is that the human brain utilizes oxygen to continuously supply neurons with energy used for vital body functioning. In the absence of oxygen, as is the case during ischemic stroke or desanguination, cognitive and functional impairment resulting in death often occurs. NIRS technology makes it possible to apply critical safety thresholds with regards to cerebral tissue saturation in order to avoid dangerously low levels with the primary goal being to reduce mortality rates and cognitive deficits due to cerebral hypoxemia.

Prior to 1977, and the advent of commercially available fiber optic cables, the quantification of hemoglobin concentrations in the human body was only possible using cuvette tubes containing sampled blood and large spectrophotometer units. These spectrometers, utilized the theoretical work of Karl Vierodt in 1873, to measure the absorbance of a colored solution based on the magnitude of "visible light" attenuation per unit of the colored solution. The limitation however, was that visible light was not able to penetrate superficial human tissue, making it impossible to quantify hemoglobin concentration changes in living tissue under any circumstance and was often done using bulky expensive spectrometers. Fiber optic cables transmitting near-infrared light however, made it possible for researchers and clinicians to safely penetrate skin, bone and other tissues with minimal incident light loss and ultimately shining a literal light on cerebral tissue oxygenation. This breakthrough paved the way for multiple methods of measuring near-infrared light absorbance in oxygenated and deoxygenated hemoglobin molecules found in cerebral tissues.

The improved resolution of living tissue provided by using near-infrared light, and the additional modification of theoretical models (Beer-Lambert law, Monte Carlo technique), is proving that the NIRS technique, is quickly becoming a useful and invaluable tool in monitoring tissue hemodynamics.

2. Physical principles of NIRS

The basis of NIRS relies upon two principles: (1) that tissue is relatively transparent to near-infrared light and (2) that there are compounds in tissue in which absorption of light is dependent on the oxygenation status of the tissue (Elwell & Phil, 1995).

The propagation of light in tissue depends on the combination of absorption, scattering, and reflection properties of photons. Absorption and scatter in tissue is dependent on the wavelength. Scatter decreases with increasing wavelengths; thereby favoring the transmission of near-infrared light compared to visible light. Reflection, in contrast, is generally a function of the angle of the light beam and the tissue surface (Jöbsis, 1977).

2.1 Absorption of light

When light is absorbed its energy is dissipated as thermal energy throughout the absorber (Elwell & Phil, 1995). Absorption occurs at specific wavelengths, determined by the molecular properties of the materials in the light path (Jöbsis, 1977; Wray et al., 1988). The primary light-absorbing compounds in tissue within the near-infrared range are called chromophores (Jöbsis, 1977). Most chromophores can be considered to have stable concentrations during a measurement period (~10 min), however, there presence adds to the total light attenuation (i.e. melanin, bilirubin, water). The primary chromophores of interest are oxyhemoglobin (HbO_2), deoxyhemoglobin (Hb) and cytochrome c oxidase, because the concentration of these chromophores varies with time and oxygenation status (Elwell & Phil, 1995). Each chromophore has a unique absorption spectrum, where the specific extinction coefficient[1] (ε) is expressed as a function of the wavelength (Horecker, 1942; Pellicer & Bravo, 2011). ε describes how strongly a chromophore absorbs light at a particular wavelength. In Fig. 1 the absorption spectra for Hb, HbO_2, cytochrome c oxidase and water (H_2O) are given.

Cytochrome c oxidase changes with oxygenation status. However, it does not have a significant effect on the measurement because the effect on the attenuation signal is ten times smaller than hemoglobin (Madsen & Secher, 1999). Cytochrome c oxidase is a mitochondrial enzyme and therefore describes the intracellular oxygenation (Heekeren et al., 1999), its concentration is not entirely the result of changes in oxygen availability. Therefore, in monitoring tissue oxygenation with NIRS the chromophores Hb and HbO_2 are of interest. Hb and HbO_2 are responsible for the transport, delivery and removal of oxygen (O_2) and carbon dioxide (CO_2) throughout human body. NIRS instruments utilize light in the 700-1000 nm wavelength range to transilluminate cerebral and muscular tissues. This range follows from the increased absorption bands of H_2O above 1000 nm and increased scattering and more intense absorption bands of Hb below 700 nm. In the 700-1000 nm

[1] In literature the term specific extinction coefficient is often confused with the terms molar absorption coefficient, molar extinction coefficient and the absorption coefficient. The molar absorption coefficient describes how strongly a *chemical species* absorbs light at a particular wavelength, whereas the molar extinction coefficient describes how strongly a *substance* absorbs light at a particular wavelength. The specific extinction coefficient (in $\mu molar^{-1}cm^{-1}$) is the molar extinction coefficient multiplied by the molar mass of the compound, describing how strongly a specific chromophore absorbs light at a particular wavelength. Whereas the absorption coefficient is the specific extinction coefficient multiplied by the concentration of the compound (Elwell & Phil, 1995).

range Hb and HbO_2 have unique absorption spectra, which allows emitted light to propagate through tissue for several centimeters. The attenuation of the emitted light can be related to the change in chromophore concentration using the Beer-Lambert law as described in section 2.3.

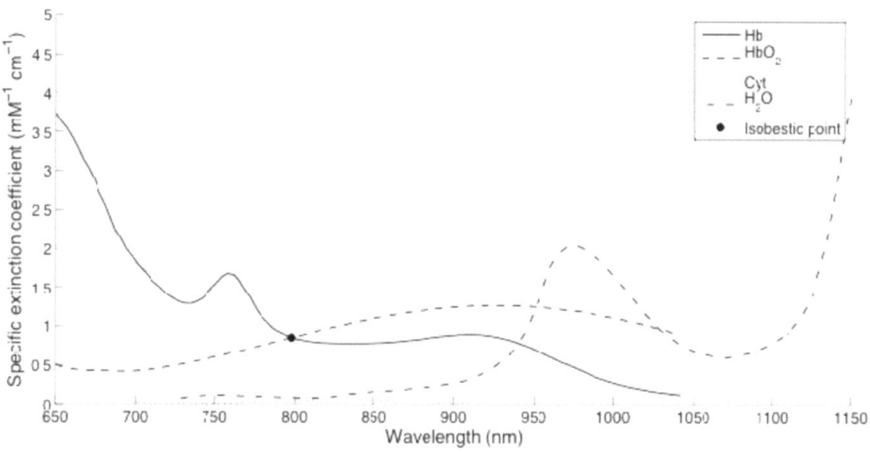

Fig. 1. Absorption spectra for deoxyhemoglobin (Hb), oxyhemoglobin (HbO_2), cytochrome c oxidase (Cyt), and water (H_2O) in the near-infrared range. The isobestic point near 800 nm is the point where the absorptivity of Hb and HbO_2 are equal (Palmer & Williams, 1974; Wray et al., 1988).

2.2 Scattering of light

In addition to the attenuation of light by absorption, scatter also causes attenuation of light. When NIR light is scattered in tissue the collisions are elastic, implicating that no energy is lost and the photon merely changes direction. The direction in which the scattered photon travels is dependent upon the wavelength, the different refractive indices of the tissue layers through which the photon is travelling and the size of the scattering particle (Elwell & Phil, 1995).

A complex structure such as the human head consists of multiple layers of tissue each with varying thicknesses and densities, resulting in varying degrees of scatter. These include cell membranes, transitions between different fluids and various organelles within the cell, large blood vessels as well as the boundaries between bone and soft tissue. The most important source of scatter in tissue are cell membranes since they account for a large proportion of the solid content of the tissue. However, red blood cells only account for approximately 1.5% of the solid content of tissue and as such the attenuation by scattering due to red blood cells is low (Cope, 1991; Elwell & Phil, 1995). Highly scattering tissues include bone, cerebral white matter and skin dermis (Elwell & Phil, 1995).

2.3 Attenuation by light

When light travels through tissue it is attenuated due to the effects of both absorption and scatter, hence the effects of both parameters being considered during spectroscopic measurements. The attenuation of light caused by tissue can be related to the concentration of chromophores in tissue by the Beer-Lambert law.

$$A = \log(\frac{I}{I_0}) = \varepsilon \cdot C \cdot d \tag{1}$$

Attenuation (A) is the logarithmic ratio of two intensities, the intensity of the incident light (I_0) and the transmitted light (I). ε is the molar extinction coefficient, as shown in Fig. 1, expressed in $mM^{-1}cm^{-1}$. C is the concentration of a chromophore and d is the direct path-length of the photon from the emitting to the receiving optode, i.e. the inter-optode or geometrical distance.

Considering that there are more chromophores in tissue, the Beer-Lambert law can be written using that the absorption coefficient of each chromophore is additive (Wray et al., 1988), i.e.

$$A = [\varepsilon_1 \cdot C_1 + \varepsilon_2 \cdot C_2 + ... + \varepsilon_n \cdot C_n] \cdot d \tag{2}$$

The typical application of the Beer-Lambert law is that A is experimentally measured (at n wavelengths for n chromophores of interest), Assuming that d is the inter-optode distance and $\varepsilon_1 ... \varepsilon_n$ has been found previously for each chromophore, the objective is to find $C_1 ... C_n$ (Pellicer & Bravo, 2011). Accurate estimation of chromophore concentration requires (at a minimum) the same number of wavelengths, as there are chromophores in the given tissue. A similar specific extinction coefficient of Hb and HbO_2 in the near-infrared spectrum makes measuring at a single wavelength difficult and confounds the interpretation of changes in concentration of the chromophores. Simultaneous measurements of two wavelengths can be used to separate the changes for both Hb and HbO_2 (Strangman et al., 2002). To increase the sensitivity of the estimation, two wavelengths should be chosen in order to distinguish between Hb and HbO_2 molar extinction coefficients, such that HbO_2 has the highest molar extinction coefficient at one wavelength and the lowest at the other (Klungsøyr & Støa, 1954; Refsum, 1957; Siggaard-Andersen et al., 1972). These wavelengths are normally found around the isobestic point, i.e. the wavelength at which the specific extinction coefficient of Hb and HbO_2 are equal (near 800 nm[1]). In Fig. 1 the isobestic point of Hb and HbO_2 in the near-infrared spectrum is displayed. The isobestic point can be used to calculate hemoglobin concentration independent of oxygen saturation (Elwell & Phil, 1995). When three or more wavelengths are used, the changes can be extracted in other, less-absorbing chromophores such as cytochrome c oxidase and H_2O or the accuracy of the measurements of Hb and HbO_2 can be improved (Heekeren et al., 1999; Matcher & Cooper, 1994), by using multilinear regression to fit each chromophore spectrum to the measurements and performing a residual analysis to determine systematic errors (Cope, 1991).

However, if d is not equal to the inter-optode distance, the hemoglobin changes cannot be quantified and comparisons between different subjects or NIRS regions cannot be made. d depends on subjects, the measured region and the wavelength of the light. Due to scattering d will increase in an unknown manner. Approximately 80% of the total attenuation of near-infrared light in tissue is due to scattering, and the remaining 20% to absorption (Cope, 1991). Scattering is thus the biggest problem when attempting quantitative measurements with NIRS. In a highly scattering medium, photons travel a mean distance that is far greater than *d*, which has been defined as the differential path-length (*DP*), i.e. the true optical distance between the optodes. Delpy et al. (1988) defined a scaling factor to correct for the path-length; the differential path-length factor (*DPF*).

$$A = \log(\frac{I}{I_0}) = \varepsilon \cdot C \cdot d \tag{3}$$

Therefore, the modified Beer-Lambert law incorporates the additions

$$A = \log(\frac{I}{I_0}) = \mathrm{e} \times \mathrm{C} \times d \times \mathrm{DPF} + \mathrm{G} \tag{4}$$

The attenuation and the specific extinction coefficient in the modified Beer-Lambert law are no longer strictly linearly related, the degree of non-linearity is a function of the scattering coefficients. The scattering coefficient of the tissue together with the geometry of the optodes are described in the term *G*. *G* is unknown and therefore an absolute calculation of chromophore concentration cannot be derived from Eq. 4. This is a fundamental problem in tissue NIRS, making the determination of absolute concentrations of Hb, HbO_2 and cytochrome c oxidase problematic. Assuming that *G* has the same value for all chromophores in the medium, by using a differential equation between two chromophores, *G* is cleared. As a consequence, only changes in concentration of chromophores can be measured with NIRS (Matcher & Cooper, 1994). Assuming that *DPF* and *d* remain constant during the measuring period, and *d* and *DPF* are known, quantitative data on changes in the concentration of chromophores can be derived.

$$\Delta(A) = \varepsilon \cdot \Delta(C) \cdot d \cdot DPF \tag{5}$$

The changes in the concentration of chromophores can be calculated using a different wavelength for each chromophore, writing a Beer-Lambert equation for each, and solving the simultaneous equations through matrix inversion (Wahr et al., 1996). The NIRS technique can still be applied as an oxygenation trend monitor if the *DPF* is unknown, such as the continuous wave NIRS. There are several techniques available that can be used to calculate the *DPF*, i.e. by time domain (Delpy et al., 1988), frequency domain (Chance, 1990) or derivative spectroscopy (Matcher et al., 1994; Wray et al., 1988), which allow for oxygenation changes to be measured. However, without the knowledge of the term G the absolute chromophore concentration cannot be measured. Though, oxygenation trend monitoring and the measurement of absolute changes in concentration are very useful measurements as well.

2.4 NIRS device

A NIRS device exists out of a light source (emitting optode) to deliver light to the tissues at a known intensity and at two (or more) wavelengths surrounding the isobestic point, and a light detector (receiving optode), which measures the intensity of the exiting light. A computer translates the change in light intensity to clinical useful information.

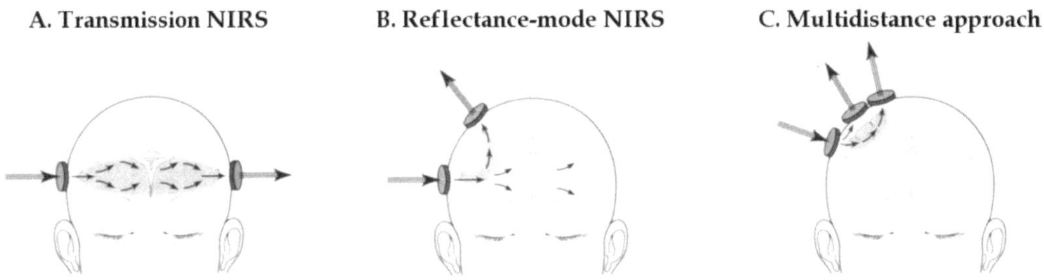

Fig. 2. Different type of NIRS set-ups: (a) transmission NIRS, (b) reflectance-mode NIRS, (c) multi-distance approach NIRS with several receiving optodes to differ between oxygenation changes in different tissue layers (modified from Wahr et al., 1996).

The receiving optode can be either contralateral (transmission NIRS) or ipsilateral (reflectance-mode NIRS) located to the receiver, see Fig. 2A and B. Transmission cerebral NIRS, in which a near-infrared light source is placed contralateral to the receiver, is most frequently used in infants. In adults this is not believed to be sensitive enough, primarily because of the reduced intensity of the exiting near-infrared light (Jöbsis, 1977) and poor signal-to-noise ratio (Germon et al., 1999). In reflectance-mode NIRS the near-infrared light source is placed ipsilateral to the receiver, it has been developed to overcome the problems of transmission NIRS. This approach assumes that there is homogeneous light absorption and constant optical scattering effects. If these assumptions are correct, then the mean path-length of the travelling photons should describe an ellipse whose mean depth is proportional (i.e. 1/3) to the optode spacing (Germon et al., 1999; Strangman et al., 2002).

In Fig. 2C a NIRS device that uses two receiving optodes is displayed. This device attempts to differentiate between light attenuation caused by skull and overlying tissues and light attenuation caused by cerebral tissue. This is called the multi-distance approach and is used in several types of spectrometer, such as spatially resolved spectroscopy and functional NIRS. In most of the NIRS instruments, the distance between source and detector on the surface of the tissue varies between 3 and 5 cm. Measurements at larger distances are difficult because of the fast decay of the signals with the inter-optode distance (Liebert et al., 2011).

3. Types of spectrometer

Three main categories of near-infrared light spectrometers have been developed: continuous wave, time domain and frequency domain spectrometers. The type of information one needs to collect basically determines the choice of spectrometer. The principles, advantages and disadvantages are discussed per category instrument; also other types of spectrometers are discussed.

3.1 Continuous wave NIRS

Continuous wave (CW) NIRS instruments are the earliest and most common commercial NIRS devices. These instruments generally employ either a multiple discrete wavelength source or a filtered white light source, they measure the light attenuation using either a photomultiplier, photodiode or a avalanche photodiode detector (Delpy & Cope, 1997).

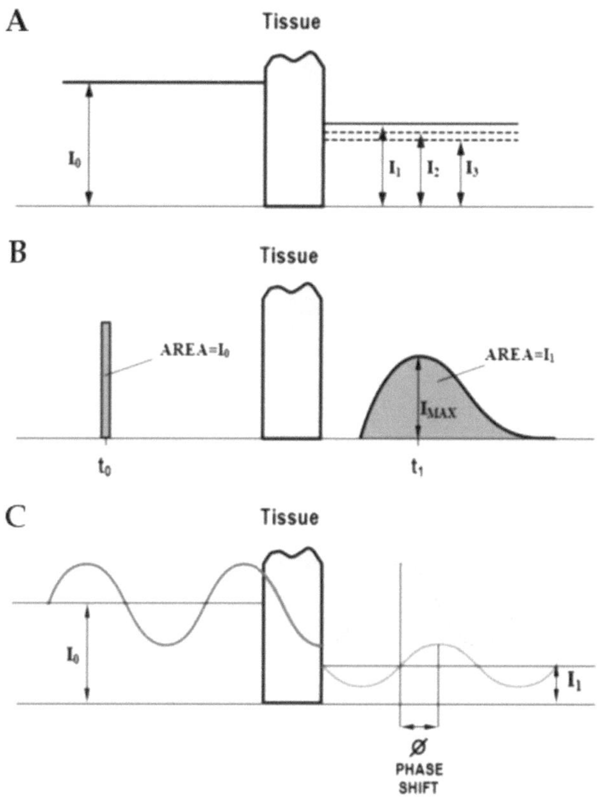

Fig. 3. Schematic presentation of the three main categories of NIRS. (a) Continuous wave NIRS, (b) time domain NIRS (c) and frequency domain NIRS (modified from Pellicer & Bravo, 2011).

The measured attenuation (*A*) at the receiving optode cannot be quantified in CW NIRS, as it contains an unknown light loss due to tissue scattering, increased path-length and thereby increased absorption. However, the changes in measured attenuation (ΔA) can be linearly related to the specific extinction coefficient (ε), according to the Beer-Lambert law, see Eq. 6. Which assumes that the direct path-length (*d*) is a constant value and that changes in attenuation can only arise from variations in the concentrations (ΔC) of Hb, HbO_2 and the cytochrome c oxidase. Considering this, the changes in concentration of these chromophores can be separately identified (but not quantified) from measurements of ΔA made at three different wavelengths (Delpy & Cope, 1997).

$$\Delta A = \varepsilon \cdot d \cdot \Delta C \tag{6}$$

The main advantages of CW NIRS are the sampling rate, the size of the instrument, the weight, the simplicity and the cost, which makes CW NIRS ideal for bedside monitoring. However, CW NIRS has a few disadvantages, including the penetration depth and the difficulty to separate absorption and scattering effects. CW NIRS is only fit to do oxygenation trend monitoring, however, over the years several possibilities to quantify the changes in concentrations of chromophores were investigated. Applications of CW NIRS as a concentration monitor are for example second derivative spectroscopy and spatially resolved spectroscopy, which are described in the next sections. In section 3.1.3 functional NIRS is described which allows for three-dimensional reconstruction of the oxygenation in the brain.

3.1.1 Second derivative spectroscopy

Wray et al. (1988) suggested that CW NIRS could also yield estimates of the differential path-length factor (*DPF*) and thereby quantifies the measured changes in concentration. Its principles are that in the near infrared range, the water spectrum contains three major features, a prominent peak centered around 965 nm and two other small peaks around 820 and 740 nm. The 965 peak is large enough to allow accurate curve-fitting of its shape to the known spectrum of water. The concentration of water in the brain is usually known to within 2% to 3%; therefore it is possible to estimate the *DPF* at 965 nm using the ratio of the peak amplitudes and the known inter-optode spacing (Delpy & Cope, 1997; Wray et al., 1988).

The actual comparison is performed on the second derivative of the spectra, which will eliminate most of the effects of tissue scattering (Wahr et al., 1996). The principle of this technique is that if the measured spectrum has an unknown constant attenuation, this can be removed by taking the first derivative of the spectrum with respect to wavelength. If there is an additional unknown, but linearly wavelength-dependent, attenuation present, this will appear as a constant in the first derivative, which can be removed by taking the second derivative. This should leave a flat spectrum containing only features corresponding to the second derivative of the absorption spectra of any chromophores in the tissue. In the near infrared, the second derivative of the water spectrum has three components corresponding to the previous named peaks. Hb has a large peak at 760 nm, but HbO_2 and cytochrome c oxidase have negligible features (Delpy & Cope, 1997). Therefore, it is possible to calculate the ratio of the Hb concentration to the water concentration and thereby obtain an absolute measure of changes in the Hb concentration (Wahr et al., 1996).

The advantage of this technique is that it uses CW NIRS, which are easy to use on the bedside. Additionally, changes in chromophore concentrations can be measured. However, at shorter wavelengths the *DP* is underestimated (Matcher et al., 1994).

3.1.2 Spatially resolved spectroscopy

Spatially resolved spectroscopy (SRS) is one of the most used NIRS systems. The SRS system incorporates several detectors housed in a single probe, with an inter-optode distance of 4–5 cm. The combination of the multi-distance measurements of optical attenuation allows calculation of the relative concentrations of HbO_2 and Hb in the illuminated tissue. This calculation is derived from the relative absorption coefficients obtained from the slope of light attenuation at different wavelengths over a distance measured at several focal points from the light emission. The opinion about NIRS in adults has been influenced by the additive effect of the extracerebral tissues on the light attenuation. By using a SRS approach, the superficial layers of brain tissue affect all the light bundles similarly and therefore the influence of the extracerebral tissues on the light attenuation cancel out. Only deeper tissue layers have an effect on the values (Choi et al., 2004).

The main advantage of spatially resolved spectroscopy is that it also uses the small, light CW NIRS technology. Additionally it can measure online hemoglobin concentration changes and the TIO. However, the scattering factor included in the TIO calculation make spatially resolved spectroscopy less reliable for multilayered structure like in cerebral oxygenation measurements. However, Al-Rawi et al. (2001) showed that the NIRO 300, a spatially resolved spectrometer, has a high degree of sensitivity and specificity to intracranial and extracranial changes. SRS is technically simpler than TRS and provides measurements with a good signal-to-noise ratio and a high time resolution (Perrey, 2008).

3.1.3 Functional NIRS

After the development of multichannel CW NIRS imaging systems, which allow the generation of images of a larger area of the subject's head with high temporal resolution, and thereby the production of maps of cortical oxygenation changes (Quaresima et al., 2002), functional NIRS was developed. In multichannel CW NIRS multiple source-detector probes are used, which for example can result in a 7 by 7 cm measurement surface. The development of three-dimensional reconstruction methods resulted in the present functional NIRS (fNIRS) (Quaresima et al., 2002). If a sufficient number of sources and detectors are placed around the head it is feasible to generate cross-sectional or three-dimensional (3D) images of the optical properties of the brain. This approach, known as either functional NIRS, diffuse optical imaging (DOI) diffuse optical tomography (DOT) or near-infrared imaging (NIRI), requires sophisticated image reconstruction algorithms to convert the transmittance measurements into 3D images (Minagawa-Kawai et al., 2008).

However, fNIRS is far from routine use, mainly because of its slow acquisition and reconstruction speed, and high cost. Optical tomography of the entire brain is also limited to newborn infants, since the attenuation of light across a larger head is too great to sample the inner regions of the brain. Because of the high attenuation, data acquisition is relatively slow, and imaging of evoked response requires averaging over several activations (Gibson et al., 2005).

3.2 Time domain NIRS

Time domain spectrometers are also called time-of-flight or time-resolved systems. They generally employ a semiconductor or solid state laser to generate ultrashort pulses. They measure the attenuation by either a synchroscan streak camera or a time-correlated single photon counting in which a photon counting detector detects and sorts the received photons by their time of arrival (Delpy & Cope, 1997).

In time domain spectrometers a light pulse of a few picoseconds long propagates in the tissue and, as a result of scattering, the timeline of photons exiting the tissues has a broad distribution, this distribution is called the temporal point spread function (TPSF). A typical tissue TPSF is characterized by a relatively rapidly rising intensity, peaking around 600-1000 ps and then a slow decay often several nanoseconds in duration (Chance et al., 1988b), see Fig. 3. The TPSF data can be analyzed in four different ways; (1) The DP can be derived from the mean of the integrated TPSF (Delpy et al., 1988). (2) When the TPSF data is plotted on a logarithmic scale, the slowly decaying final slope is observed to be almost linear and, from diffusion theory, a simple relationship between the asymptotic limit of this final slope and the specific extinction coefficients of the chromophores can be obtained (Chance et al.,

1988a). (3) The TPSF of the tissue is measured at two different wavelengths and then the ratio of the intensities at corresponding times calculated. As time can be related to distance (knowing the speed of light and tissue refractive index), the resulting plot is essentially attenuation ratio as a function of distance. Changes in chromophore concentration can be calculated from these if the difference in the chromophore specific extinction coefficients is known and assuming that the scattering coefficient is constant over the wavelength measurement range (Oda et al., 1996). (4) A variant of this technique takes the above attenuation ratio versus time data and then extrapolates the resulting linear relation back to a time when the first light, which can be considered as unscattered light, would have exited the tissues (Yamada et al., 1993). The attenuation at this point is theoretically the absorption ratio one would obtain in the absence of scattering. This is the so-called temporally extrapolated absorbance method (TEAM) (Yamada, 1993).

The main advantages of time domain spectrometers are the spatial resolution; the penetration depth and that time domain spectrometers are the most accurate spectrometers in separating absorption and scattering effects. However, there are several disadvantages including the sampling rate, the instrument size, the instrument weight, the necessity for cooling, the lack of stabilization and the cost.

3.3 Frequency domain NIRS

Frequency domain spectrometers are also called frequency-resolved or intensity modulated systems. They generally employ a laser diode, LED or modulated white light sources. They measure the attenuation, phase shift (Φ) and modulation depth (M) of the exiting light by either a photon counting detector or gain modulated area detector (Chance et al., 1990; Delpy & Cope, 1997).

In frequency domain spectrometers radio frequency modulated light propagates through tissue. The resulting signal is the Fourier transform of the TPSF, relating time domain results to frequency domain results. Therefore, the same information as measured with the time domain spectrometers can be found with the frequency domain spectrometers. There are three different principles of frequency domain spectrometers, which are all based on diffusion theory. The frequency domain spectrometers perform measurements of changes in intensity, phase and modulation using either (1) a single wavelength and a fixed inter-optode distance. (2) multiple wavelengths and a fixed inter-optode distance. (3) Or a single wavelength and multiple inter-optode distances (Delpy & Cope, 1997).

The main advantages of frequency domain spectrometers are the sampling rate and the relative accurate separation of absorption and scattering effects. A limitation of frequency domain spectrometers is that the radio frequency modulated light cannot exceed 200 MHz, because a linear relationship between phase shift and path-length no longer applies above 200 Mhz (Arridge et al., 1992). However, the main disadvantage is the penetration depth of frequency domain spectrometers.

4. Utility of NIRS

Cerebral injury due to hypoxic/ischemic and hyperperfusion are common issues associated with clinical and surgical practice. Monitoring of cerebral oxygenation during surgery, eg;

cardiac and cerebral endarterectomy, has been shown to improve patient outcomes and reduce the risk of negative surgical outcomes. In addition to surgical monitoring, NIRS technology provides useful insight into cerebral hemodynamics when used in combination of other cerebral monitoring systems. NIRS monitoring and comparisons have been made with transcranial Doppler (TCD) and electroencephalography (EEG) in its ability to accurately predict cerebral ischemia and hyperperfusion. In addition to peri-operative monitoring in clinical settings, many researchers utilize the various NIRS systems to reflect on the cerebral tissue oxygenation status during environmental and exercise interventions despite strong evidence and proper analytical techniques. The following sections will outline the above utilities associated with NIRS technology.

4.1 Cardiovascular procedures

Post surgical outcomes of cardiac surgeries like are often confounded with poor neurological outcomes. Despite advanced techniques in the operation protocol, (ie: arterial line filtering and aortic arch ultrasound) complications still arise. Stroke occurs in 1-3% of patients during these surgeries, with an increasing number of those who undergo cardiovascular procedures developing cognitive impairments (Murkin et al., (2007)). A study performed by Murkin et al., (2007) demonstrated that prolonged cerebral de-saturation in the control group of a coronary artery bypass surgical population resulted in a higher incidence of peri-operative stroke, and longer post surgical ICU durations. Additionally, the control group while suffering from longer time spent de-saturated below the experimental mean of 84% also had a higher frequency of organ morbidity and death compared to the intervention group who remained above or near the 84% cerebral saturation point. The NIRS device, although apparent in its usefulness in reducing intra and post surgery complications, is further exalted in its ability to guide cardiac surgeons with temporally targeted cerebral de-saturation limits while maintaining a non-invasive and relatively viable and cost effective technology.

4.2 Cerebrovascular procedures

The neurological outcome of a patient undergoing cerebrovascular surgery, which often requires the supplementary artery blood flow to the brain, is dependent on the successful management of brain oxygenation. Carotid endarterectomy (CEA) is a surgery involving intra-operative clamping of the carotid artery, resulting in a change in blood supply to the brain via the ipsilateral vertebral artery and contralateral vertebral and carotid arteries (European Carotid Surgery Trialists' Collaborative Group, 1998). Since the first CEA surgery in 1954, there have been regular incidences of peri-operative stroke. Approximately 3-5% of all subjects undergoing this procedure in the aforementioned study suffered either embolic or ischemic stroke. Peri-operative monitoring of cerebral oxygenation enables surgeons to set ischemic thresholds, typically in the range of 12-20% reduction in cerebral oxygenation, aimed at identifying crucial periods when implementing a cerebral shunt. To allow for measurement of adequate oxygenation levels during the implementation of the shunt, it requires a highly specific and sensitive monitoring device to correctly identify ischemic conditions. Implementing a carotid shunt too early can increase the risk of an embolic stroke, thereby reducing the benefit of using the peri-operative monitoring device (Botes et al., 2007; Matsumoto et al., 2009; Samra et al., 2000). In the literature, three primary methods of non-invasive monitoring of cerebral oxygenation and perfusion can be found: transcranial Doppler (TCD), electroencephalography (EEG) and (NIRS). Each technique has its own limitations and advantages. In TCD it is possible to monitor bilateral anterior and posterior cerebral perfusion with good specificity and sensitivity to changes in blood pressure, but remains to have implementation issues as not every patient has optimal temporal acoustic windows. Approximately 15% of all subjects do not have ecogenic cerebral arteries (Willie et al. (2011)). EEG on the other hand remains a highly specific monitoring tool, yet it fails to be as sensitive to changes in BP and ischemia as TCD and NIRS during peri-operative monitoring, additionally it often requires trained operators thereby decreasing the cost effectiveness and efficiency. Botes et al., 2007 compared the ability of EEG and NIRS during CEA surgery, and demonstrated that NIRS was able to recognize changes in brain perfusion earlier than EEG (Botes et al., 2007). However, the low specificity and high sensitivity may also have resulted in false positive ischemic findings and could possibly lead to a premature carotid shunt. Since the application of continuous peri-operative monitoring during CEA, incidences of intra-operative stroke have decreased, however few multisurgical designs investigating the combined and individual use of NIRS as an improved device over TCD and EEG have been done. Although it may be cost-effective and useful on occasion, little direct evidence supporting the wide spread use of NIRS as a CEA technique is available.

4.3 Exercise and cerebral tissue oxygenation

In addition to practical clinical applications, researchers have attempted to use the NIRS device to measure and quantify the differences between muscular, cerebral, and respiratory tissue oxygenation during exercise. However, NIRS as a stand-alone device to quantify cerebral tissue oxygen kinetics have not been validated. The use of NIRS as a sports medicine and exercise tool should be used with caution as studies are often time consuming and frequently difficult to interpret. One example of how to utilize NIRS during exercise can be seen in a study performed by Nielsen et al. (1999) where the authors had world-class rowers perform two 6-min bouts of all out rowing on a rowing ergometer while breathing two different mixtures of oxygen. Cerebral tissue saturation during normal exercise (normoxic inpired fraction of oxygen, F_IO_2=0.21) as measured by NIRS indicated that the frontal lobe of the brain dropped from 80 to 63% cerebral saturation. However, when subject performed the same trial while inspiring a higher O_2 mixture (F_IO_2=0.30) cerebral saturation was maintained at baseline levels. The authors of the study suggested that the high F_IO_2 resulted in a reversal of the exercise induced cerebral de-saturation. The study provided a unique look into the brain's response to exercise, however issues with measuring the NIRS signal during exercise continue to arise. The primary difficulty stems from the knowledge that hyper and hypoventilatory responses associated with exercise result in Cerebral blood flow and volume. CBF and cerebral blood volume changes may interfere with accurate signal interpretation due to issues with arterial-venous differences which are to be discussed in the oncoming sections.

5. NIRS limitations

NIRS, like most technology, has various limitations. The most important of those limitations are as follows: interference from non targeted chromophores; indefinite differential path-length; unknown scattering loss factor; and complicated signal interpretation.

5.1 Influence of other chromophores

Before the NIR light reaches the brain it must first pass through the different tissue layers, see Fig. 4. In some of these layers there are chromophores present, which will cause light attenuation independent of brain oxygenation.

The skin is composed of the epidermis and the dermis. The epidermis contains melanin, at near-infrared wavelengths melanin has a constant specific extinction coefficient. Melanin also has a significant optical effect on skin reflectance. Caucasian skin causes two times more reflection than negroid skin in the 600-1000 nm region. Attenuation by melanin only increases the sensitivity required of the instrument. Since its absorption is constant and oxygenation independent, it does not produce attenuation changes that are time dependent (Cope, 1991).

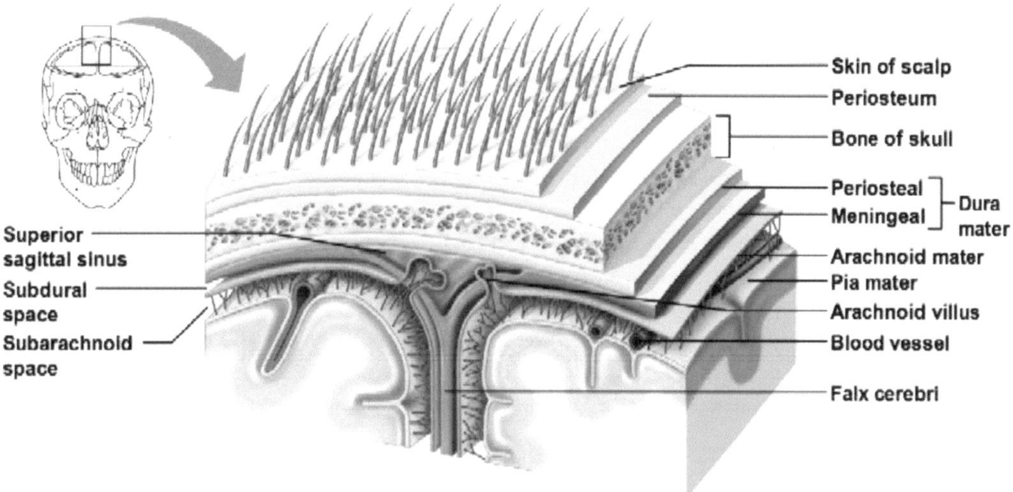

Fig. 4. Different tissue layers of the human head (modified from Hammoudi, 2011).

The dermis and the skull contain the chromophores *bilirubin*, *hemoglobin* and *cytochrome c oxidase*. Overall, the skin and the skull provide a barrier which must be penetrated before light enters the brain tissues. The attenuation caused by this region will also change with oxygenation (due to the presence of hemoglobin), the magnitude of this effect being proportional to its thickness and chromophore concentration. It is recommended that the thickness of brain tissue illuminated is therefore much greater than that of the surface tissues. Bilirubin can be found in blood plasma. Bilirubin systematically lowers brain oxygenation and attenuates the detection of changes in cerebral oxygenation (Madsen & Secher, 1999). In liver disease the bilirubin level can be increased in severe manners, so that the NIRS signal is seriously confounded (Murkin & Arango, 2009).

In the surface layers covering the skull a small amount of muscle can sometimes be found, the thickness of which is spatially dependent. This is important because muscle additionally contains the chromophore myoglobin. NIRS is unable to differentiate between the signal attenuation from hemoglobin and myoglobin; the absorbency signals of these two chromophores overlap in the NIR range. Myoglobin is much less sensitive to tissue oxygenation than hemoglobin; therefore oxygen delivery must be greatly reduced before the myoglobin spectrum is affected (Doornbos et al., 1999; Ferrari et al., 2004).

In the brain water and lipids are present together with bilirubin, hemoglobin, and cytochrome c oxidase. The average water content of neonatal brain is 90% (Fillerup & Mead, 1967) and 80% (Woodard & White, 1986) for an adult brain. This obviously implies that any absorption band of water will have a large optical effect. An infant's brain consists of about 80% of water, lipids constitute about 5% of the total wet weight. This percentage increases to 8% of the grey matter and 17% of the white matter in adulthood (Fillerup & Mead, 1967). The extinction coefficient for lipids is similar in magnitude to that of water. Lipids will not significantly add to the overall extinction coefficient of brain tissue as it is only present at approximately one tenth the proportion compared to water, although it is possible that lipids have a significant effect on the light attenuation (Cope, 1991).

5.2 Differential path-length

There are several factors influencing the optical path-length including tissue type, wavelength, scattering coefficients, optode geometry and blood volume changes. In reality there is no unique optical path through a scattering medium but rather a distribution of paths (Cope, 1991). The DPF is mainly influenced by scatter. It increases the optical path-length in an unknown manner, which leads to an increased absorption. With several techniques an estimation of the mean optical path-length can be made. However, this is not very accurate for the whole measurement. Further, the differential path-length factor generally decreases with increasing wavelength (Essenpreis et al., 1993). For this reason it is always important when quoting DPF values to also quote the wavelength at which the measurements have been made (Elwell & Phil, 1995). Also, the DPF depends on the geometry of the optodes, i.e. the angular position of the optodes on a spherical object, such as the human head (van der Zee et al., 1990).

The brain can move or expand to a limited degree in the skull, and it is possible that the thickness of the cerebrospinal fluid (CSF) layer varies during the NIRS measurements or because of changes in posture. Changes in the thickness of the CSF layer alter the intensity of detected light, therefore any brain movement and expansion during the measurement would affect the NIRS signal. The optical path length in the brain for a certain inter-optode distance depends to a great extent on the thickness of the skull whereas the thickness of the CSF layer scarcely affects the optical path-length in the brain (Okada & Delpy, 2003).

When the DPF is not determined accurately cross talk might occur, i.e., a change in the concentration of one chromophore might yield an artifactual change in the concentration of another unless the algorithms for deconvoluting the spectral contributions were without error (Heekeren et al., 1999).

5.3 Scattering loss factor

The main reason why concentrations in chromophores cannot be quantified is the unknown loss due to scattering. Several models have been developed for prediction of near-infrared light through tissue; (1) To seek an analytical solution of the diffusion equation. However, this has only succeeded under restricted geometries and in a homogeneous medium. (2) The MC method, which can be applied to an inhomogeneous medium, has the advantage of being able to calculate the path-length directly and can offer the individual photon histories, but which requires considerable computation time. (3) To solve the diffusion equation numerically by the finite-difference method, which has been successful under restricted conditions for an inhomogeneous medium. (4) To solve the diffusion equation by the finite-element method, which can be applied to the complex geometries of an inhomogeneous medium and has the advantage of fast calculation time, but it does not calculate individual photon histories (Hiraoka et al., 1993).

However, these models can only approximate the scattering loss factor. There is still an uncertainty in every model because it will not predict unlinearities, which will probably arise in human tissue.

5.4 Interpretation of the NIRS signal

The measured attenuation of near-infrared light is influenced by many factors. Although the NIRS signal can be related to the regional oxygenation, it cannot differentiate between venous, arterial or capillary blood, or between an increase utilization of oxygen or decreased saturation. Also, the changes in Hb and HbO_2 concentrations in the blood flow of the skin or additional to the total attenuation. These issues are addressed in the next sections.

5.4.1 A/V ratio

An advantage of NIRS is that it measures the regional saturation. However, this also comes with a disadvantage because the regional blood flow consists of venous, arterial and capillary blood flow. Cerebral NIRS devices measure mean tissue oxygen saturation and, as such, reflect hemoglobin saturation in venous, capillary, and arterial blood comprising the sampling volume. For cerebral cortex, average tissue hemoglobin is distributed in a proportion of 70% venous and 30% arterial (McCormick et al., 1991), based on correlations between position emission tomography (PET) and NIRS (Ohmae et al., 2006). However, clinical studies have demonstrated that there can be considerable biological variation in individual cerebral arterial/venous (A/V) ratios between patients, further underscoring that the use of a fixed ratio can produce significant divergence from actual in vivo tissue oxygen saturation, thus confounding even 'absolute' measures of changes in cerebral oxygenation (Watzman et al., 2000).

NIRS results are not only influenced by oxygenation changes. For example, an increase in arterial oxygen saturation causes an equal increase and decrease in the cerebral HbO_2 and Hb concentration respectively (and visa versa). However, an increase in cerebral oxygen consumption would lead to an equal decrease and increase in the cerebral HbO_2 and Hb concentration respectively (and visa versa). Note that an arterial saturation monitor would allow the changes in arterial and venous systems to be differentiated from each other. Further, an increase in cerebral blood flow leads to an increase in cerebral blood volume, which is largely taken up by the HBO_2 concentration (and visa versa). However, an increase in blood pressure in the venous system (i.e. blocking venous return) would lead to an increase in blood volume in the venules, a much larger fraction of which would be made up of Hb compared to the case of increased cerebral blood volume. Deliberately increasing venous pressure has been suggested as a method of measuring absolute venous saturation (Cope, 1991). This suggests that the NIRS results are not only influenced by oxygenation changes but other factors are also of importance. This should be considered when the interpretation of the results is done, especially in critical care situations.

5.4.2 Cerebral vs extracerebral blood flow

A serious problem connected with the application of the NIRS technique is contamination of the measured signals with the components originating from the extracerebral tissue layers (Liebert et al., 2011). An increase of inter-optode distance leads to better determination of intracerebral changes in tissue absorption, i.e. the volume of cerebral tissue which is interrogated by NIRS increases (Germon et al., 1999). Also, when using the multi-distance approach, see Fig 2C, the oxygenation changes in cerebral and extracerebral tissue can be separated.

Since mean depth of photon penetration approximates 1/3 of the transmitter/receiver separation, by utilizing two differentially spaced receiving optodes—one spaced more closely and the other spaced farther from the transmitter—a degree of spatial resolution can be achieved. The closer receiver (e.g. 3 cm separation) detects primarily extracerebral tissue, whereas the farther optode (e.g. 4 cm separation) reflects extracerebral and cerebral tissue. Incorporation of a subtraction algorithm enables calculation of the difference between the two signals and thus a measure of deeper, cortical tissue saturation. Thus the multi-distance approach can provide spatial resolution to distinguish signals from cerebral vs extracerebral tissue. Approximately 85% of cerebral regional oxygen saturation is derived from cerebral tissue with the remaining 15% derived from the extracerebral tissue (Murkin & Arango, 2009).

However, most NIRS devices do not incorporate the multi-distance approach and therefore do not differentiate between cerebral and extracerebral blood flow. An increase in extracerebral blood flow, as can occur, during exercise, induces an unknown change in the total attenuation due to extracerebral blood flow, while cerebral blood flow might not have changed.

5.5 Hospital setting

Practical optical measurements are commonly contaminated by constant (or temporally uncorrelated) background illumination. Frequency domain systems are able to reject uncorrelated signals by the use of lock-in amplifiers, while time domain systems reject photons that reach the detector outside a finite temporal window. However, frequency domain systems are unable to identify unwanted light that is temporally correlated with the measurement, such as light that has leaked around the object being imaged. In the time domain inspection of the TPSF can enable these contaminated measurements to be rejected (Hebden et al., 2004).

6. Future directions

NIRS has various limitations as discussed in section 5, which result in the possibility to measure only the quantitative changes in chromophore concentration. These results should be analyzed carefully to exclude other causes of altered attenuation. In contradiction to the inability of NIRS to measure absolute chromophore concentrations, it can measure cerebral blood volume (CBV) and cerebral blood flow (CBF) with the use of a dye, indocyanine green, and without using radioisotopes or X-rays, as is used in CBF measurements with single-photon emission computed tomography (SPECT) or positron emission tomography (PET).

Another future direction is brain mapping using multimodality approaches; this could enhance the knowledge about neurovascular coupling. Simultaneous measurements of EEG or fMRI with fNIRS results provide more information about cerebrovascular responses to neural stimuli.

6.1 Indocyanine green

As mentioned earlier, NIRS cannot quantify the chromophore concentrations in tissue, however, when using NIRS in combination with indocyanine green (ICG) cerebral blood volume (CBV) and cerebral blood flow (CBF) can be determined. ICG is a highly absorbing intravascular chromophore. It is a tricarbocyanine dye that binds to albumin and therefore remains in the plasma. It shows strong absorption in the NIR range with maximal absorption at 805 nm. Because ICG is normally not present in the human tissue, a zero-concentration reference point is available before any dye is administered. This enables NIRS to quantify absolute tissue concentrations of ICG (Hopton et al., 1999).

6.1.1 CBV

The ratio between the blood and tissue concentration of ICG over a measurement period can be used to derive a mean CBV, by using blood and tissue time integrals. Thereby minimizing changes due to alterations in blood pressure and $paCO_2$.

$$CBV = \frac{\int_{t_1}^{t_2} [ICG_{tissue}]dt}{\int_{t_1}^{t_2} [ICG_{blood}]dt} \tag{7}$$

Where $[ICG]_{tissue}$ is the concentration of ICG in the tissue measured by NIRS, $[ICG]_{blood}$ is the concentration of ICG in cerebral blood estimated by analysis of a peripheral venous sample, compensating for the Fahraeus effect and t_1 and t_2 are respectively the start and finish times of the measurement period. After administration of a bolus of ICG, ICG concentration decreases, as there is hepatic uptake and biliary excretion (Kuebler et al., 1998). The integrated tissue and blood concentrations over a period of time (usually from 3 to 20 minutes after the ICG bolus) are determined by calculating the areas under the elimination curves for NIRS tissue measurements and peripheral venous concentration measurements of ICG (for a more detailed explanation see Hopton et al., 1999).

6.1.2 CBF

The measurement of CBF is based on the principles of the direct Fick method (Fick, 1870) and the later adapted Kety-Schmidt technique (Kety & Schmidt, 1945), i.e. the rate of proportionality, or the balancing of venous content and arterial content, of an inert gas dependent upon the volume of blood flowing through the brain (Kety & Schmidt, 1945). ICG can act as a Fick tracer, similar to that of an inert gas. The rate of arrival of ICG in the brain, a few seconds after the rapid injection of ICG, can be observed by NIRS (Gora et al., 2002). ICG is introduced rapidly and its rate of accumulation is measured over time. Blood flow can be measured as a ratio of ICG accumulated to the quantity of ICG introduced over a given time (Perrey, 2008). The accumulation of ICG in the brain will be dependent on both arterial inflow and venous outflow (Gora et al., 2002). The method of measuring CBF relies on several assumptions: first, blood flow must be constant for the period of measurement. Second, there must be linearity and stability of the tracer dose response in tissue. Third, the tracer must not be metabolized or permanently retained in the tissue during the period of measurement (Perrey, 2008). And finally, the measurements should be made within the cerebrovascular transit time (four to six seconds), because then the venous outflow is negligible and the measured increase in cerebral ICG concentration can be assumed to be entirely the result of arterial inflow of the tracer. ICG meets up with these assumptions and can thus be used as the specific tracer in CBF measurements (Gora et al., 2002). The amount of tracer delivered to the brain can be calculated from the area under the curve of the arterial ICG concentration change measured by the dye–densitometer

A disadvantage of CBV and CBF determinations with NIRS in combination with ICG is that it is invasive since it requires arterial cannulation, repeated blood withdrawals, and reinfusions (Guenette et al., 2011). It is still less invasive than SPECT or PET (radioisotopes and X-rays, respectively), but nonetheless invasive. However, NIRS in combination with ICG could be feasible on the bedside, in contradiction to SPECT or PET. Exploring and validating this technique should be an aim in the nearby future.

6.2 Multimodal approach

Human brain mapping by multimodality approaches has been proposed as an integrated methodology towards a deeper understanding of cortical response and neurovascular coupling. Integration of functional magnetic resonance imaging (fMRI) or electroencephalography (EEG) with functional near-infrared spectroscopy (fNIRS) has the potential to monitor neuronal and vascular response and provide new insights into the origin and development of cortical activation (Torricelli et al., 2011; Wallois et al., 2011).

6.2.1 EEG-fNIRS

Since electrical and hemodynamic changes involve subtle, complex mechanisms, EEG-fNIRS coregistration is a promising approach to study language related, neural and cerebral functional activity (Wallois et al., 2011). NIRS combined with video EEG is a promising upcoming development for the evaluation of epileptic patients. fNIRS in combination with EEG could become an essential tool for the management of epileptic patients in daily clinical routine, particularly in neonates and children (Wallois et al., 2010).

EEG has very high temporal resolution whereas fNIRS is not affected by electromagnetic interference and is not as susceptible to movement artefact as EEG. By using both modalities on the same area of cortex, extra information about the cortical activity can be recorded. As this implements a combined electrical and hemodynamic recording of cortical activity, we are making direct observations of neurovascular coupling. Such information may prove to be vital for research into stroke rehabilitation, epilepsy and language related studies. An advantage of a multimodal approach is that for the same measurement space on the head, more information about the underlying neurovascular relationship is being recorded. An EEG of fNIRS alone system can only record the electrical or hemodynamic response in an area of cortex. A multimodal approach records fNIRS and EEG but also records information about the relationship between them, even if that relationship is not fully understood. Investigation into dual-modality measurement is of importance due to the potential gains in classification accuracy while utilizing the same area of cortex (Leamy et al., 2011).

6.2.2 fMRI-fNIRS

fMRI is the golden standard to image neuronal processes in the brain in-vivo, The golden standard to detect activation in the brain during neural stimulation is fMRI. It relies on an indirect signal, the blood oxygenation level-dependent (BOLD) contrast, which is caused by an increase in oxygen delivery (Steinbrink et al., 2006; Toyoda et al., 2007).

However, the details of the translation of firing neurons to an increase in focal cerebral blood flow remains controversial. fNIRS has the potential to resolve some of the key issues concerning the basis of the vascular response, since it measures the physiological changes of total hemoglobin, Hb and HbO_2 concentration. The BOLD signal correlates with changes in Hb, HbO_2 and total hemoglobin concentration (Steinbrink et al., 2006).

NIRS offers superior temporal resolution (40 ms versus 2000 ms), whereas BOLD offers superior spatial resolution and whole brain coverage (Tong & Frederick, 2010). Combined fMRI-fNIRS studies have been used to elucidate the biophysics of the BOLD response. However, most studies have focused on the correlation of the BOLD signal to the changes in the hemoglobin concentrations, but there is a lack in studies of the transient effects of the BOLD signal. For example, the interplay of the vascular dynamics in flow, volume and oxygen extraction and the origin of the BOLD signal due to the differential behavior in CBV and Hb concentration (Steinbrink et al., 2006).

Multimodal fMRI-fNIRS may provide a novel contrast mechanism that can be exploited as a tool for characterizing cerebral blood flow directly. And that further optimatization of the technique may allow for quantification of other blood flow parameters (Tong & Frederick, 2010), for example, the oxygen extraction fraction and CBV (Toyoda et al., 2007).

7. References

Al-Rawi, P. G., Smielewski, P., & Kirkpatrick, P. J. (2001). Evaluation of a Near-Infrared Spectrometer (NIRO 300) for the Detection of Intracranial Oxygenation Changes in the Adult Head. *Stroke,* 32, 11, (July 2001), pp. (2492-2500), 0039-2499

Arridge, S. R., Cope, M., & Delpy, D. T. (1992). The theoretical basis for the determination of optical path-lengths in tissue: temporal and frequency analysis. *Physics in medicine and biology,* 37, 7, (March 1992), pp. (1531-1560), 0031-9155

Botes, K., Roux, D. A. Le, & Marle, J. van. (2007). Cerebral monitoring during carotid endarterectomy -a comparison between electroencephalography, transcranial cerebral oximetry and carotid stump pressure. *South African Journal of Surgery,* 45, 2, (May 2007), pp. (43-46), 0038-2361

Chance, B., Leigh, J., Miyake, H., Smith, D. S., Nioka, S., Greenfeld, R., Finander, M., Kaufmann, K., Levy, W., & Young, M. (1988a). Comparison of time-resolved and -unresolved measurements of deoxyhemoglobin in brain. *Proceedings of the National Academy of Sciences of the United States of America,* 0027-8424, USA, July 1988

Chance, B., Nioka, S., Kent, J., McCully, K. K., Fountain, M., Greenfeld, R., & Holtom, G. (1988b). Time-resolved spectroscopy of hemoglobin and myoglobin in resting and ischemic muscle. *Analytical biochemistry,* 174, 2, (April 1988), pp. (698-707), 0003-2697

Chance, B., Maris, M. B., Sorge, J., & Zhang, M. Z. (1990). Phase modulation system for dual wavelength difference spectroscopy of hemoglobin deoxygenation in tissues, *Proceedings of SPIE,* 0277-786X, Los Angeles, CA, USA, January 1990

Choi, J. H., Wolf, M., Toronov, V., Wolf, U., Polzonetti, C., Hueber, D., Safonova, L. P., Gupta, R., Michalos, A., Mantulin, W., & Gratton, E. (2004). Noninvasive determination of the optical properties of adult brain: near-infrared spectroscopy approach. *Journal of biomedical optics,* 9, 1, (May 2003), pp. (221-229), 1083-3668

Cope, M. (April 1991). *The application of near infrared spectroscopy to non invasive monitoring of cerebral oxygenation in the newborn infant,* University College London, Retrieved from <http://www.medphys.ucl.ac.uk/research/borl/docs/mcope.pdf>

Delpy, D. T., Cope, M., Zee, P. van der, Arridge, S. R., Wray, S., & Wyatt, J. S. (1988). Estimation of optical path-length through tissue from direct time of flight measurement. *Physics in medicine and biology,* 33, 12, (July 1988), pp. (1433-1442), 0031-9155

Delpy, D. T., & Cope, M. (1997). Quantification in tissue near-infrared spectroscopy. *Philosophical Transactions of the Royal Society B: Biological Sciences,* 352, 1354, (June 1997), pp. (649-659), 0962-8436

Doornbos, R. M. P., Lang, R., Aalders, M. C., Cross, F. W., & Sterenborg, H. J. C. M. (1999). The determination of in vivo human tissue optical properties and absolute chromophore concentrations using spatially resolved steady-state diffuse reflectance spectroscopy. *Phys. Med. Biol..* 44, (December 1999), pp. (967-981), 0031-9155

Elwell, C. E., & Phil, M. (1995). *A practical users guide to near infrared spectroscopy* (1st edition), Hamatsu Phototonics KK, London

Essenpreis, M., Elwell, C. E., Cope, M., Zee, P. van der, Arridge, S. R., & Delpy, D. T. (1993). Spectral dependence of temporal point spread functions in human tissues. *Applied optics,* 32, 4, (February 1993), pp. (418-425), 0003-6935

European Carotid Surgery Trialists' Collaborative Group. (1998), Randomised trial of endarterectomy for recently symptomatic carotid stenosis: final results of the MRS European Carotid Surgery Trial (ECST). *Lancet,* 351, 9713, (May 1998), p. (1379), 0140-6736

Fick A. (1870) Ueber die Messung des Blutquantums in den Herzventrikeln. *Verh Phys Med Ges Wurzburg* 2: 16–28

Ferrari, M., Mottola, L., & Quaresima, V. (2004). Principles, techniques, and limitations of near infrared spectroscopy. *Canadian journal of applied physiology,* 29, 4, (August 2004), pp. (463-487), 1066-7814

Fillerup, D. L., & Mead, J. F. (1967). The lipids of the aging human brain. *Lipids,* 2, 4, (July 1967), pp. (295-328), 0024-4201

Germon, T. J., Evans, P. D., Barnett, N. J., Wall, P., Manara, A. R., & Nelson, R. J. (1999). Cerebral near infrared spectroscopy: emitter-detector separation must be increased. *British journal of anaesthesia,* 82, 6, (January 1999), pp. (831-837), 0007-0912

Gibson, A. P., Hebden, J. C., & Arridge, S. R. (2005). Recent advances in diffuse optical imaging. *Physics in Medicine and Biology,* 50, 4, (February 2005), pp. (R1-R43), 0031-9155

Gora, F., Shinde, S., Elwell, C. E., Goldstone, J. C., Cope, M., Delpy, D. T., & Smith, M. (2002). Noninvasive Measurement of Cerebral Blood Flow in Adults Using Near-Infrared Spectroscopy and Indocyanine Green: A Pilot Study. *Computer,* 14, 3, (March 2002), pp. (218-222), 0898-4921

Guenette, J. A., Henderson, W. R., Dominelli, P. B., Querido, J. S., Brasher, P. M., Griesdale, D. E. G., Boushel, R., & Sheel, A. W. (2011). Blood flow index using near-infrared spectroscopy and indocyanine green as a minimally invasive tool to assess respiratory muscle blood flow in humans. *American journal of physiology,* 300, 4, (February 2011), pp. (R984-R992), 1522-1490

Hammoudi, D. (DATE). Meninges, In: *The Brain,* August 1, 2011, Available from: < http://sinoemedicalassociation.org/AP/brainspinalreflexe.pdf>

Hebden, J. C., Gibson, A., Austin, T., Yusof, R., Everdell, N., Delpy, D. T., Arridge, S. R., Meek, J. H., & Wyatt, J. S. (2004). Imaging changes in blood volume and oxygenation in the newborn infant brain using three-dimensional optical tomography. *Physics in Medicine and Biology,* 49, 7, (March 2004), pp. (1117-1130), 0031-9155

Heekeren, H. R., Kohl, M., Obrig, H., Wenzel, R., Pannwitz, W. von, Matcher, S. J., Dirnagl, U., Cooper, C. E., & Villringer, A. (1999). Noninvasive assessment of changes in cytochrome-c oxidase oxidation in human subjects during visual stimulation. *Journal of cerebral blood flow and metabolism,* 19, 6, (September 1999), pp. (592-603), 0271-678X

Hiraoka, M., Firbank, M., Essenpreis, M., Cope, M., Arridge, S. R., van der Zee, P., & Delpy, D. T. (1993). A Monte Carlo investigation of optical path-length in inhomogeneous tissue and its application to near-infrared spectroscopy. *Physics in medicine and biology,* 38, 12, (August 1993), pp. (1859-1876), 0031-9155

Hopton, P., Walsh, T. S., & Lee, A. (1999). Measurement of cerebral blood volume using near-infrared spectroscopy and indocyanine green elimination. *Journal of applied physiology,* 87, 5, (November 1999), pp. (1981-1987), 8750-7587

Horecker, B. L. (1942). The absorption spectra of hemoglobin and its derivatives in the visible and near infra-red regions. *Journal of Biological Chemistry,* (December 1942), pp. (173-183), 0021-9258

Jöbsis, F. F. (1977). Noninvasive, Infrared Monitoring of Cerebral and Myocardial Oxygen Sufficiency and Circulatory Parameters. *Science,* 198, 4323, (December 1977), pp. (1264-1267), 0036-8075

Kety SS and Schmidt CF (1945). The determination of cerebral blood flow in man by the use of nitrous oxide in low concentrations. *Am J Physiol* 143: 53- 66

Klungsøyr, L., & Støa, K. F. (1954). Spectrophotometric determination of hemoglobin oxygen saturation. *Scandinavian journal of clinical and laboratory investigation,* 74, 5, (May 1954), pp. (270-276), 0036-5513

Kuebler, W. M., Sckell, A., Habler, O., Kleen, M., Kuhnle, G. E., Welte, M., Messmer, K., & Goetz, A.E. (1998). Noninvasive measurement of regional cerebral blood flow by near-infrared spectroscopy and indocyanine green. *Journal of cerebral blood flow and metabolism,* 18, 4, (October 1998), pp. (445-456), 0271-678X

Leamy, D. J., Collins, R., & Ward, T. E. (2011). Combining fNIRS and EEG to Improve Motor Cortex Activity Classification during an Imagined Movement-Based Task. In: *Foundations of Augmented Cognition. Directing the Future of Adaptive Systems,*

Schmorrow, D. D., & Fidopiastis, C. M., pp. (177-185), Springer-Verlag, 0302-9743, Berlin

Liebert, A., Sawosz, P., Milej, D., Kacprzak, M., Weigl, W., Botwicz, M., Maczewska, J., Fronczewska, K., Mayzner-Zawadzka, E., Krolicki, L., & Maniewski, R. (2011). Assessment of inflow and washout of indocyanine green in the adult human brain by monitoring of diffuse reflectance at large source-detector separation. *Journal of Biomedical Optics,* 16, 4, (April 2011), pp. (046011-1-7), 1560-2281

Madsen, P. L., & Secher, N. H. (1999). Near-infrared oximetry of the brain. *Progress in Neurobiology,* 58, (October 1999), pp. (541-560), 0301-0082

Matcher, S. J., & Cooper, C. E. (1994). Absolute quantification of deoxyhaemoglobin concentration in tissue near infrared spectroscopy. *Physics in medicine and biology,* 39, 8, (June 1994), pp. (1295-1312), 0031-9155

Matcher, S. J., Cope, M., & Delpy, D. T. (1994). Use of the water absorption spectrum to quantify tissue chromophore concentration changes in near-infrared spectroscopy. *Physics in medicine and biology,* 39, 1, (September 1994), pp. (177-196), 0031-9155

Matsumoto, S., Nakahara, I., Higashi, T., Iwamuro, Y., Watanabe, Y., Takahashi, K., Ando, M., Takezawa, M., & Kira, J. I. (2009). Near-infrared spectroscopy in carotid artery stenting predicts cerebral hyperperfusion syndrome. *Neurology,* 72, 17, (April 2009), pp. (1512-1518), 1526-632X

McCormick, P. W., Stewart, M., Goeting, M. G., & Balakrishnan, G. (1991). Regional cerebrovascular oxygen saturation measured by optical spectroscopy in humans. *Stroke,* 22, (January 1991), pp. (596-602), 1524-4628

Minagawa-Kawai, Y., Mori, K., Hebden, J. C., & Dupoux, E. (2008). Optical imaging of infants' neurocognitive development: recent advances and perspectives. *Developmental neurobiology,* 68, 6, (March 2008), pp. (712-728), 1932-8451

Moosmann, M., Ritter, P., Krastel, I., Brink, A., Thees, S., Blankenburg, F., Taskin, B., Obrig, H., & Villringer, A. (2003). Correlates of alpha rhythm in functional magnetic resonance imaging and near infrared spectroscopy. *NeuroImage,* 20, 1, (May 2003), pp. (145-158), 1053-8119

Murkin, J. M., & Arango, M. (2009). Near-infrared spectroscopy as an index of brain and tissue oxygenation. *British journal of anaesthesia,* 103, (December 2009), pp. (i3-i13), 1471-6771

Murkin, J. M., Adams, S. J., Novick, R. J., Quantz, M., Bainbridge, D., Iglesias, I., Cleland, A., et al. (2007). Monitoring brain oxygen saturation during coronary bypass surgery: a randomized, prospective study. *Anesthesia and analgesia, 104*(1), 51-8. doi:10.1213/01.ane.0000246814.29362.f4

Nielsen, H. B., Boushel, R., Madsen, P., & Secher, N. H. (1999). Cerebral desaturation during exercise reversed by O2 supplementation. *The American journal of physiology, 277*(3 Pt 2), H1045-52. Retrieved from http://www.ncbi.nlm.nih.gov/pubmed/10484427

Oda, M., Yamashita, Y., Nishimura, G.. & Tamura, M. (1996), A simple and novel algorithm for time-resolved multiwavelength oximetry. *Physics in medicine and biology,* 41, (October 1996), pp. (551-562), 0031-9155

Ohmae, E., Ouchi, Y., Oda, M., Suzuki, T., Nobesawa, S., Kanno, T., Yoshikawa, E., Futsatsubashi, M., Ueda, Y., Okada, H., & Yamashita, Y. (2006). Cerebral hemodynamics evaluation by near-infrared time-resolved spectroscopy: correlation with simultaneous positron emission tomography measurements. *NeuroImage,* 29, 3, (August 2006), pp. (697-705), 1053-8119

Okada, E., & Delpy, D. T. (2003). Near-infrared light propagation in an adult head model. II. Effect of superficial tissue thickness on the sensitivity of the near-infrared spectroscopy signal. *Applied optics,* 42, 16, (September 2003), pp. (2915-2922), 0003-6935

Palmer, K. F., & Williams, D. (1974). Optical properties of water in the near infrared. *Journal of the Optical Society of America,* 64, 8, (August 1974), pp. (1107-1110), 0030-3941

Pellicer, A., & Bravo, M. D. C. (2011). Near-infrared spectroscopy: a methodology-focused review. *Seminars in fetal & neonatal medicine,* 16, 1, (February 2011), pp. (42-49), 1744-165X

Perrey, S. (2008). Non-invasive NIR spectroscopy of human brain function during exercise. *Methods,* 45, 4, (June 2008), pp. (289-299), 1095-9130

Quaresima, V., Ferrari, M., Sluijs, M. C. P. van der, Menssen, J., & Colier, W. N. J. M. (2002). Lateral frontal cortex oxygenation changes during translation and language switching revealed by non-invasive near-infrared multi-point measurements. *Brain research bulletin,* 59, 3, (May 2002), pp. (235-243), 0361-9230

Refsum, H. E. (1957). Spectrophotometric determination of hemoglobin oxygen saturation in hemolyzed whole blood by means of various wavelength combinations. *Scandinavian journal of clinical and laboratory investigation,* 9, 2, (October 1957), pp. (190-193), 0036-5513

Samra, S. K., Dy, E. A., Welch, K., Dorje, P., Zelenock, G. B., & Stanley, J. C. (2000). Evaluation of a cerebral oximeter as a monitor of cerebral ischemia during carotid endarterectomy. *Anesthesiology,* 93, 4, (May 2000), pp. (964-970), 0003-3022

Siggaard-Andersen, O., Norgaard-Pedersen, B., & Rem, J. (1972). Hemoglobin pigments, spectrophotometric determination of oxy-, carboxy-, met-, and sulfhemoglobin in capillary blood. *Clinica Chimica Acta,* 42, (July 1972), pp. (85-100), 0009-8981

Steinbrink, J., Villringer, A., Kempf, F., Haux, D., Boden, S., & Obrig, H. (2006). Illuminating the BOLD signal: combined fMRI-fNIRS studies. *Magnetic resonance imaging,* 24, 4, (December 2006), pp. (495-505), 0730-725X

Strangman, G., Boas, D. A., & Sutton, J. P. (2002). Non-invasive neuroimaging using near-infrared light. *Biological psychiatry,* 52, 7, (July 2002), pp. (679-693), 0006-3223

Tong, Y., & Frederick, B. D. (2010). Time lag dependent multimodal processing of concurrent fMRI and near-infrared spectroscopy (NIRS) data suggests a global circulatory origin for low-frequency oscillation signals in human brain. *NeuroImage,* 53, (June 2010), pp. (553-564), 1095-9572

Torricelli, A., Contini, D., Caffini, M., Zucchelli, L., Cubeddu, R., Spinelli, L., Molteni, E., Bianchi, A. M., Baselli, G., Cerutti, S., Visani, E., Gilioli, I., Rossi Sebastiano, D., Schiaffi, E., Panzica, F., & Franceschetti, S. (2011). Assessment of cortical response during motor task in adults by a multimodality approach based on fNIRS-EEG, fMRI-EEG, and TMS, *Proceedings of the SPIE,* 1605-7422, Munich, Germany, June 2011

Toyoda, H., Kashikura, K., Okada, T., Nakashita, S., Honda, M., Yonekura, Y., Kawaguchi, H., Maki, A., & Sadato, N. (2007). Source of nonlinearity of the BOLD response revealed by simultaneous fMRI and NIRS. *NeuroImage,* 39, 3, (September 2007), pp. (997-1013), 1053-8119

Wahr, J. A., Tremper, K. K., Samra, S. K., & Delpy, D. T. (1996). Near-infrared spectroscopy: theory and applications. *Journal of Cardiothoracis and Vascular Anesthesia,* 10, 3, (April 1996), pp. (406-418), 1053-0770

Wallois, F., Patil, A., Héberlé, C., & Grebe, R. (2010). EEG-NIRS in epilepsy in children and neonates. *Clinical Neurophysiology,* 40, 5-6, (August 2010), pp. (281-292), 1769-7131

Wallois, F., Mahmoudzadeh, M., Patil, A., & Grebe, R. (2011). Usefulness of simultaneous EEG-NIRS recording in language studies. *Brain & Language,* In Press, (March 2011), 1090-2155

Watzman, H. M., Kurth, C. D., Montenegro, L. M., Rome, J., Steven, J. M., & Nicolson, S. C. (2000). Arterial and venous contributions to near-infrared cerebral oximetery. *Anesthesiology,* 93, (April 2000), pp. (947-953), 1708-5381

Woodard, H. Q., & White, D. R. (1986). The composition of body tissues. *The British Journal of Radiology,* 59, (June 1986), pp. (1209-1219), 0007-1285

Wray, S., Cope, M., Delpy, D. T., Wyatt, J. S., & Reynolds, E. O. R. (1988). Characterization of the near infrared absorption spectra of cytochrome aa3 and haemoglobin for the non-invasive monitoring of cerebral oxygenation. *Biochimica et biophysica acta,* 933, 1, (December 1988), pp. (184-192), 0006-3002

Yamada, Y. (1993). Simulation of time-resolved optical computer tomography imaging. *Optical Engineering,* 32, 3, (March 1993), pp. (634-641), 0091-3286

Yamada, Y., Hasegawa, Y., & Yamashita, Y. (1993). Simulation of fan-beam-type optical computed-tomography imaging of strongly scattering and weakly absorbing media. *Applied optics,* 32, 25, (September 1993), pp. (4808-4814), 0003-6935

Zee, P. van der, Arridge, S. R., Cope, M. & Delpy, D. T. (1990) The effect of optode positioning on optical path-length in near infrared spectroscopy of the brain. *Advanced Experimental Medicine & Biology,* 277, (1990), pp. (79-84), 0065-275X

5

Assessment of Endothelial Function Using Ultrasound

Lee Stoner and Manning J. Sabatier
[1]*Massey University,*
[2]*Clayton State University,*
[1]*New Zealand*
[2]*USA*

1. Introduction

The pathological complications of atherosclerosis, namely heart attacks and strokes, remain the leading cause of mortality in the Western world (Lloyd-Jones & Adams *et al.* 2010). Preceding atherosclerosis is endothelial dysfunction (Ross 1993; Cohn 1999; Quyyumi 2003). The endothelium comprises a continuous monolayer of cells which separate the vascular wall from the circulation (Lerman & Zeiher 2005). Disruption of this essential monolayer is thought to occur early in the pathogenesis of cardiovascular disease (CVD). There is, therefore, interest in the application of non-invasive clinical tools to assess the function and health of this essential monolayer.

The flow-mediated dilation (FMD) test is the standard tool used to assess endothelial function (Celermajer & Sorensen *et al.* 1992). Reduced FMD is an early marker of atherosclerosis (Celermajer & Sorensen *et al.* 1992), has been noted for its capacity to predict future CVD events (Schroeder & Enderle *et al.* 1999; Neunteufl & Heher *et al.* 2000; Heitzer & Schlinzig *et al.* 2001; Murakami & Arai 2001; Yoshida & Kawano *et al.* 2006; Inaba & Chen *et al.* 2010), and an impaired vascular response has also been demonstrated in children as young as 7 years old with familial hypercholesterolemia (Sorensen & Celermajer *et al.* 1994). This review discusses the measurement of endothelial function, with a focus on the FMD technique.

2. The vascular endothelium

From the lumen to the outer wall all arteries are composed of an intima, media, and adventitia (see Fig. 1). The adventitia is the outer most layer, and is mainly composed of connective tissue that maintains vessel shape and limits distention. The media is comprised mainly of vascular smooth muscle cells that regulate blood flow by vasoconstriction or vasodilation. The intima is the inner most lining of the vessel, and consists of the endothelium and underlying connective tissue.

Vascular endothelial cells essentially have the same characteristics as all the cells of the human body: cytoplasm and organelles surrounding a nucleus and contained by the cellular membrane. Endothelial cells form a continuous flat mono-layer that cover the vascular lumina throughout the arterial tree. The endothelium is mechanically and metabolically strategically located, separating the vascular wall from the circulation and the blood components (Lerman & Zeiher 2005).

The vascular endothelium utilizes autocrine, paracrine, and classical endocrine signaling to promote vascular homeostasis (Luscher & Barton 1997). These cells are capable of producing a variety of agonistic and antagonistic molecules, including vasodilators and vasoconstrictors, pro-coagulants and anti-coagulants, inflammatory and anti-inflammatory, fibrinolytics and anti-fibrinolytics, oxidizing and anti-oxidizing, and many others (Luscher & Barton 1997).

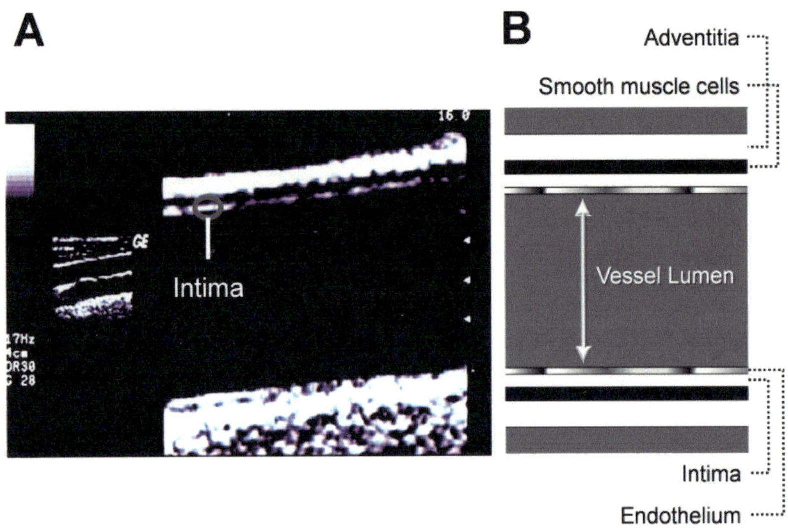

Fig. 1. *Anatomy of the arterial wall.* (A) A conduit artery imaged in the longitudinal plane using ultrasound. (B) The layers comprising the wall of an artery. Endothelial cells form a continuous layer lining the intima throughout the arterial tree.

2.1 Endothelial dysfunction and atherosclerosis

Upsetting the delicate balance of functions performed by the endothelium initiates a number of events that promote atherosclerosis, the precursor to CVD. Although atherosclerosis is commonly described as the presence of plaques that obstruct the lumen of the conduit arteries, endothelial dysfunction precedes plaque formation (Gibbons & Dzau 1994; Ross 1999; Nissen & Yock 2001). Reduced endothelial responses can be observed early in the course of atherogenesis, preceding angiographic or ultrasonic evidence of atherosclerotic plaque (Luscher & Barton 1997).

Disruption of the functional integrity of the vascular endothelium plays an integral role in all stages of atherogenesis, ranging from lesion initiation to plaque rupture. Endothelial dysfunction leads to increased permeability to lipoproteins, foam cell formation, T-cell activation, and smooth muscle migration into the arterial wall (Ross 1999). The first step in the formation of the plaque occurs when the inflammatory response is incited and fatty streaks appear. If these conditions persist, fatty streaks progress and the plaques become vulnerable to rupture.

Parameter	Recommendations
Subject preparation	Fast overnight prior to testing, and avoid exercise during the preceding 24 hrs.
	Refrain from taking drugs with known vascular effects.
	Rest supine for 20 mins in a quiet, temperature controlled room at 21 °C.
	Test conducted with subjects in the supine position.
	Artery segment of interest must remain at or below heart level.
	Women should be tested during the early follicular phase of the ovarian cycle (i.e., day 7-14 of the ovarian cycle).
	For successive tests, subjects should report at the same time of day to reduce error associated with circadian variation.
Probe selection	A higher frequency probe (12MHz) should be used for superficial arteries (e.g., brachial, radial or posterior tibialis).
	A lower frequency probe (7.5MHz) should be used for deeper arteries (e.g., common femoral).
	The same transducer should be used for all subjects in a given study.
Probe placement	Mark anatomical placement for studies with repeated measurements.
	Use a probe holding device to maintain image focus.
Ultrasound Settings	Standardize ultrasound global (acoustic output, gain, dynamic range, gamma, rejection) and probe-dependent (zoom factor, edge enhancement, frame averaging, target frame rate) settings.
Artery	Artery selection should be made based on the population of interest, e.g., lower limb arteries should be measured in patients with SCI.
Diameters (general)	Extend across the entire imaging plane to minimize skewing prior to focusing.
	Use automated or semi-automated image analysis software.
	Use mean or end-diastolic diameters.
Baseline diameters	Collect prior to cuff inflation.
	Subject should hold breath during measurement.
	Collect and average 3 * 10 sec measurements.
Peak diameters	Capture diameters continuously to ensure true peak diameter.
Blood velocity	The beam-vessel angle must be $\leq 60°$.
	Measure continuously.
	Time-averaged maximum velocities are more accurate and reproducible than time-averaged mean velocities.
Shear Stimulus	Shear rate is a suitable substitute for shear stress.
	Diameters and velocities must be captured continuously to estimate shear.
	Shear rates should be presented as an integral, we recommend 40 secs post-ischemia.
	Attention should be paid to secondary flow phenomena, e.g., turbulence and velocity acceleration.
Analysis	Present FMD in absolute (mm) and relative (%) terms.
	The shear rate stimuli should be presented for each research setting.
	Do not normalize FMD to shear rate as ratio or using ANCOVA.
	HLM can be used to statistically account for shear rate in the evaluation of FMD.

Table 1. *Recommendations for FMD Testing*

2.2 Stimuli regulating endothelial function

The haemodynamic conditions inside blood vessels lead to the development of superficial stress near the vessel walls which can be divided into two categories: 1) circumferential stress due to pulse pressure variation inside the vessel, and 2) shear stress (Nerem 1992; Papaioannou & Stefanadis 2005; Papaioannou & Karatzis *et al.* 2006). Circumferential stress acts perpendicular to the vessel wall, whereas shear stress acts at a tangent to the wall to create a frictional force at the surface of the endothelium. Circumferential stress applies stress to all layers of the vessel wall (intima, media and adventia), while shear stress is applied principally at the endothelial surface. Shear stress is considered to be the primary stimulus regulating endothelial cell function.

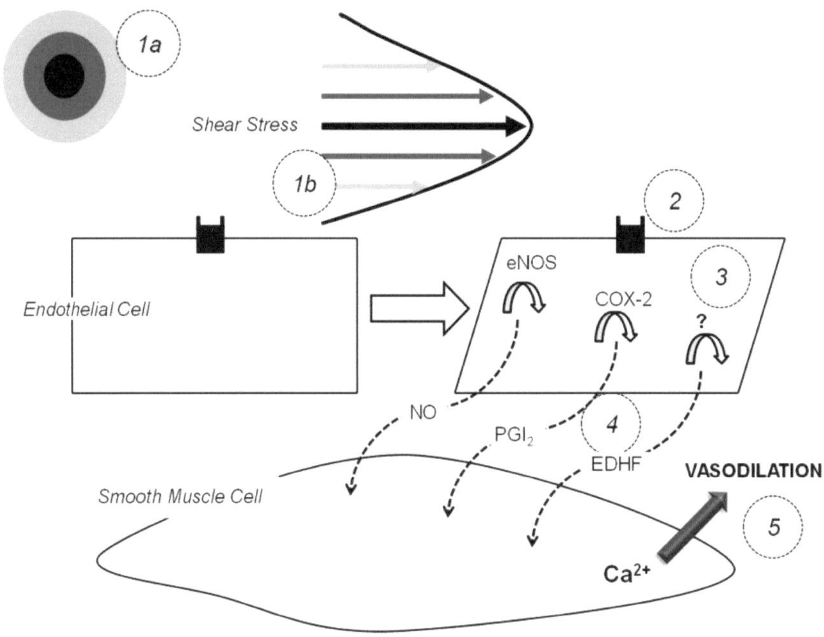

Fig. 2. *Endothelium-dependent dilation.* (1) Blood flowing through an artery creates a shearing stress at the endothelial surface. A composite of superimposed concentric circles is shown in 1a (i.e., transverse plane) to correspond with the gradient of increasing RBC velocity from the periphery to the center of the lumen. RBC velocity is represented as a parabola (i.e., longitudinal plane) in 1b using the same color coding as in 1a. The magnitude of the parabola (left to right) corresponds with the gradient of increasing RBC velocity from the periphery to the center of the lumen. (2) Shear stress-induced deformation of the endothelial cells is detected by mechanoreceptors on the cell membrane. (3) In response to mechanotransduced shear stress, a signaling cascade results in the production of NO, PGI_2 and EDHF . (4) The vasodilators diffuse cross the interstitial space and enter the vascular smooth muscle cells. (5) A signaling cascade is initiated which lowers Ca^{2+} concentration and results in smooth muscle cell relaxation (i.e., vasodilation). Ca^{2+} = calcium; eNOS = endothelial NO synthase; COX-2 = cyclooxygenase; EDHF = endothelial-derived hyperpolarizing factor; NO = nitric oxide; PGI_2 = prostaglandins; RBC = red blood cell.

Shear stress is primarily related to movement of red blood cells close to the endothelial layer (represented by bottom and top-most arrows in Fig. 2.1b). As fluid particles "travel" parallel to the vessel wall, their average velocity increases from a minimum at the wall to a maximum value at some distance from the wall, resulting in a gradient of velocities that form concentric circles in the lumen of the vessel (Fig. 2.1a). This shearing stress therefore acts at a tangent to the wall to create a frictional force at the surface of the endothelium. Although shear stress has a very small magnitude in comparison to circumferential stress, the endothelial cells are equipped with numerous mechanosensors to detect this stress (Olesen & Clapham *et al.* 1988; Davies 1995; Barakat & Leaver *et al.* 1999; Shyy & Chien 2002; Fleming & Busse 2003; Labrador & Chen *et al.* 2003). To maintain physiological levels of vessel wall shear stress, vascular tissues respond to changes in shear stress with acute adjustments in vascular tone (through vasodilation) (Langille & O'Donnell 1986). Vasodilation reflects alterations in the rate of production of endothelial-derived mediators, including nitric oxide (NO), prostacyclin (PGI_2) and endothelium derived hyperpolarizing factor (EHRF), which act locally to modulate vascular smooth muscle tone (see Fig. 2).

3. Flow-mediated dilation testing

In 1970, Rodbard (Rodbard 1970) proposed that the endothelium may sense and respond to shear stress generated by flowing blood. In 1980, Furchgott and Zawadski (Furchgott & Zawadzki 1980) discovered that agonist-mediated vasodilation requires participation by the endothelium. The dependence of FMD on an intact endothelium was subsequently shown to occur in large-conduit arteries as well as in resistance-sized vessels (Rubanyi & Romero *et al.* 1986). More recent studies have demonstrated that vasodilation is directly proportional to increases in shear stress (Koller & Sun *et al.* 1993; Moncada & Higgs 1993).

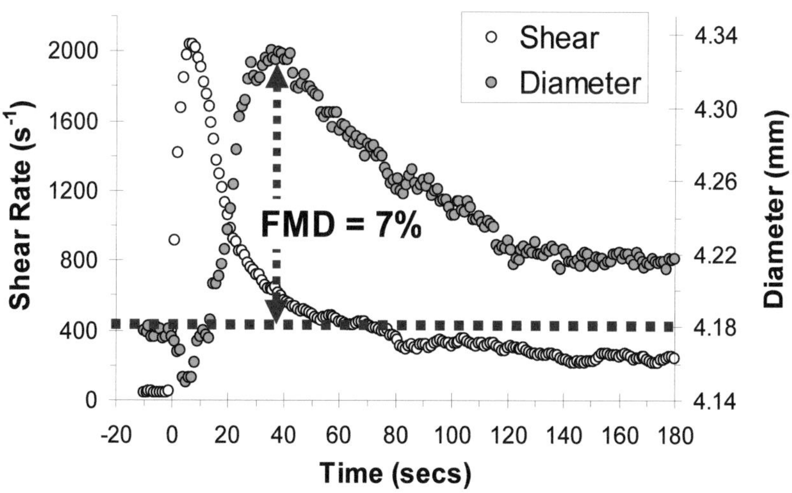

Fig. 3. *Shear rate and diameter responses to 5 minutes ischemia.* The horizontal line represents resting diameter. Flow-mediated dilation (FMD) is typically represented as the peak percentage increase in diameter above rest. Note that the peak diameter occurs ~40 sec whereas the bulk of the hyperemic (shear) response occurs within the initial 20 sec.

Endothelium-dependent agonists, such as acetylcholine, can be used to induce a dilatory response (Furchgott & Zawadzki 1980). However, such practice is invasive and often unpractical, especially for use within clinical settings. Alternatively, the FMD test is a *non-invasive* method (Fig. 3). Typically, a pneumatic tourniquet will be placed around the forearm approximately 5cm below the olecranon process and inflated to a super-systolic blood pressure for 5 minutes. Rapid deflation of the tourniquet instigates increased blood flow (reactive hyperemia) to the oxygen starved forearm muscles, with a subsequent increase in flow through the upstream brachial artery. The flow-induced increase in shear stress results in vasodilation. FMD is typically expressed as the percentage increase in the artery diameter above baseline. Table 1 provides a list of recommendations to consider when conducting this test.

4. Ultrasound

Arndt (Arndt & Klauske *et al.* 1968), in 1968, was the first to apply ultrasound to [carotid] arterial measurements. Since then, the advancement of ultrasound technology has had a profound impact on the capacity of researchers and clinicians alike to non-invasively assess endothelial function and health. Most commercial ultrasound machines now provide duplex Doppler functionality; that is, they can simultaneously image and measure blood velocity in conduit arteries in real-time. Duplex Doppler functionality offers immense potential for tracking vascular mechanical and functional changes.

4.1 Arterial diameter measurements

Conventionally, two-dimensional brightness mode (B-mode) is used to visualize, in real-time, the ultrasound echo amplitude distribution in a tomographic plane. The arteries of interest, except for the aorta, are typically within a depth range of 30 mm; a high carrier frequency (typically 7–13 MHz) is used to provide detailed images of peripheral arteries, in both longitudinal and cross-sectional views (Hoeks & Brands *et al.* 1999). Ultrasound wave reflections will only have a prominent amplitude if they originate from acoustic interfaces with a substantial change in acoustic impedance and, are oriented perpendicular (i.e., at a 90 degree angle) to the ultrasound beam direction. Therefore, in the cross-sectional view the lateral segments of the artery wall are blurred, with relatively low amplitude for the anterior and posterior lumen-wall transitions. In the longitudinal view, both walls will show up distinctly over a certain range, provided that the arterial segment considered is straight and without branches (Fig. 1). The transition of the inner layer of the wall, the intima to the lumen, induces a weak signal while the outer layer, the adventitia, results in reflections with high amplitude. The layer in between, the media, has a relatively low reflectivity and appears as a hypo-echoic band in images obtained with ultrasound systems with sufficient resolution.

A number of laboratories, using commercial or custom edge-detection software, are now able to make semi-automated diameter measurements (Woodman & Playford *et al.* 2001; Craiem & Chironi *et al.* 2007; Peretz & Leotta *et al.* 2007; Padilla & Johnson *et al.* 2008; Pyke & Jazuli 2011; Thijssen & Tinken *et al.* 2011). The authors of this chapter, using custom edge-detection software, are able to make thirty diameter measurements per second. A video capture device is used to make recordings at a rate of 30 frames / second. These video files are broken down and converted into JPEG (Joint Photographic Experts Group) images, which provides comparable accuracy for ultrasound image measurements compared to the DICOM (Digital Image and Communications in Medicine) standard (Hangiandreou & James *et al.* 2002). The images are analyzed offline using semi-automated edge-detection software (Fig. 4) custom written to interface with National Instruments LabVIEW software (National Instruments, Austin, TX, USA) (Sabatier & Stoner *et al.* 2006; Stoner & Sabatier *et al.* 2006). Custom-written Visual Basic Code is used to fit peaks and troughs to diameter waveforms in order to calculate diastolic, systolic, and mean diameters. The authors use mean diameters for analysis. Traditionally, end-diastolic diameters were used to calculate FMD, owing to: 1) FMD measurements that incorporate non-end-diastolic diameters may introduce measurement errors due to fixed vessel structural issues, and 2) prior to the advent of automated image analysis software, mean diameter measurements were beyond the technical capabilities of most research units. A recent study indicates that calculating FMD based on mean diameters yields comparable results to calculations based on end-diastolic diameters (Kizhakekuttu & Gutterman *et al.* 2010). The within-session $SEM_{3,1}$ for the described set-up is 0.046 mm; between-day coefficients of variation are 2.4-2.7% (Stoner & Sabatier *et al.* 2004).

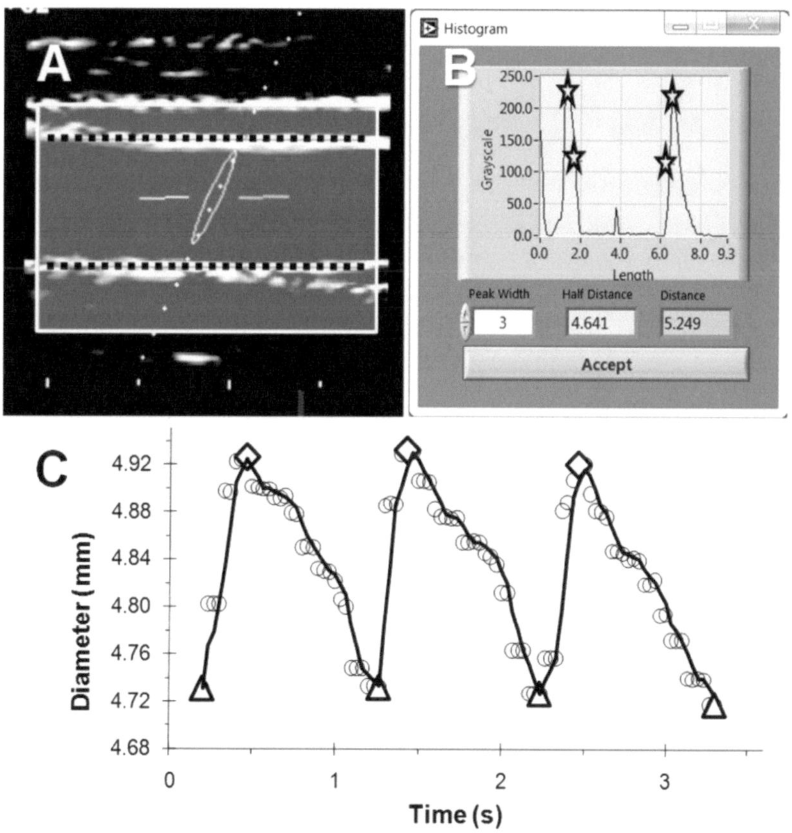

Fig. 4. *Semi-automated diameter analysis.* (A) B-mode image of the brachial artery with a region of interest (ROI) denoted by a selection box. The histogram (B) corresponds with the average pixel brightness of rows in the ROI in (A). The peaks (stars) correspond with the vessel walls. (C) Diameter waveforms from three cardiac cycles. Triangles represent diastole and diamonds represent systole.")

4.1.1 Measurement protocol

When imaging a vessel care should be taken to ensure that the vessel clearly extends across the entire [un-zoomed] plane to minimize likelihood of skewing the vessel walls. The ultrasound transducer should then be adjusted until the vessel walls appear thickest. Ultrasound global (acoustic output, gain, dynamic range, gamma, rejection) and probe-dependent (zoom factor, edge enhancement, frame averaging, target frame rate) settings should be standardized, especially for a given study. Alterations to probe selection and optimization settings - particularly probe selection - can have a significant impact on measurement precision (Stoner, in press). Figure 5 shows two diameter waveforms, both measured on the same subject within 10 minutes, albeit with different probes (11MHz and 6.6MHz); despite all other global and probe-dependent settings being equal, the 6.6mhz resulted in bias for smaller diameters. To ensure image focus is maintained and that diameter waveforms are stable, the ultrasound probe needs to be fixed in place using a probe holding device. The stability of diameter waveforms is also affected by rhythmic breathing patterns; to ensure optimal quality of diameter waveforms, the subject should ideally hold their breath during image acquisition.

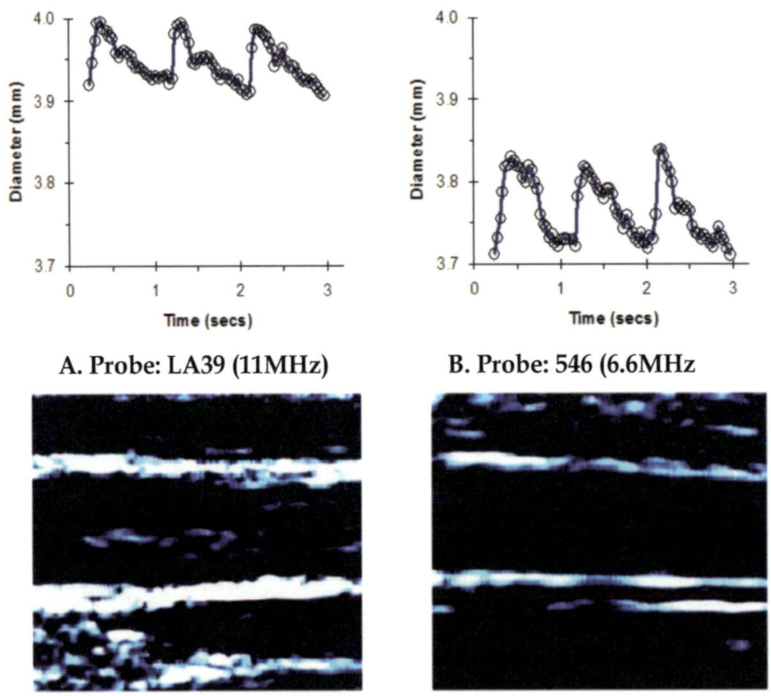

Fig. 5. *Brachial artery diameter waveforms using a GE 11MHz (A) and 6.6MHz (B) probe.* Measurements were taken from the same subjects within 10 minutes of one another. Note the bias towards smaller diameters using the 6.6Mhz probe.

4.1.2 Probe selection

Selection of the appropriate ultrasound probe is dependent on the vessel being imaged. The higher the probe frequency the greater the axial resolution, but this comes at the cost of tissue penetration (Roelandt & van Dorp *et al.* 1976; Lieu 2010). The operator should use the highest frequency that has adequate tissue penetration to clearly resolve the structure of interest. For superficial arteries, e.g., brachial, radial and posterior tibialis, a 12Mhz probe will allow adequate penetration and will provide optimal axial resolution. When imaging deeper arteries, e.g., common femoral, a 12MHz probe will not provide sufficient penetration, and a lower frequency probe (e.g., 7.5MHz) is recommended. However, the use of a lower frequency probe will yield a lower axial resolution, and will limit the capacity to discern small changes in vessel diameter. The same transducer should be used across subjects for a given study to maximize statistical power (see Fig. 5).

4.2 Blood velocity measurements

Ultrasound assessments of blood velocity have been favorably compared to magnetic resonance imaging, which is capable of higher resolution but is much more costly (Nesbitt & Schmidt-Trucksass *et al.* 2000). With ultrasound, blood velocity is calculated by measuring the Doppler shift, which results from a change in the frequency of a wave due to the motion of the wave source or receiver, or in the case of a reflected wave, motion of the reflector. The Doppler shift is dependent on the insonating frequency, the velocity of moving blood, and the angle between the sound beam and direction of moving blood, as expressed in the Doppler equation:

$$Df = \frac{2 \cdot f \cdot v \cdot \cos q}{c} \tag{1}$$

where: *Df* is the Doppler shift frequency (the difference between transmitted and received frequencies), *f* is the transmitted frequency, *v* is the blood velocity, *q* is the angle between the sound beam and the direction of moving blood, and *c* is the speed of sound. The equation can be rearranged to solve for blood velocity, and this is the value calculated by the ultrasound machine:

$$v^{\circ} = \frac{Df \cdot c}{2 \cdot f \cdot \cos q} \tag{2}$$

Since red blood cells travel at different speeds, even for a small measuring volume, there will be a range of blood velocities for a given unit of time. Per cardiac cycle, Doppler ultrasound systems measure minimum, maximum, and mean blood velocities. The maximum velocities represent the fastest moving blood cells flowing through the center of the vessel, whereas mean-velocities represent the average speed of blood cells from across the vessel. Mean velocities tend to be limited by incomplete sampling of Doppler shifts across the full width of the artery (Thrush & Hartshorne 2004). Time-averaged maximum velocities are more accurate and reproducible, even though they may lead to overestimations of blood flow by approximately 40% (Olive & Slade *et al.* 2003).

4.2.1 Measurement protocol

Most commercial ultrasound units come equipped with software to automatically calculate blood velocities. These automated calculations are typically limited to each heart beat. When making simultaneous diameter and blood velocity measurements, a compromise has to be made. An optimal B-Mode image is obtained when the ultrasound probe is perpendicular (90 degrees) to the imaged vessel, whereas an optimal velocity signal is obtained with a beam-vessel angel $\leq$60°. Error associated with incorrect estimation of insonation angle increases exponentially with angles $\geq$60° (Thrush & Hartshorne 2004). For further discussion on this topic see Thijssen et al. 2011 (Thijssen & Black *et al.* 2011).

4.3 Measurement location

For two decades brachial artery FMD has been widely used as a global endothelial health index (Celermajer & Sorensen *et al.* 1992). However, the brachial artery may not adequately characterize global endothelial health for all populations. For instance, given the incidence of CVD following spinal cord injury (SCI), it may be surprising that normal brachial artery FMD has been reported (De Groot & Poelkens *et al.* 2004). The current authors previously reported decreased FMD in the legs (posterior tibialis) compared to the arms (radial) for patients with SCI (Stoner & Sabatier *et al.* 2006). The retention of upper-extremity function likely explains the lack of deterioration for SCI radial arteries. Patients with paraplegia mostly rely on upper-body function for performing daily activities. Since individuals with SCI actively use their upper extremities, blood flow patterns may be such that the blood vessels retain their functional status due to normal shear stressor activity (Zarins & Zatina *et al.* 1987; Gnasso & Carallo *et al.* 1996). Notably, we subsequently found that 18 weeks of self-administered neuromuscular electrical stimulation-induced resistance exercise therapy significantly increased FMD and arterial range of the posterior tibial artery in male patients with chronic, complete SCI (Stoner & Sabatier *et al.* 2007).

5. Limitations of the FMD test

Despite its potential, validity of the FMD test has been questioned due to lack of normalization to the primary stimulus (Mitchell & Parise *et al.* 2004; Pyke & Tschakovsky 2005; Stoner & McCully 2011). Despite the term *flow*-mediated dilatation, shear stress is the established stimulus for FMD (Koller & Sun *et al.* 1993). The magnitude of the shear stimulus created with reactive hyperemia is influenced by several factors; subsequently, the shear stimulus may differ significantly between individuals. Therefore, in order to efficaciously compare groups of individuals the shear stimulus should be considered (see below for further discussion). For instance, Mitchell *et al.* (Mitchell & Parise *et al.* 2004) demonstrated that reduced FMD may be attributable not only to impaired endothelial release of dilatory molecules, but also as a result of a lesser shear stimulus. Fortunately, the ultrasound technology used to conduct the FMD test can also provide estimates of shear stress.

6. Shear stress estimation

Clinical studies in humans, including FMD studies, typically estimate shear stress by employing a simplified mathematical model based on Poiseuille's law. More sophisticated approaches are available, but are beyond the reach of most clinical studies since such approaches are not readily available, too expensive, technically challenging and time-consuming (Oyre & Pedersen *et al.* 1997; Gatehouse & Keegan *et al.* 2005; Reneman & Arts *et al.* 2006). Based on Poiseuille's law shear stress is calculated as the product of *shear rate* and blood viscosity, where shear rate equals:

$$\text{Shear rate }(\gamma)=\frac{2(2+n)v}{d} \tag{3}$$

where d is the internal arterial diameter, v is the time-averaged mean blood velocity, and n represents the shape of the velocity profile. For a fully developed parabolic profile, n is 2; this is the normal assumption when estimating shear rate.

Poiseuille's law assumes that: 1) the fluid (blood) is Newtonian, 2) blood flows through a rigid tube, 3) whole blood viscosity represents viscosity at the vessel wall and is linearly proportional to shear rate, 4) the velocity profile is parabolic, and 5) mean blood velocity adequately defines the shear stimulus. First, although blood is a non-Newtonian fluid at low shear rates (smaller than approx 100 reciprocal seconds (s^{-1})) (Chien & Usami *et al.* 1966) *in vivo*, shear rates in large arteries, particularly at the endothelial surface, are generally considerably larger than this threshold value so that the effect of the non-Newtonian behavior does not appear to be pronounced. Second, blood vessels are distensible, meaning that increases in arterial cross-section occur during the cardiac cycle. Wall shear rate may be ~ 30% less in a distensible artery as compared to a rigid tube (Duncan & Bargeron *et al.* 1990).

Third, to estimate shear stress from shear rate, invasive measures of blood viscosity are required. This potentially adds an additional source of error (Tangelder & Teirlinck *et al.* 1985). Human *in vivo* studies are usually limited to whole blood measurements of viscosity. These measurements overestimate the viscosity at the wall of the vessel. Less red blood cells travel along the artery wall, where, in addition to a thin layer of plasma, blood platelets are traveling (Tangelder & Teirlinck *et al.* 1985). Red blood cells tend to stream in the center of the vessel. The result is higher viscosity in the center of the vessel, thereby reducing the shear stress gradients at the vessel wall. It is worth noting that shear stress assessments do not seem to result in conclusions different from shear rate assessments alone (Padilla & Johnson *et al.* 2008). This may be explained by two factors: 1) sources of error from whole blood viscosity estimates, and 2) for a given population, viscosity changes little. Shear rate can therefore be used as an adequate surrogate measure (Gnasso & Carallo *et al.* 1996; Joannides & Bakkali el *et al.* 1997; Betik & Luckham *et al.* 2004; Pyke & Dwyer *et al.* 2004; Padilla & Johnson *et al.* 2008).

Fourth, in arteries, the velocity profile will not form a well-defined parabola as a consequence of flow unsteadiness and short vessel entrance lengths. In both arteries and arterioles, the velocity profiles are actually flattened parabolas (Reneman & Arts et al. 2006). In the common carotid artery, mean wall shear stress is underestimated by a factor of two when assuming a parabolic velocity profile since the velocity difference is smaller between the innermost column of flow and the outermost circumferential layer (Dammers & Stifft *et al.* 2003). However, in the brachial artery - at least under baseline conditions - the underestimation is less pronounced - likely due to a more parabolic velocity profile in this artery (Dammers & Stifft *et al.* 2003).

Despite the aforementioned limitations, shear rate assessments can be reliably made using ultrasound (Samijo & Willigers *et al.* 1997). However, little attention has been given to the most appropriate blood velocity parameter(s) for calculating shear rate (see below).

6.1 Peak or integrated shear rates?

Recently, we conducted a study to determine which shear rate expression explained the most variation in FMD. Seven shear rate expressions were calculated: peak, change (peak hyperemia minus baseline), integrated over 10, 20, 30, and 40 seconds after tourniquet deflation, and integrated to peak diameter time (Stoner & McCully). Shear rates integrated for 40 seconds after tourniquet deflation (i.e., post-ischemia) explained the greatest portion of variation for change in diameter. However, the addition of *peak* shear rate to *time-integrated* shear rate was significant. This suggests that peak shear rate may be an additional important independent predictor of FMD. It is worth noting that while peak shear positively correlated with peak diameter when regressed independently, the addition of 40 seconds integrated shear rate led to a negative relationship between peak shear rate and peak diameter. A greater peak shear rate for a given integrated shear rate is indicative of a more transitory hyperemic response. A less sustained increase in shear rate may result in a lower stimulus mechanotransduced to the endothelial cells. This study was conducted on young, healthy males. Therefore, further study is warranted to confirm these findings on other cohorts.

6.2 Importance of the velocity profile

The earliest studies investigating the implications of shear stress on endothelial function did so by assessing endothelial cell responses to high versus low shear stress. This was until Davies et al. (Davies & Remuzzi *et al.* 1986), in 1986, provided evidence that the time-averaged shear stress alone could not explain the pathological behavior of endothelial cells exposed to complex flow patterns. Subsequent studies (Helmlinger & Geiger *et al.* 1991; Waters & Chang *et al.* 1997; Lum & Wiley *et al.* 2000; McAllister & Du *et al.* 2000; Peng & Recchia *et al.* 2000; Apodaca 2002; Blackman & Garcia-Cardena *et al.* 2002; Cullen & Sayeed *et al.* 2002; Barakat & Lieu 2003) have shown that vascular endothelial cells respond not only to the time-averaged shear stress, but respond differently to different patterns of flow.

The cyclic nature of the beating heart creates pulsatile flow conditions in all arteries. The heart ejects blood during systole, and fills during diastole. These cyclic conditions create relatively simple *mono-phasic* flow pulses in the upper region of the aorta (Wootton & Ku 1999). However, pressure and flow characteristics are substantially altered as blood circulates through the arterial tree. Figure 6 shows an example of a typical brachial artery blood velocity profile. The normal brachial arterial signal is *tri-phasic*, corresponding to 1) rapid blood flow during systole, 2) initial reversal of blood flow in diastole, and 3) gradual return of forward flow during late diastole.

The blood flow profile in the aorta is predominately governed by the force of blood ejected from the heart (Wang & Parker 2004). However, in the periphery the blood flow profile becomes more complex as a result of the energy transfer between the heart and arteries. The heart generates forward-traveling wave energy that propagates through the arteries to maintain tissue and organ perfusion for metabolic homeostasis. An individual forward-traveling waveform, generated by the heart at the beginning of systole, initiates flow and increases pressure in the arteries. Although most of the wave energy in this initial compression wave travels distally into smaller arteries, some is reflected back towards the heart at sites of impedance mismatch. Interactions between forward- and backward-traveling waves result in complex blood flow patterns. Wave reflections result from arterial geometry, arterial wall compliance, and downstream resistance created by resistance arteries (Perktold & Rappitsch 1995; Barakat & Lieu 2003).

Complex flow characteristics have a profound impact on the shear stress distribution to which vascular endothelial cells are exposed. While human *in vivo* studies typically describe shear stress as a mean construct, numerous secondary phenomena associated with flow, including pulsatile flow, reversing flow, and flow turbulence, can influence the regulation of endothelial cells.

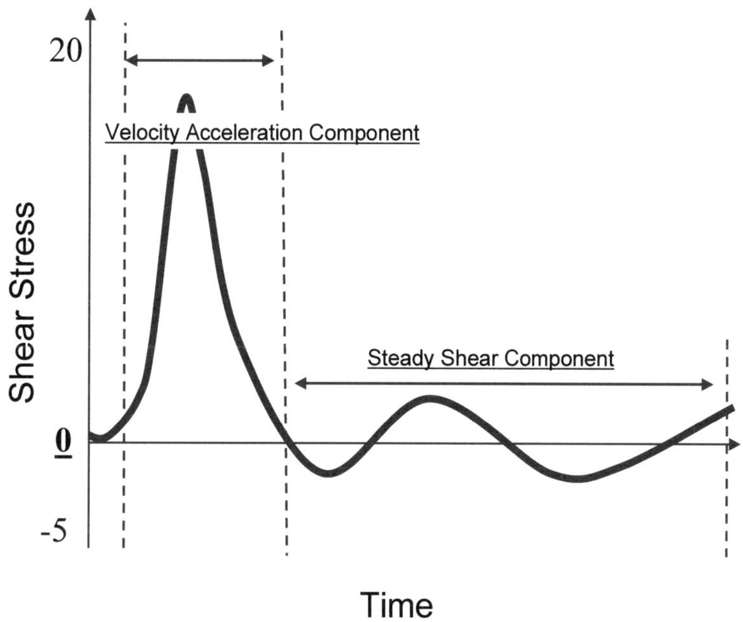

Fig. 6. *Acceleration and steady shear components.* The normal brachial arterial signal is *tri-phasic*, corresponding to the: 1) rapid blood flow during systole, resulting in velocity acceleration, 2) initial reversal of blood flow in diastole, and 3) gradual return of forward flow during late diastole, resulting in steady shear component.

6.2.1 Velocity acceleration and endothelial function

The pulsatile nature of blood flow exposes the endothelial cells to two distinct shear stimuli during the cardiac cycle: a large rate of change in shear at the onset of flow (velocity acceleration), followed by a steady shear component (Fig. 6). *In vitro* studies suggest that these two distinct fluid stimuli (velocity acceleration vs. steady shear) regulate short- and long-term endothelial function via independent biomechanical pathways (Ojha 1994; Bao & Lu et al. 1999; White & Haidekker et al. 2001; Hsiai & Cho et al. 2002 DePaola, 1992). Studies have shown that the rate of velocity acceleration can affect the progression of atherosclerosis

(Ojha 1994; Bao & Lu *et al.* 1999; Hsiai & Cho *et al.* 2001), endothelial cell function (White & Haidekker *et al.* 2001 ; Hsiai & Cho *et al.* 2002), mechanotransduction (Hsieh & Li *et al.* 1993; Bao & Clark *et al.* 2000), calcium kinetics (Helmlinger & Berk *et al.* 1995; Blackman & Barbee *et al.* 2000), and vascular tone (Frangos & Eskin *et al.* 1985; Noris & Morigi *et al.* 1995). Conditions which affect velocity acceleration include ventricular ischemia (Sabbah & Przybylski *et al.* 1987), acute myocardial infarction (Kezdi & Stanley *et al.* 1969), stenosis (Bassini & Gatti *et al.* 1982), hypertension (Sainz & Cabau *et al.* 1995), and hyperthyroidism (Chemla & Levenson *et al.* 1990). Velocity acceleration is also influenced by aging (Sainz & Cabau *et al.* 1995) and physical activity (Bonetti & Barsness *et al.* 2003; Shechter & Matetzky *et al.* 2003).

Recently, we studied the effect of velocity acceleration on FMD in a group of 14 healthy, young, male subjects (Stoner & McCully). FMD was measured prior to, and following, increases in velocity acceleration. Velocity acceleration (see Fig. 6) was increased by inflating a tourniquet around the forearm to 40 mmHg. We found that a 14% increase in velocity acceleration attenuated FMD by 11%. This finding suggests that mean blood velocity alone may not adequately characterize the shear stimulus. Attention to secondary flow phenomena may be particularly important when comparing groups with known secondary flow abnormalities.

6.3 Statistical analysis

Studies using the FMD test (i.e., using 5 minutes ischemia) should *consider* both time integrated- and peak-shear parameters, particularly when attempting to detect differences between experimental groups. Emphasis is placed on *consider* since the FMD test should not be normalized to shear rate using conventional approaches. A number of studies have attempted to account for the effect of shear stimulus on FMD by evaluating the quotient of FMD and shear, rather than FMD alone, or by using an analysis of covariance (ANCOVA), with shear stimulus as the cofactor (De Groot & Poelkens *et al.* 2004; Parker & Ridout *et al.* 2006; Padilla & Johnson *et al.* 2008; Atkinson & Batterham *et al.* 2009; Thijssen & Bullens *et al.* 2009; Pyke & Jazuli 2011). The techniques described above require use of the General Linear Model (GLM) for determining statistical probabilities associated with the differences found between groups or experimental treatments. However, when using a GLM the following assumptions must hold true: 1) there must be at least a moderate correlation between the two variables (i.e., shear and FMD), 2) the relationship between shear and diameter must be linear, 3) the intercept for the regression slope must be zero, 4) variance must be similar between groups, and 5) data must be normally distributed (Allison & Paultre *et al.* 1995; Atkinson & Batterham *et al.* 2009). A recent study found that all assumptions for reliable use of shear-diameter ratios were violated (Atkinson & Batterham *et al.* 2009).

Another alternative is to normalize the FMD response (i.e., change in diameter) to shear using hierarchical linear modeling (HLM) (Raudenbush & Bryk 2001). HLM is a more advanced form of multiple linear regression that accounts for hierarchical (i.e., successive inter-related levels) effects on the outcome variable. This is accomplished in HLM by including a complex random subject effect which can appropriately account for correlations among the data. This approach models different patterns in the data by allowing for the intercepts (initial diameter) and slopes (shear rate-diameter) to randomly vary. A third level may also be specified; this may be the specification of groups (e.g., to delineate differences in endothelial function), an intervention or a modifiable risk factor such as smoking. This approach has been used to compare upper vs. lower extremity arterial health in persons with spinal cord injury (SCI) (Stoner & Sabatier *et al.* 2006), to assess improvements in arterial health following electrical stimulation-evoked resistance exercise therapy in persons with SCI (Stoner & Sabatier *et al.* 2007), and to assess the effects of occasional cigarette smoking on arterial health (Stoner & Sabatier *et al.* 2008). The disadvantage of this approach is that multiple stimuli (preferably ranging from minimal to maximal shear stimuli) are required to generate a reliable shear-diameter relationship.

7. Improving reliability of the FMD test

The within-subject variability of FMD has been reported to be as low as approximately 50% (De Roos & Bots *et al.* 2003), which helps to explain why FMD is related to low but not medium or high CVD risk (Witte & Westerink *et al.* 2005). Within any given study, FMD tests can consistently demonstrate a smaller degree of dilation in subjects with atherosclerotic/risk factors versus controls. However, subtle changes in FMD are more difficult to detect. Patients with only one CVD risk factor report FMD values of approximately 7% (Accini & Sotomayor *et al.*). For a typical brachial artery with a 4 mm diameter at baseline, this translates to a 0.28 mm increase in diameter. The pixel resolution of a typical ultrasound unit is 0.04 * 0.04 mm. Measurements of 0.28 mm are within the standard error of measurement. To compound the issue maximal diameters in response to reactive hyperemia are short lived and, therefore, hard to capture. Aside from standardizing measurement protocols, measurement reproducibility can be improved by considering the following suggestions.

7.1 Automate diameter measurements

Studies using edge detection software to automate diameter measurement when calculating FMD have reported intersession coefficients of variation of approximately 14-18% (Hijmering & Stroes *et al.* 2001; Woodman & Playford *et al.* 2001).

7.2 Use ANCOVA to account for measurable covariates

FMD can be calculated as: 1) post-only score, 2) change score, 3) fraction, or 4) co-varied for resting diameter. A simulation study found the greatest statistical power for the ANCOVA approach out of the four methods listed above, with fraction scores resulting in the lowest power (Vickers 2001). Expressing FMD as a percentage effectively squares the variation due to resting diameter, and may result in a non-normally distributed statistic from normally distributed data. Using resting diameters as a covariate is most likely to adjust for the bias due to baseline values (Vickers 2001; Twisk & Proper 2004; Tu & Blance et al. 2005)

7.3 Normalize to the stimulus

While FMD is certainly attenuated in a number of disease states, FMD may also be "attenuated" if the magnitude of hyperemia (Mitchell & Parise *et al.* 2004) or the blood velocity profile is altered, including the rate of velocity acceleration (Stoner & McCully).

Further study is required to comprehensively quantify the appropriate expression of the shear stimulus. At present, shear rate can be calculated as described above and used to normalize to FMD through HLM, but not by using ANCOVA or presenting as a ratio.

7.4 Use multiple FMD measurements when possible

The peak diameter in response to reactive hyperemia is short lived and, therefore, hard to capture (see Fig. 3). Variance in peak diameter measurements may be attributable to differences in the stimulus (i.e., shear stress) or to measurement error (see see Fig. 7). Variance due to change in the stimulus can be accounted for by normalizing FMD to shear stress. To account for measurement error, according to laws governing regression to the mean (Shephard 2003), the FMD test would need to be repeated multiple times in order to obtain a "true" response. Alternatively, a more accurate assessment of endothelial function can be achieved by estimating shear rate-diameter dose-response curves (see Fig. 8).

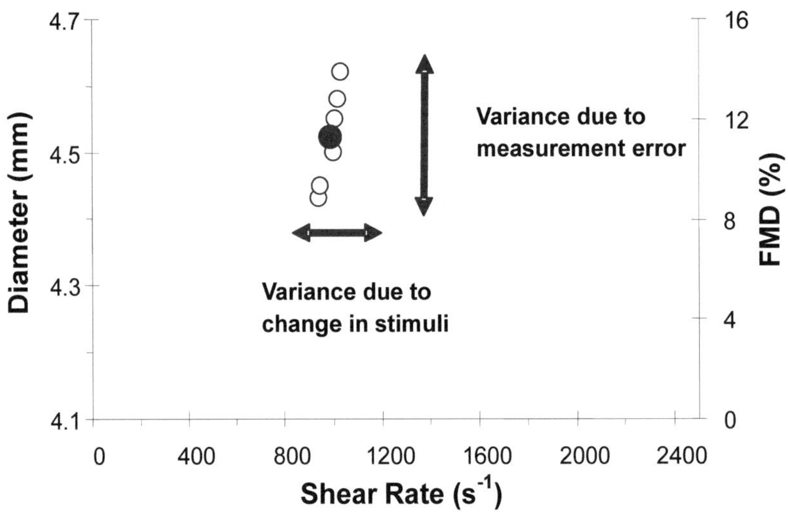

Fig. 7. *Flow-mediated dilation (FMD) measurement variance.* Open circles represent multiple FMD measurements. The closed circle represents mean FMD. Variance due to change in stimuli (shear rate) can be accounted for by normalizing to shear rate. Variance due to measurement error can be minimized by multiple FMD measurements (or by calculating a shear rate : diameter dose response curve).

7.5 Shear rate: Diameter dose response curves

Capturing shear rate-diameter dose-response curves (Stoner & Sabatier *et al.* 2004; Stoner & Sabatier *et al.* 2006; Stoner & Sabatier *et al.* 2007; Stoner & Sabatier *et al.* 2008) will decrease the likelihood of making erroneous conclusions. A standard dose-response curve (Fig. 8) is defined by three parameters: the baseline response (Bottom), the maximum response (Top), and the slope. The slope (i.e., change in diameter per one unit change in shear rate) would most accurately reflect endothelial function. The maximum response reflects the degree of arterial stiffness (Harris & Faggioli *et al.* 1995; Black & Vickerson *et al.* 2003; Sabatier & Stoner *et al.* 2006; Stoner & Sabatier *et al.* 2006).

There are a number of advantages to this approach, namely: 1) the stimulus (shear) is directly accounted for in a manner that does not violate statistical assumptions, 2) improved sensitivity, i.e., the slope (endothelial function) can be clearly identified (with the standard FMD test it cannot be ascertained at which point on the slope endothelial function is being estimated), 3) improved reliability, i.e., the dose-response slope is more resistant to measurement error when compared to a single measurement (Shephard 2003), and 4) more information is provided, i.e., the slope isolates endothelial function whereas the maximum response more likely reflects the degree of arterial stiffness (Harris & Faggioli *et al.* 1995; Black & Vickerson *et al.* 2003; Sabatier & Stoner *et al.* 2006; Stoner & Sabatier *et al.* 2006).

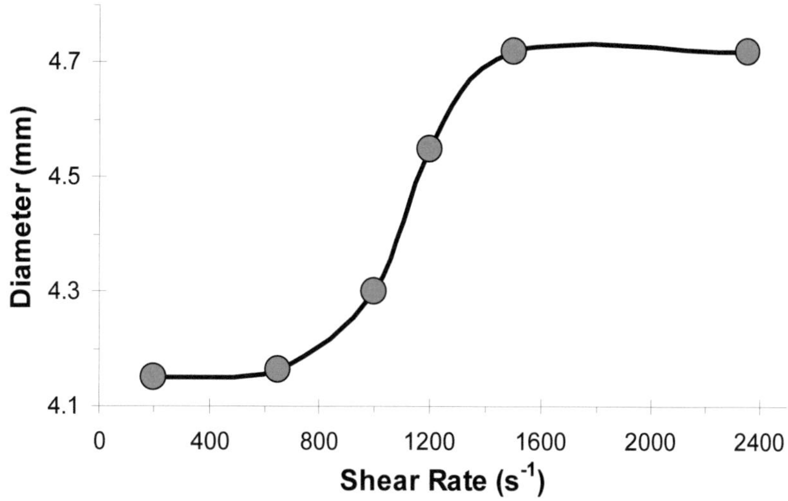

Fig. 8. *Theoretical shear rate-diameter dose-response curve.* Six data points are shown: baseline, and the responses to 5 durations of ischemia.

7.6 Transient versus steady-state shear stress

To overcome the short lived reactive hyperemia response, and hence short lived change in diameter, endothelial function can be evaluated by using sustained increases in shear stress, e.g., through local hand warming and low-intensity handgrip exercise (Mullen & Kharbanda *et al.* 2001; Joannides & Costentin *et al.* 2002; Pyke & Dwyer *et al.* 2004; Stoner & Sabatier *et al.* 2004). This approach would also allow for more accurate assessment of shear rate since the assumptions of Poiseuille's law are less likely to be violated (full description provided above).

Recently, we found that the relationship between shear rate and vasodilatation is comparable when shear rate is increased transiently (ischemia-induced) or in a sustained manner (local hand warming- and handgrip exercise-induced) (Stoner & McCully). This is consistent with a recent study by Pyke et al. (Pyke & Jazuli 2011), who similarly found a significant relationship between ischemia-induced FMD and handgrip exercise-induced FMD when the FMD responses were normalized to shear rate. Consideration has to be given to the mechanism(s) inducing FMD; the mechanisms regulating vascular tone may be dependent on the duration of the shear stimulus (Frangos & Eskin *et al.* 1985; Macarthur &

Hecker *et al.* 1993; Kuchan & Jo *et al.* 1994; Frangos & Huang *et al.* 1996; Mullen & Kharbanda *et al.* 2001), with FMD in response to sustained shear rate likely being less NO-dependent (Doshi & Naka *et al.* 2001). Nonetheless, the endothelium is still thought to primarily govern vasodilation under steady-state shear rate conditions. For instance, studies have shown that hand warming has no effect on brachial artery diameter when flow is not allowed to rise (Joannides & Bakkali el *et al.* 1997; Mullen & Kharbanda *et al.* 2001; Pyke & Dwyer *et al.* 2004). Furthermore, pharmacological blockade of the autonomic nervous system has no effect on radial artery FMD in response to hand warming (Mullen & Kharbanda *et al.* 2001), consistent with animal studies showing that FMD is preserved after surgical or pharmacological denervation (Hilton 1959; Lie & Sejersted *et al.* 1970).

A recent meta-analysis by Inaba et al. (Inaba & Chen *et al.* 2010), which was subsequently re-analyzed by Green et al. (Green & Jones *et al.* 2011), assessed the CVD prognostic strength of FMD by conducting a meta-analysis of observational studies which examined the association between brachial artery FMD and future cardiovascular events. Green et al. found that FMD resulting from more intense and prolonged shear stimuli using proximal cuff placement, which has been demonstrated to be less NO-dependent (Doshi & Naka *et al.* 2001), provides a better prognosis for CVD risk. Further study is needed to confirm these findings and determine whether FMD in response to sustained increases in shear rate provides greater prognostic strength for detecting future CVD events.

8. Conclusions

Assessments of endothelial function offer the potential to predict and track individuals at risk for CVD complications. However, despite the obvious potential, the reliability of this test has been questioned. Recently, a range of practices has been adopted to improve test reliability, including consideration of the shear stimulus and automated diameter measurements. However, the standard approach for inducing the shear stimuli, i.e., reactive hyperemia following ischemia, has inherent limitations, namely: 1) the peak diameter in response to reactive hyperemia is short lived and, therefore, hard to capture, and, 2) there is no consensus on the appropriate calculation of shear stress/rate. These limitations can be overcome with the following strategies: 1) repeat the FMD test multiple times to obtain a more reliable estimate of the "true" response, 2) calculate the shear rate-diameter dose-response to decrease the likelihood of erroneous conclusions, and, 3) use sustained increases in shear stress. Further study is required to determine: 1) whether shear-rate diameter dose-response curves offer greater statistical power, 2) whether FMD in response to sustained increases in shear rate provides greater prognostic strength, and, 3) the importance of secondary flow phenomena to estimations of shear rate.

9. References

Accini, J.L.; Sotomayor, A.; Trujillo, F.; Barrera, J.G.; Bautista, L. & Lopez-Jaramillo, P. (2001). Colombian study to assess the use of noninvasive determination of endothelium-mediated vasodilatation (CANDEV). Normal values and factors associated, *Endothelium*, Vol.8, No.2, pp.157-166

Allison, D.B.; Paultre, F.; Goran, M.I.; Poehlman, E.T. & Heymsfield, S.B. (1995). Statistical considerations regarding the use of ratios to adjust data, *Int J Obes Relat Metab Disord,* Vol.19, No.9, pp.644-652

Apodaca, G. (2002). Modulation of membrane traffic by mechanical stimuli, *Am J Physiol Renal Physiol,* Vol.282, No.2, pp.F179-190

Arndt, J.O.; Klauske, J. & Mersch, F. (1968). The diameter of the intact carotid artery in man and its change with pulse pressure, *Pflugers Arch Gesamte Physiol Menschen Tiere,* Vol.301, No.3, pp.230-240

Atkinson, G.; Batterham, A.M.; Black, M.A.; Cable, N.T.; Hopkins, N.D.; Dawson, E.A.; Thijssen, D.H.; Jones, H.; Tinken, T.M. & Green, D.J. (2009). Is the ratio of flow-mediated dilation and shear rate a statistically sound approach to normalization in cross-sectional studies on endothelial function?, *J Appl Physiol,* Vol.107, No.6, pp.1893-1899

Bao, X.; Clark, C.B. & Frangos, J.A. (2000). Temporal gradient in shear-induced signaling pathway: Involvement of MAP kinase, c-fos, and connexin 43, *Am J Physiol Heart Circ Physiol,* Vol.278, No.5, pp.H1598-1605

Bao, X.; Lu, C. & Frangos, J.A. (1999). Temporal gradient in shear but not steady shear stress induces PDGF-A and MCP-1 expression in endothelial eells : Role of NO, NF{kappa}B, and egr-1, *Arterioscler Thromb Vasc Biol,* Vol.19, No.4, pp.996-1003

Barakat, A. & Lieu, D. (2003). Differential responsiveness of vascular endothelial cells to different types of fluid mechanical shear stress, *Cell Biochem Biophys,* Vol.38, No.3, pp.323-343

Barakat, A.I.; Leaver, E.V.; Pappone, P.A. & Davies, P.F. (1999). A flow-activated chloride-selective membrane current in vascular endothelial cells, *Circ Res,* Vol.85, No.9, pp.820-828

Bassini, M.; Gatti, E.; Longo, T.; Martinis, G.; Pignoli, P. & Pizzolati, P.L. (1982). In vivo recording of blood velocity profiles and studies in vitro of profile alterations induced by known stenoses, *Tex Heart Inst J,* Vol.9, No.2, pp.185-194

Betik, A.C.; Luckham, V.B. & Hughson, R.L. (2004). Flow-mediated dilation in human brachial artery after different circulatory occlusion conditions, *Am J Physiol Heart Circ Physiol,* Vol.286, No.1, pp.H442-448

Black, C.D.; Vickerson, B. & McCully, K.K. (2003). Noninvasive assessment of vascular function in the posterior tibial artery of healthy humans, *Dyn Med,* Vol.2, No.1, pp.1

Blackman, B.R.; Barbee, K.A. & Thibault, L.E. (2000). In vitro cell shearing device to investigate the dynamic response of cells in a controlled hydrodynamic environment, *Ann Biomed Eng,* Vol.28, No.4, pp.363-372

Blackman, B.R.; Garcia-Cardena, G. & Gimbrone, M.A., Jr. (2002). A new in vitro model to evaluate differential responses of endothelial cells to simulated arterial shear stress waveforms, *J Biomech Eng,* Vol.124, No.4, pp.397-407

Bonetti, P.O.; Barsness, G.W.; Keelan, P.C.; Schnell, T.I.; Pumper, G.M.; Kuvin, J.T.; Schnall, R.P.; Holmes, D.R.; Higano, S.T. & Lerman, A. (2003). Enhanced external counterpulsation improves endothelial function in patients with symptomatic coronary artery disease, *J Am Coll Cardiol,* Vol.41, No.10, pp.1761-1768

Celermajer, D.S.; Sorensen, K.E.; Gooch, V.M.; Spiegelhalter, D.J.; Miller, O.I.; Sullivan, I.D.; Lloyd, J.K. & Deanfield, J.E. (1992). Non-invasive detection of endothelial dysfunction in children and adults at risk of atherosclerosis, *Lancet,* Vol.340, No.8828, pp.1111-1115

Chemla, D.; Levenson, J.; Valensi, P.; LeCarpentier, Y.; Pourny, J.C.; Pithois-Merli, I. & Simon, A. (1990). Effect of beta adrenoceptors and thyroid hormones on velocity and acceleration of peripheral arterial flow in hyperthyroidism, *Am J Cardiol*, Vol.65, No.7, pp.494-500

Chien, S.; Usami, S.; Taylor, H.M.; Lundberg, J.L. & Gregersen, M.I. (1966). Effects of hematocrit and plasma proteins on human blood rheology at low shear rates, *J Appl Physiol.*, Vol.21, No.1, pp.81-87

Cohn, J. (1999). Vascular wall function as a risk marker for cardiovascular disease, *Journal of Hypertension*, Vol.17, pp.S41-S44

Craiem, D.; Chironi, G.; Gariepy, J.; Miranda-Lacet, J.; Levenson, J. & Simon, A. (2007). New monitoring software for larger clinical application of brachial artery flow-mediated vasodilatation measurements, *J Hypertens*, Vol.25, No.1, pp.133-140

Cullen, J.P.; Sayeed, S.; Sawai, R.S.; Theodorakis, N.G.; Cahill, P.A.; Sitzmann, J.V. & Redmond, E.M. (2002). Pulsatile Flow-Induced Angiogenesis: Role of Gi Subunits, *Arteriosclerosis, Thrombosis, and Vascular Biology*, Vol.22, No.10, pp.1610-1616

Dammers, R.; Stifft, F.; Tordoir, J.H.; Hameleers, J.M.; Hoeks, A.P. & Kitslaar, P.J. (2003). Shear stress depends on vascular territory: comparison between common carotid and brachial artery, *J Appl Physiol*, Vol.94, No.2, pp.485-489

Davies, P.F. (1995). Flow-mediated endothelial mechanotransduction, *Physiol Rev*, Vol.75, No.3, pp.519-560

Davies, P.F.; Remuzzi, A.; Gordon, E.J.; Dewey, C.F. & Gimbrone, M.A. (1986). Turbulent Fluid Shear Stress Induces Vascular Endothelial Cell Turnover in vitro, *PNAS*, Vol.83, No.7, pp.2114-2117

De Groot, P.C.; Poelkens, F.; Kooijman, M. & Hopman, M.T. (2004). Preserved Flow Mediated Dilation in the inactive legs of spinal cord-injured individuals, *Am J Physiol Heart Circ Physiol*, Vol.287, No.1, pp.H374-380

De Roos, N.M.; Bots, M.L.; Schouten, E.G. & Katan, M.B. (2003). Within-subject variability of flow-mediated vasodilation of the brachial artery in healthy men and women: implications for experimental studies, *Ultrasound Med Biol*, Vol.29, No.3, pp.401-406

Doshi, S.N.; Naka, K.K.; Payne, N.; Jones, C.J.; Ashton, M.; Lewis, M.J. & Goodfellow, J. (2001). Flow-mediated dilatation following wrist and upper arm occlusion in humans: the contribution of nitric oxide, *Clin Sci (Lond)*, Vol.101, No.6, pp.629-635.

Duncan, D.D.; Bargeron, C.B.; Borchardt, S.E.; Deters, O.J.; Gearhart, S.A.; Mark, F.F. & Friedman, M.H. (1990). The effect of compliance on wall shear in casts of a human aortic bifurcation, *J Biomech Eng*, Vol.112, No.2, pp.183-188

Fleming, I. & Busse, R. (2003). Molecular mechanisms involved in the regulation of the endothelial nitric oxide synthase, *Am J Physiol Regul Integr Comp Physiol*, Vol.284, No.1, pp.R1-12

Frangos, J.A.; Eskin, S.G.; McIntire, L.V. & Ives, C.L. (1985). Flow effects on prostacyclin production by cultured human endothelial cells., *Science*, Vol.227, No.4693, pp.1477-1479

Frangos, J.A.; Huang, T.Y. & Clark, C.B. (1996). Steady shear and step changes in shear stimulate endothelium via independent mechanisms--superposition of transient and sustained nitric oxide production, *Biochem Biophys Res Commun*, Vol.224, No.3, pp.660-665

Furchgott, R.F. & Zawadzki, J.V. (1980). The obligatory role of endothelial cells in the relaxation of arterial smooth muscle by acetylcholine., *Nature*, Vol.299, pp.373-376

Gatehouse, P.D.; Keegan, J.; Crowe, L.A.; Masood, S.; Mohiaddin, R.H.; Kreitner, K.F. & Firmin, D.N. (2005). Applications of phase-contrast flow and velocity imaging in cardiovascular MRI, *Eur Radiol,* Vol.15, No.10, pp.2172-2184

Gibbons, G.H. & Dzau, V.J. (1994). The emerging concept of vascular remodeling, *N Engl J Med,* Vol.330, No.20, pp.1431-1438.

Gnasso, A.; Carallo, C.; Irace, C.; Spagnuolo, V.; De Novara, G.; Mattioli, P.L. & Pujia, A. (1996). Association between intima-media thickness and wall shear stress in common carotid arteries in healthy male subjects, *Circulation,* Vol.94, No.12, pp.3257-3262

Green, D.J.; Jones, H.; Thijssen, D.; Cable, N.T. & Atkinson, G. (2011). Flow-mediated dilation and cardiovascular event prediction: does nitric oxide matter?, *Hypertension,* Vol.57, No.3, pp.363-369

Hangiandreou, N.J.; James, E.M.; McBane, R.D.; Tradup, D.J. & Persons, K.R. (2002). The effects of irreversible JPEG compression on an automated algorithm for measuring carotid artery intima-media thickness from ultrasound images, *J Digit Imaging,* Vol.15, No.Suppl 1, pp.258-260

Harris, L.M.; Faggioli, G.L.; Shah, R.; Koerner, N.; Lillis, L.; Dandona, P.; Izzo, J.L.; Snyder, B. & Ricotta, J.J. (1995). Vascular reactivity in patients with peripheral vascular disease, *Am J Cardiol,* Vol.76, No.3, pp.207-212

Heitzer, T.; Schlinzig, T.; Krohn, K.; Meinertz, T. & Munzel, T. (2001). Endothelial dysfunction, oxidative stress, and risk of cardiovascular events in patients with coronary artery disease, *Circulation,* Vol.104, No.22, pp.2673-2678

Helmlinger, G.; Berk, B.C. & Nerem, R.M. (1995). Calcium responses of endothelial cell monolayers subjected to pulsatile and steady laminar flow differ, *Am J Physiol,* Vol.269, No.2 Pt 1, pp.C367-375

Helmlinger, G.; Geiger, R.V.; Schreck, S. & Nerem, R.M. (1991). Effects of pulsatile flow on cultured vascular endothelial cell morphology, *J Biomech Eng,* Vol.113, No.2, pp.123-131

Hijmering, M.L.; Stroes, E.S.; Pasterkamp, G.; Sierevogel, M.; Banga, J.D. & Rabelink, T.J. (2001). Variability of flow mediated dilation: consequences for clinical application, *Atherosclerosis,* Vol.157, No.2, pp.369-373

Hilton, S.M. (1959). A peripheral arterial conducting mechanism underlying dilatation of the femoral artery and concerned in functional vasodilatation in skeletal muscle, *J Physiol,* Vol.149, pp.93-111

Hoeks, A.P.; Brands, P.J.; Willigers, J.M. & Reneman, R.S. (1999). Non-invasive measurement of mechanical properties of arteries in health and disease, *Proc Inst Mech Eng [H],* Vol.213, No.3, pp.195-202.

Hsiai, T.K.; Cho, S.K.; Honda, H.M.; Hama, S.; Navab, M.; Demer, L.L. & Ho, C.M. (2002). Endothelial cell dynamics under pulsating flows: Significance of high versus low shear stress slew rates (d(tau)/dt), *Ann Biomed Eng,* Vol.30, No.5, pp.646-656

Hsiai, T.K.; Cho, S.K.; Reddy, S.; Hama, S.; Navab, M.; Demer, L.L.; Honda, H.M. & Ho, C.M. (2001). Pulsatile flow regulates monocyte adhesion to oxidized lipid-induced endothelial cells, *Arteriosclerosis, Thrombosis, and Vascular Biology,* Vol.21, No.11, pp.1770-1776

Hsieh, H.J.; Li, N.Q. & Frangos, J.A. (1993). Pulsatile and steady flow induces c-fos expression in human endothelial cells, *J Cell Physiol,* Vol.154, No.1, pp.143-151

Inaba, Y.; Chen, J.A. & Bergmann, S.R. (2010). Prediction of future cardiovascular outcomes by flow-mediated vasodilatation of brachial artery: a meta-analysis, *Int J Cardiovasc Imaging,* Vol.26, No.6, pp.631-640

Joannides, R.; Bakkali el, H.; Richard, V.; Benoist, A.; Moore, N. & Thuillez, C. (1997). Evaluation of the determinants of flow-mediated radial artery vasodilatation in humans, *Clin Exp Hypertens,* Vol.19, No.5-6, pp.813-826

Joannides, R.; Costentin, A.; Iacob, M.; Compagnon, P.; Lahary, A. & Thuillez, C. (2002). Influence of vascular dimension on gender difference in flow-dependent dilatation of peripheral conduit arteries, *Am J Physiol Heart Circ Physiol,* Vol.282, No.4, pp.H1262-1269

Kezdi, P.; Stanley, E.L.; Marshall, W.J., Jr. & Kordenat, R.K. (1969). Aortic flow velocity and acceleration as an index of ventricular performance during myocardial infarction, *Am J Med Sci,* Vol.257, No.1, pp.61-71

Kizhakekuttu, T.J.; Gutterman, D.D.; Phillips, S.A.; Jurva, J.W.; Arthur, E.I.; Das, E. & Widlansky, M.E. (2010). Measuring FMD in the brachial artery: how important is QRS gating?, *J Appl Physiol,* Vol.109, No.4, pp.959-965

Koller, A.; Sun, D. & Kaley, G. (1993). Role of shear stress and endothelial prostaglandins in flow- and viscosity-induced dilation of arterioles in vitro, *Circ Res,* Vol.72, No.6, pp.1276-1284

Kuchan, M.J.; Jo, H. & Frangos, J.A. (1994). Role of G proteins in shear stress-mediated nitric oxide production by endothelial cells, *Am J Physiol,* Vol.267, No.3, pp.C753-758

Labrador, V.; Chen, K.D.; Li, Y.S.; Muller, S.; Stoltz, J.F. & Chien, S. (2003). Interactions of mechanotransduction pathways, *Biorheology,* Vol.40, No.1-3, pp.47-52

Langille, B.L. & O'Donnell, F. (1986). Reductions in arterial diameter produced by chronic decreases in blood flow are endothelium-dependent, *Science,* Vol.231, No.4736, pp.405-407

Lerman, A. & Zeiher, A.M. (2005). Endothelial function: cardiac events, *Circulation,* Vol.111, No.3, pp.363-368

Lie, M.; Sejersted, O.M. & Kiil, F. (1970). Local regulation of vascular cross section during changes in femoral arterial blood flow in dogs, *Circ Res,* Vol.27, No.5, pp.727-737

Lieu, D. (2010). Ultrasound physics and instrumentation for pathologists, *Arch Pathol Lab Med,* Vol.134, No.10, pp.1541-1556

Lloyd-Jones, D.; Adams, R.J.; Brown, T.M.; Carnethon, M.; Dai, S.; De Simone, G.; Ferguson, T.B.; Ford, E.; Furie, K.; Gillespie, C.; Go, A.; Greenlund, K.; Haase, N.; Hailpern, S.; Ho, P.M.; Howard, V.; Kissela, B.; Kittner, S.; Lackland, D.; Lisabeth, L.; Marelli, A.; McDermott, M.M.; Meigs, J.; Mozaffarian, D.; Mussolino, M.; Nichol, G.; Roger, V.L.; Rosamond, W.; Sacco, R.; Sorlie, P.; Stafford, R.; Thom, T.; Wasserthiel-Smoller, S.; Wong, N.D.; Wylie-Rosett, J.; Committee, o.b.o.t.A.H.A.S. & Stroke Statistics Subcommittee (2010). Heart disease and stroke statistics--2010 update: a report from the American Heart Association, *Circulation,* Vol.121, No.7, pp.e46-215

Lum, R.M.; Wiley, L.M. & Barakat, A.I. (2000). Influence of different forms of fluid shear stress on vascular endothelial TGF-beta1 mRNA expression, *Int J Mol Med,* Vol.5, No.6, pp.635-641

Luscher, T.F. & Barton, M. (1997). Biology of the endothelium, *Clin Cardiol,* Vol.20, pp.3-10

Macarthur, H.; Hecker, M.; Busse, R. & Vane, J.R. (1993). Selective inhibition of agonist-induced but not shear stress-dependent release of endothelial autacoids by thapsigargin, *Br J Pharmacol,* Vol.108, No.1, pp.100-105

McAllister, T.N.; Du, T. & Frangos, J.A. (2000). Fluid shear stress stimulates prostaglandin and nitric oxide release in bone marrow-derived preosteoclast-like cells, *Biochem Biophys Res Commun,* Vol.270, No.2, pp.643-648

Mitchell, G.F.; Parise, H.; Vita, J.A.; Larson, M.G.; Warner, E.; Keaney, J.F., Jr.; Keyes, M.J.; Levy, D.; Vasan, R.S. & Benjamin, E.J. (2004). Local shear stress and brachial artery flow-mediated dilation: the Framingham Heart Study, *Hypertension,* Vol.44, No.2, pp.134-139

Moncada, S. & Higgs, A. (1993). The L-arginine-nitric oxide pathway, *N Engl J Med,*No.329, pp.2002-2012

Mullen, M.J.; Kharbanda, R.K.; Cross, J.; Donald, A.E.; Taylor, M.; Vallance, P.; Deanfield, J.E. & MacAllister, R.J. (2001). Heterogenous nature of flow-mediated dilatation in human conduit arteries in vivo: relevance to endothelial dysfunction in hypercholesterolemia, *Circ Res,* Vol.88, No.2, pp.145-151

Murakami, T. & Arai, Y. (2001). Relationship between non-invasively evaluated endothelial dysfunction and future cardiovascular events., *ACC Conference,* Vol.Session 1263,

Nerem, R.M. (1992). Vascular fluid mechanics, the arterial wall, and atherosclerosis, *J Biomech Eng,* Vol.114, No.3, pp.274-282

Nesbitt, E.; Schmidt-Trucksass, A.; Il'yasov, K.A.; Weber, H.; Huonker, M.; Laubenberger, J.; Keul, J.; Hennig, J. & Langer, M. (2000). Assessment of arterial blood flow characteristics in normal and atherosclerotic vessels with the fast Fourier flow method, *Magma,* Vol.10, No.1, pp.27-34.

Neunteufl, T.; Heher, S.; Katzenschlager, R.; Wolfl, G.; Kostner, K.; Maurer, G. & Weidinger, F. (2000). Late prognostic value of flow-mediated dilation in the brachial artery of patients with chest pain, *Am J Cardiol,* Vol.86, No.2, pp.207-210

Nissen, S.E. & Yock, P. (2001). Intravascular Ultrasound : Novel Pathophysiological Insights and Current Clinical Applications, *Circulation,* Vol.103, No.4, pp.604-616

Noris, M.; Morigi, M.; Donadelli, R.; Aiello, S.; Foppolo, M.; Todeschini, M.; Orisio, S.; Remuzzi, G. & Remuzzi, A. (1995). Nitric oxide synthesis by cultured endothelial cells is modulated by flow conditions, *Circ Res,* Vol.76, No.4, pp.536-543

Ojha, M. (1994). Wall shear stress temporal gradient and anastomotic intimal hyperplasia, *Circ Res,* Vol.74, No.6, pp.1227-1231

Olesen, S.P.; Clapham, D.E. & Davies, P.F. (1988). Haemodynamic shear stress activates a K+ current in vascular endothelial cells, *Nature,* Vol.331, No.6152, pp.168-170

Olive, J.L.; Slade, J.M.; Dudley, G.A. & McCully, K.K. (2003). Blood flow and muscle fatigue in SCI individuals during electrical stimulation, *J Appl Physiol,* Vol.94, No.2, pp.701-708

Oyre, S.; Pedersen, E.M.; Ringgaard, S.; Boesiger, P. & Paaske, W.P. (1997). In vivo wall shear stress measured by magnetic resonance velocity mapping in the normal human abdominal aorta, *Eur J Vasc Endovasc Surg,* Vol.13, No.3, pp.263-271

Padilla, J.; Johnson, B.D.; Newcomer, S.C.; Wilhite, D.P.; Mickleborough, T.D.; Fly, A.D.; Mather, K.J. & Wallace, J.P. (2008). Normalization of flow-mediated dilation to shear stress area under the curve eliminates the impact of variable hyperemic stimulus, *Cardiovasc Ultrasound,* Vol.6, pp.44

Papaioannou, T.G.; Karatzis, E.N.; Vavuranakis, M.; Lekakis, J.P. & Stefanadis, C. (2006). Assessment of vascular wall shear stress and implications for atherosclerotic disease, *Int J Cardiol,*

Papaioannou, T.G. & Stefanadis, C. (2005). Vascular wall shear stress: basic principles and methods, *Hellenic J Cardiol,* Vol.46, No.1, pp.9-15

Parker, B.A.; Ridout, S.J. & Proctor, D.N. (2006). Age and flow-mediated dilation: a comparison of dilatory responsiveness in the brachial and popliteal arteries, *Am J Physiol Heart Circ Physiol,* Vol.291, No.6, pp.H3043-3049

Peng, X.; Recchia, F.A.; Byrne, B.J.; Wittstein, I.S.; Ziegelstein, R.C. & Kass, D.A. (2000). In vitro system to study realistic pulsatile flow and stretch signaling in cultured vascular cells, *Am J Physiol Cell Physiol,* Vol.279, No.3, pp.C797-805

Peretz, A.; Leotta, D.F.; Sullivan, J.H.; Trenga, C.A.; Sands, F.N.; Aulet, M.R.; Paun, M.; Gill, E.A. & Kaufman, J.D. (2007). Flow mediated dilation of the brachial artery: an investigation of methods requiring further standardization, *BMC Cardiovasc Disord,* Vol.7, pp.11

Perktold, K. & Rappitsch, G. (1995). Mathematical modeling of arterial blood flow and correlation to atherosclerosis, *Technol Health Care,* Vol.3, No.3, pp.139-151

Pyke, K.E.; Dwyer, E.M. & Tschakovsky, M.E. (2004). Impact of controlling shear rate on flow-mediated dilation responses in the brachial artery of humans, *J Appl Physiol,* Vol.97, No.2, pp.499-508

Pyke, K.E. & Jazuli, F. (2011). Impact of repeated increases in shear stress via reactive hyperemia and handgrip exercise: no evidence of systematic changes in brachial artery FMD, *Am J Physiol Heart Circ Physiol,* Vol.300, No.3, pp.H1078-1089

Pyke, K.E. & Tschakovsky, M.E. (2005). The relationship between shear stress and flow-mediated dilatation: implications for the assessment of endothelial function, *J Physiol,* Vol.568, No.Pt 2, pp.357-369

Quyyumi, A.A. (2003). Prognostic value of endothelial function, *Am J Cardiol,* Vol.91, No.12A, pp.19H-24H.

Raudenbush, S.W. & Bryk, A.S. (2001). *Hierarchical Linear Models: Applications and Data Analysis Methods (Advanced Quantitative Techniques in the Social Sciences).* SAGE Publications, Thousand Oaks, CA

Reneman, R.S.; Arts, T. & Hoeks, A.P.G. (2006). Wall Shear Stress -- an Important Determinant of Endothelial Cell Function and Structure -- in the Arterial System in vivo, *Journal of Vascular Research,* Vol.43, No.3, pp.251-269

Rodbard, S. (1970). Negative feedback mechanisms in the architecture and function of the connective and cardiovascular tissues, *Perspect Biol Med,* Vol.13, No.4, pp.507-527

Roelandt, J.; van Dorp, W.G.; Bom, N.; Laird, J.D. & Hugenholtz, P.G. (1976). Resolution problems in echocardiology: a source of interpretation errors, *Am J Cardiol,* Vol.37, No.2, pp.256-262

Ross, R. (1993). The pathogenesis of atherosclerosis: A perspective for the 1990s, *Nature,* Vol.362, No.6423, pp.801-809

Ross, R. (1999). Atherosclerosis -- An Inflammatory Disease, *N Engl J Med,* Vol.340, No.2, pp.115-126

Rubanyi, G.M.; Romero, J.C. & Vanhoutte, P.M. (1986). Flow-induced release of endothelium-derived relaxing factor, *Am J Physiol,* Vol.250, No.6 Pt 2, pp.H1145-1149

Sabatier, M.J.; Stoner, L.; Reifenberger, M. & McCully, K. (2006). Doppler ultrasound assessment of posterior tibial artery size in humans, *J Clin Ultrasound,* Vol.34, No.5, pp.223-230

Sabbah, H.N.; Przybylski, J.; Albert, D.E. & Stein, P.D. (1987). Peak aortic blood acceleration reflects the extent of left ventricular ischemic mass at risk, *Am Heart J*, Vol.113, No.4, pp.885-890

Sainz, A.; Cabau, J. & Roberts, V.C. (1995). Deceleration vs. acceleration: a haemodynamic parameter in the assessment of vascular reactivity. A preliminary study, *Med Eng Phys*, Vol.17, No.2, pp.91-95

Samijo, S.K.; Willigers, J.M.; Brands, P.J.; Barkhuysen, R.; Reneman, R.S.; Kitslaar, P.J. & Hoeks, A.P. (1997). Reproducibility of shear rate and shear stress assessment by means of ultrasound in the common carotid artery of young human males and females, *Ultrasound Med Biol*, Vol.23, No.4, pp.583-590

Schroeder, S.; Enderle, M.D.; Ossen, R.; Meisner, C.; Baumbach, A.; Pfohl, M.; Herdeg, C.; Oberhoff, M.; Haering, H.U. & Karsch, K.R. (1999). Noninvasive determination of endothelium-mediated vasodilation as a screening test for coronary artery disease: pilot study to assess the predictive value in comparison with angina pectoris, exercise electrocardiography, and myocardial perfusion imaging., *Am Heart J*, Vol.138, No.4, pp.731-739

Shechter, M.; Matetzky, S.; Feinberg, M.S.; Chouraqui, P.; Rotstein, Z. & Hod, H. (2003). External counterpulsation therapy improves endothelial function in patients with refractory angina pectoris, *J Am Coll Cardiol*, Vol.42, No.12, pp.2090-2095

Shephard, R.J. (2003). Regression to the mean. A threat to exercise science?, *Sports Med*, Vol.33, No.8, pp.575-584

Shyy, J.Y.J. & Chien, S. (2002). Role of Integrins in Endothelial Mechanosensing of Shear Stress, *Circ Res*, Vol.91, No.9, pp.769-775

Sorensen, K.E.; Celermajer, D.S.; Georgakopoulos, D.; Hatcher, G.; Betteridge, D.J. & Deanfield, J.E. (1994). Impairment of endothelium-dependent dilation is an early event in children with familial hypercholesterolemia and is related to the lipoprotein(a) level, *J Clin Invest*, Vol.93, No.1, pp.50-55

Stoner, L. & McCully, K. (2011). *Blood Velocity Parameters that Contibute to Flow-Mediated Dilation*. LAP LAMBERT Academic Publishing, Saarbrücken, Germany

Stoner, L. & McCully, K. Peak- and time integrated-shear rates independently predict flow-mediated dilation. J Clin Ultrasound, In Press

Stoner, L. & McCully, K. Velocity acceleration as a determinant of flow-mediated dilation. *Ultrasound in Med Biol*, In Press

Stoner, L.; Sabatier, M.; Edge, K. & McCully, K. (2004). Relationship between blood velocity and conduit artery diameter and the effects of smoking on vascular responsiveness, *J Appl Physiol*, Vol.96, No.6, pp.2139-2145

Stoner, L.; Sabatier, M.; VanhHiel, L.; Groves, D.; Ripley, D.; Palardy, G. & McCully, K. (2006). Upper vs lower extremity arterial function after spinal cord injury, *J Spinal Cord Med*, Vol.29, No.2, pp.138-146

Stoner, L.; Sabatier, M.J.; Black, C.D. & McCully, K.K. (2008). Occasional cigarette smoking chronically affects arterial function, *Ultrasound Med Biol*, Vol.34, No.12, pp.1885-1892

Stoner, L.; Sabatier, M.J.; Mahoney, E.T.; Dudley, G.A. & McCully, K.K. (2007). Electrical stimulation-evoked resistance exercise therapy improves arterial health after chronic spinal cord injury, *Spinal Cord*, Vol.45, No.1, pp.49-56

Stoner, L., West, C., Cates, D & Young, J. Optimization of ultrasound assessments of arterial function. *Open Journal of Clinical Diagnostics;* In Press

Tangelder, G.J.; Teirlinck, H.C.; Slaaf, D.W. & Reneman, R.S. (1985). Distribution of blood platelets flowing in arterioles, *Am J Physiol Heart Circ Physiol,* Vol.248, No.3, pp.H318-323

Thijssen, D.H.; Black, M.A.; Pyke, K.E.; Padilla, J.; Atkinson, G.; Harris, R.A.; Parker, B.; Widlansky, M.E.; Tschakovsky, M.E. & Green, D.J. (2011). Assessment of flow-mediated dilation in humans: a methodological and physiological guideline, *Am J Physiol Heart Circ Physiol,* Vol.300, No.1, pp.H2-12

Thijssen, D.H.; Bullens, L.M.; van Bemmel, M.M.; Dawson, E.A.; Hopkins, N.; Tinken, T.M.; Black, M.A.; Hopman, M.T.; Cable, N.T. & Green, D.J. (2009). Does arterial shear explain the magnitude of flow-mediated dilation?: a comparison between young and older humans, *Am J Physiol Heart Circ Physiol,* Vol.296, No.1, pp.H57-64

Thijssen, D.H.; Tinken, T.M.; Hopkins, N.; Dawson, E.A.; Cable, N.T. & Green, D.J. (2011). The impact of exercise training on the diameter dilator response to forearm ischaemia in healthy men, *Acta Physiol (Oxf),* Vol.201, No.4, pp.427-434

Thrush, A. & Hartshorne, T. (2004). *Peripheral Vascular Ultrasound. How, Why and When.* Churchill Livingstone, New York

Tu, Y.K.; Blance, A.; Clerehugh, V. & Gilthorpe, M.S. (2005). Statistical power for analyses of changes in randomized controlled trials, *J Dent Res,* Vol.84, No.3, pp.283-287.

Twisk, J. & Proper, K. (2004). Evaluation of the results of a randomized controlled trial: how to define changes between baseline and follow-up, *J Clin Epidemiol,* Vol.57, No.3, pp.223-228.

Vickers, A.J. (2001). The use of percentage change from baseline as an outcome in a controlled trial is statistically inefficient: a simulation study, *BMC Med Res Methodol,* Vol.1, pp.6

Wang, J.J. & Parker, K.H. (2004). Wave propagation in a model of the arterial circulation, *J Biomech,* Vol.37, No.4, pp.457-470

Waters, C.M.; Chang, J.Y.; Glucksberg, M.R.; DePaola, N. & Grotberg, J.B. (1997). Mechanical forces alter growth factor release by pleural mesothelial cells, *Am J Physiol,* Vol.272, No.3 Pt 1, pp.L552-557

White, C.R.; Haidekker, M.; Bao, X. & Frangos, J.A. (2001). Temporal gradients in shear, but not spatial gradients, stimulate endothelial cell proliferation, *Circulation,* Vol.103, No.20, pp.2508-2513

Witte, D.R.; Westerink, J.; de Koning, E.J.; van der Graaf, Y.; Grobbee, D.E. & Bots, M.L. (2005). Is the association between flow-mediated dilation and cardiovascular risk limited to low-risk populations?, *J Am Coll Cardiol,* Vol.45, No.12, pp.1987-1993

Woodman, R.J.; Playford, D.A.; Watts, G.F.; Cheetham, C.; Reed, C.; Taylor, R.R.; Puddey, I.B.; Beilin, L.J.; Burke, V.; Mori, T.A. & Green, D. (2001). Improved analysis of brachial artery ultrasound using a novel edge-detection software system, *J Appl Physiol,* Vol.91, No.2, pp.929-937

Wootton, D.M. & Ku, D.N. (1999). Fluid mechanics of vascular systems, diseases, and thrombosis, *Annu Rev Biomed Eng,* Vol.1, pp.299-329

Yoshida, T.; Kawano, H.; Miyamoto, S.; Motoyama, T.; Fukushima, H.; Hirai, N. & Ogawa, H. (2006). Prognostic value of flow-mediated dilation of the brachial artery in patients with cardiovascular disease, *Intern Med,* Vol.45, No.9, pp.575-579

Zarins, C.K.; Zatina, M.A.; Giddens, D.P.; Ku, D.N. & Glagov, S. (1987). Shear stress regulation of artery lumen diameter in experimental atherogenesis, *J Vasc Surg,* Vol.5, No.3, pp.413-420

6

Ultrasonography and Tonometry for the Assessment of Human Arterial Stiffness

Graeme J. Koelwyn[1], Katharine D. Currie[2],
Maureen J. MacDonald[2] and Neil D. Eves[1]
[1]*School of Health and Exercise Sciences, University of British Columbia*
[2]*Department of Kinesiology, McMaster University*
Canada

1. Introduction

The structure and function of the human vasculature is integral to the efficacy of the cardiovascular system. In particular, arteries function as both a reservoir to dampen oscillations from the pumping heart, as well as a conduit to transport blood to the periphery. With age and disease, alterations in the composition of the arterial wall can occur. This can result in arteries becoming more resistant to wall deformation, referred to as arterial stiffness, which can have significant implications for the development of cardiovascular disease. Due to the emergence of arterial stiffness as a measure of cardiovascular disease risk, a number of non-invasive techniques have been developed, which include the use of ultrasonic assessment. These techniques are highly effective, reliable, and well validated, and consider stiffness both locally (most commonly measured at the carotid artery) as well as regionally (most commonly measured through the aorta) in the arterial tree. The assessment of arterial stiffness is critical to our understanding of the overall vascular health, and is the focus of this chapter.

2. Anatomy and physiology of the blood vessel

2.1 Anatomy of the artery

The human artery is comprised of a lumen surrounded by a series of concentric layers, which work together cohesively to assist in propagating blood from the heart to the periphery. The arterial wall itself is divided into 3 major regions: the tunica intima, media, and adventitia (Figure 1). The intima is comprised in part by the vascular endothelium, which lines the interface with the lumen. The vascular endothelium is a single layer of simple squamous epithelial cells that play a critical role in the regulation of smooth muscle tone through the release of several vasoactive substances. Adjacent to the endothelium lies a thin layer of elastin and collagen fibers, which attach to the internal elastic lamina, an elastic tissue that forms the outermost layer of the intima region. The tunica media is a more complex structure, and contains smooth muscle amidst a structure of elastin and collagen, which together act as a homogenous unit (Dobrin, 1999). A surrounding structure of thicker elastin bands wraps circumferentially with finer bands of elastin connecting them, and collagen dispersed in the intervening spaces with some inherent slack. The collagen also attaches to the smooth muscle, which lies internal to the surrounding structure. This latticework provides a flexible "safety net" for the blood vessels to prevent damage to the wall of the artery, especially at high transmural pressures. Finally the outermost region, the tunica adventitia, is separated from the tunica media by the outer elastic lamina, and is a layer of elastin and collagen that merges with the surrounding tissues.

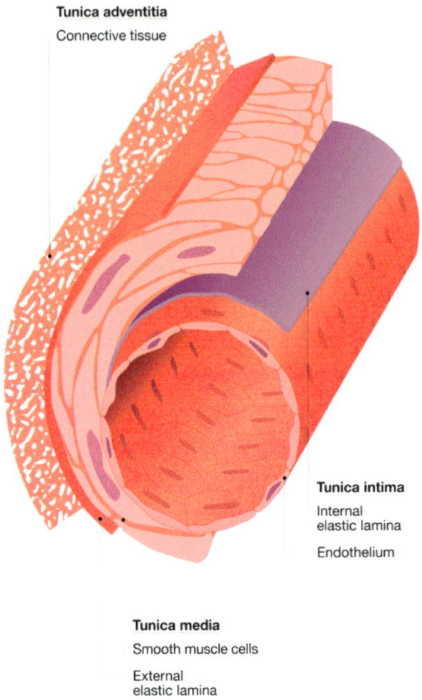

Fig. 1. Anatomy of a blood vessel

2.2 Functions of the arterial system

Arteries act as a conduit system to transport blood through the body, and dampen oscillations from the pulsatile ejection of blood to provide steady flow throughout the arterial tree. There are 3 separate anatomical arterial regions addressing these functions (Nichols & O'Rourke, 2005). First, large elastic arteries such as the aorta provide the predominant cushioning reservoir for blood flow. Second, large muscular arteries act as the conduit for blood to the periphery and actively modify wave propagation through smooth muscle tone regulation. Finally, arterioles function to alter peripheral artery resistance, and subsequently aid in the maintenance of mean arterial pressure and delivery of a continual flow to required systems and subsequent capillary beds.

Several models have been proposed for the functioning of the arterial system, with the propagative/distensible tube model considered superior (Laurent et al., 2006; O'Rourke et al., 2002). The propagative/distensible tube model consists of a single distensible tube with one end representing peripheral resistance, and the other receiving blood in pulses from the left ventricle (Nichols & O'Rourke, 2005). The pressure wave generated from the heart travels down the tube and is propagated and dampened by the viscoelastic wall of the vessel. When applying this theory to the entire arterial tree several phenomena need to be considered. As the pulse travels down the arterial tree it becomes amplified. This amplification is caused by the progressive increase in stiffness of the arteries distally from the heart (Learoyd & Taylor, 1966) and the branching, bifurcations, and non-linearity in the vascular tree that produce sites where the pressure wave can be reflected. These reflections return in the opposite direction and amplify the pressure signal. Reflection sites are closer to the pulse wave in the periphery (greater branching) than in the central arteries, and amplification is therefore greater (known as the 'amplification phenomena') (Laurent et al., 2006). Thus, the pressure wave at any given location is the result of the summation of the incident and reflected wave (Figure 2) (Davies & Struthers, 2003; O'Rourke et al., 2002), and depending on the elasticity of the vasculature, can create various pressure waveforms.

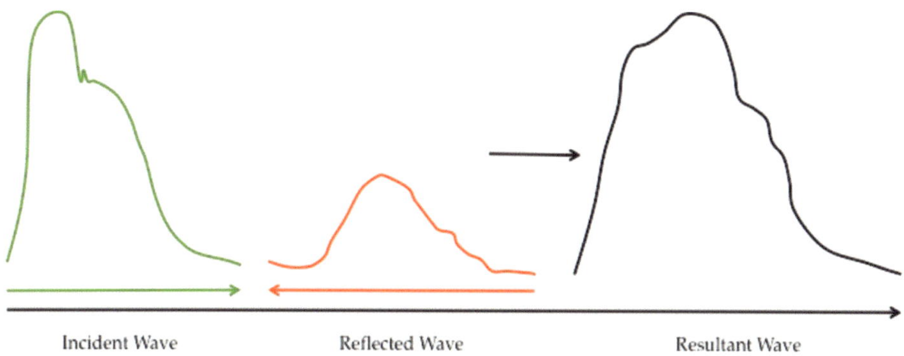

Fig. 2. The pressure waveform is a result of the summation (right) of the incident wave (left) travelling toward the periphery and combining with the reflected wave (middle) returning from the periphery.

The composition of the arterial wall, in particular the elastin and collagen content, changes from central to peripheral arteries. Starting in the proximal aorta, elastin is the dominant component. At the abdominal aorta the content of collagen and elastin appears similar, and by the periphery collagen becomes dominant (Harkness et al., 1957). As collagen is 300 times stiffer than elastin (elastic modulus 1000×10^6 dyne/cm^2 vs. 5×10^6) (Armentano et al., 1991), the altering arterial wall composition causes an increasing 'stiffness gradient' down the arterial tree. For example, in the central arteries, up to 50% of the stroke volume ejected from the heart is momentarily stored in the aorta and large elastic arteries. Approximately 10% of the energy produced by the heart is used to distend the arteries during systole. The elastic walls of the artery store the energy, and subsequently use it to recoil the vessel wall during diastole (London & Pannier, 2010), thus ensuring continuous flow to the stiffer, more collagen based, peripheral arteries. For this dampening in the central arteries to be most efficient, the energy needed to distend the wall needs to be as low as possible (London & Pannier, 2010), which not only depends on elasticity (and high elastin content), but also the geometry of the vessel walls.

Elastin and collagen cause the pressure-diameter relationship at any specific area on the arterial tree to be non linear (Figure 3) (Armentano et al., 1991). At low distensions, pressure is mainly governed by elastin fibers, which are quite compliant and the resulting curve is more linear, where at higher tensions it is governed by the supporting latticework of collagen content, which is much stiffer, resulting in a steeper slope (a greater required pressure for a given diameter change) (Lanne et al., 1992).

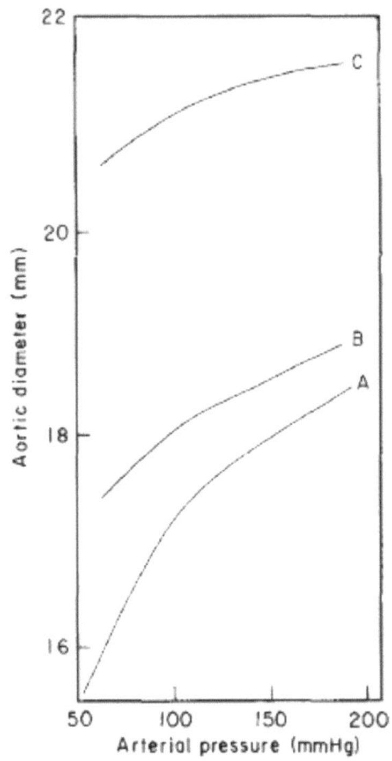

Fig. 3. Pressure-diameter relationship of the abdominal aorta in (A) young (mean 25 yrs), (B) middle aged (mean 51 yrs) and (C) elderly (mean 70 yrs) humans. Reprinted with permission (Lanne et al., 1992)

3. Arterial stiffness

3.1 Development of arterial stiffness

Considerable research supports the measurement of arterial stiffness as a highly relevant tool in the assessment of vascular structure. Degenerative stiffness of the arterial wall is considered arteriosclerosis, and is distinguishable from atherosclerosis, which is the occlusive result of endovascular inflammatory disease, lipid oxidation and plaque formation (Cavalcante et al., 2011). Even in healthy, young individuals, arterial stiffness is heterogeneous throughout the arterial tree, as amplification and the natural stiffness gradient result in more elastic central and stiffer peripheral arteries (London & Pannier, 2010). Arteries in humans, however, also stiffen with healthy ageing and disease (discussed later in the chapter), affecting predominately the aorta and proximal elastic arteries, and to a lesser degree the peripheral arteries (O'Rourke et al., 2002), and can even result in a minimization or reversing of the stiffness gradient (Benetos et al., 1993; Boutouyrie et al., 1992; Laurent et al., 2006). This regional age associated stiffening has been attributed to longstanding pulsation that induces greater cycles of stress in the central arteries (Adji et al., 2011; Lee & Oh, 2010).

With age and disease, degeneration of the media in the central arteries appears to be the primary structural change associated with chronic increases in arterial stiffness. Fatigue and fracture of elastin and collagen fibers occur. These structural changes to the elastin and collagen functional unit are determined by the extent of circumferential strain, which is greater centrally, and length of strain exposure (number of cardiac cycles) (McEniery et al., 2010). The orderly arrangement of elastic lamellae disappears, and is replaced by thinning, fragmented elastin, greater foundations of collagen (Laurent & Boutouyrie, 2007; Najjar et al., 2005; Zieman et al., 2005) and medial calcification (elastocalcinosis) (Atkinson, 2008). Other age and disease associated changes in the arterial wall include specific changes in the smooth muscle cell connections (Laurent et al., 2005), and inflammation in the form of acute systemic (Vlachopoulos et al., 2005) and chronic (Roman et al., 2005) inflammatory disease.

A stiffer artery propagates a pulse wave faster than a more compliant vessel. This leads to earlier return of the reflected wave, which amplifies systolic pressure and decreases diastolic pressure (Figure 4). Increased systolic pressure places a greater stress (distending pressure) on the wall of the vessel, which over time can accelerate the stiffening and remodeling process. A decrease in diastolic pressure can reduce coronary perfusion pressure, reducing coronary blood flow reserve, which may be a possible link to increase cardiac event risk in

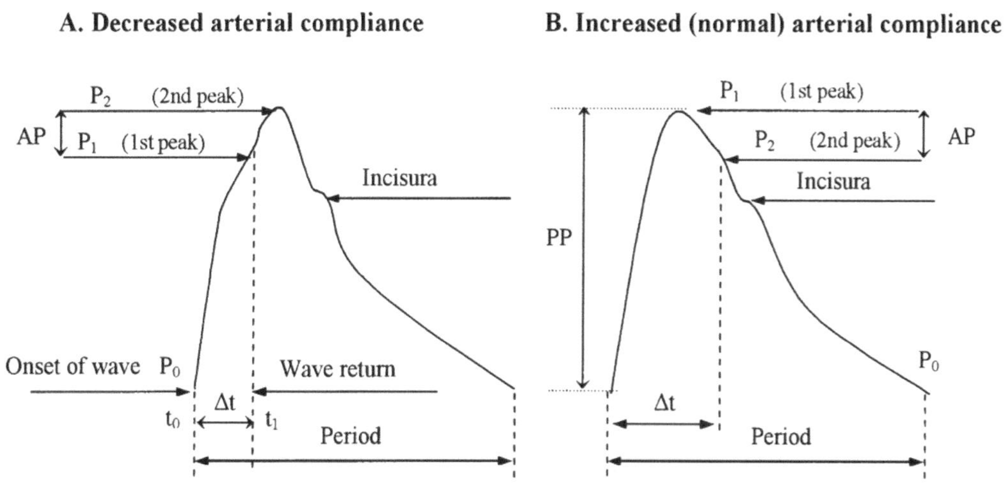

Fig. 4. Effect of decreased (A) and normal (B) arterial compliance on the pulse waveform. P_0: end-diastolic pressure; P_1: early systolic peak; P_2: late systolic peak (from reflected wave); Δt: time from onset of pressure wave (t_0) to return of reflected wave (t_1); PP: pulse pressure. Reprinted and modified with permission AP: augmentation of systolic aortic pressure (Papaioannou et al., 2004)

subjects with elevated arterial stiffness (Saito et al., 2008). Increased arterial stiffness also results in failure to suppress the pulse oscillations downstream from the central arteries. Decreased pulse suppression potentially increases the risk for damage to micro vascular beds in highly perfused organs such as the brain and kidneys (O'Rourke & Safar, 2005), and has important implications for risk of stroke and renal failure.

Increased arterial stiffness with age and disease is partially compensated for by remodeling of the arteries, through luminal enlargement (Boutouyrie et al., 1992) and wall thickening (Cheng et al., 2002; Zieman et al., 2005). It appears that endothelial dysfunction, which can occur from a decrease in nitric oxide (NO) release, increase in oxidative stress, and/or a decrease in antioxidant capacity with age or disease, is the earliest change in the vasculature that can lead to advancing vascular disease (Taddei et al., 2001; Widlansky et al., 2003). Decreased NO leads to increasing vascular tone of the small arteries responsible for major changes in total peripheral resistance (arterioles). Increasing vascular tone leads to structural and functional changes upstream in the larger arteries, resulting in stiffening and remodeling, increasing blood pressure (in particular pulse pressure), as well as atherosclerotic plaque development and additional functional abnormalities (Folkow, 1995). However, this temporal sequence in the manifestation of arterial disease is not always present, as structural changes can present without obvious functional changes, and these structural changes are not always homogenous across the vascular tree (Naghavi, 2009).

Arterial stiffness is emerging as one of the most important determinants of increased systolic blood pressure and pulse pressure in ageing and disease. It is the root cause of a number of cardiovascular complications including left ventricular hypertrophy, left ventricular failure, aneurism formation and rupture, and is a major contributor to atherosclerotic and small vessel disease, which can lead to stroke, myocardial infarction and renal failure (Nichols & O'Rourke, 2005). Central artery stiffening, in particular aortic stiffening, is strongly related to cardiovascular events, independent of age, arterial pressure, and conventional risk factors for cardiovascular disease (Adji et al., 2011), as well as future hypertension risk after correcting for systolic blood pressure, age, sex, body mass index, heart rate, total cholesterol, diabetes, smoking, alcohol and physical activity (Dernellis & Panaretou, 2005). In fact, stiffening of the aorta rather than left ventricular myocardial abnormalities appears to be the predominant cause of cardiac failure with age (Levy & Brink, 2005) as it produces higher systolic pressures in the aorta and left ventricle. These elevated systolic pressures present a high load on the ventricle, predisposing it to increased systolic wall stress and remodeling, which can progress to dysfunction and failure (Adji et al., 2011).

A variety of techniques for measuring arterial stiffness have been developed. In particular, with the use of ultrasonography, two techniques have been utilized extensively and have been validated for measuring central arterial stiffness non-invasively. In the measurement of regional arterial stiffness, pulse wave velocity has emerged as the gold standard (Laurent et al., 2006) for the noninvasive assessment of arterial stiffness, while local arterial stiffness measures, specifically at the carotid artery, have emerged as an important tool for the mechanistic study of vascular structure and function. Although researchers and clinicians extensively use arterial stiffness measures, a number of potential limitations to these techniques have been identified (Laurent et al., 2006; O'Rourke et al., 2002). Assumption of a homogenous vascular wall when it is heterogeneous in nature, the use of different locations for measures of pressure and arterial diameter, and failing to account for the altering effects of heart rate (which affects the rate that pulse pressure amplifies) (Wilkinson et al., 2002) and cardiac contractility (O'Rourke et al., 2002) are common oversights in measurement. Furthermore, nervous system activity, fluctuations in autonomic control, vasoactive substances such as nitric oxide, and hormones influence vascular smooth muscle, which can also influence arterial stiffness. Muscular arteries, particularly smaller arteries (O'Rourke et al., 2002), are also subject to spontaneous vasomotor changes that affect both diameter and stiffness (Hayoz et al., 1993). Despite these limitations, measures of arterial stiffness are considered an integral tool in the noninvasive assessment of vascular structure and function, and are an important determinant for cardiovascular risk.

3.2 Local arterial stiffness and measurement

3.2.1 Viscoelastic properties of the arterial wall

The arterial wall is considered to be viscoelastic, as it contains both elastic and viscous properties (Nichols & O'Rourke, 2005). When a stress is applied (a force that produces deformation) to a perfectly elastic material, it will regain its original form when the stress is removed. In an artery, however, wall viscosity is present, which leads to the wall retaining part of the deformation (London & Pannier, 2010). This is partially responsible for hysteresis seen in the pressure-diameter loop (Figure 5). Unfortunately the viscosity of the wall is difficult to measure in humans, and therefore the elasticity component of the arterial wall is what has been extensively evaluated.

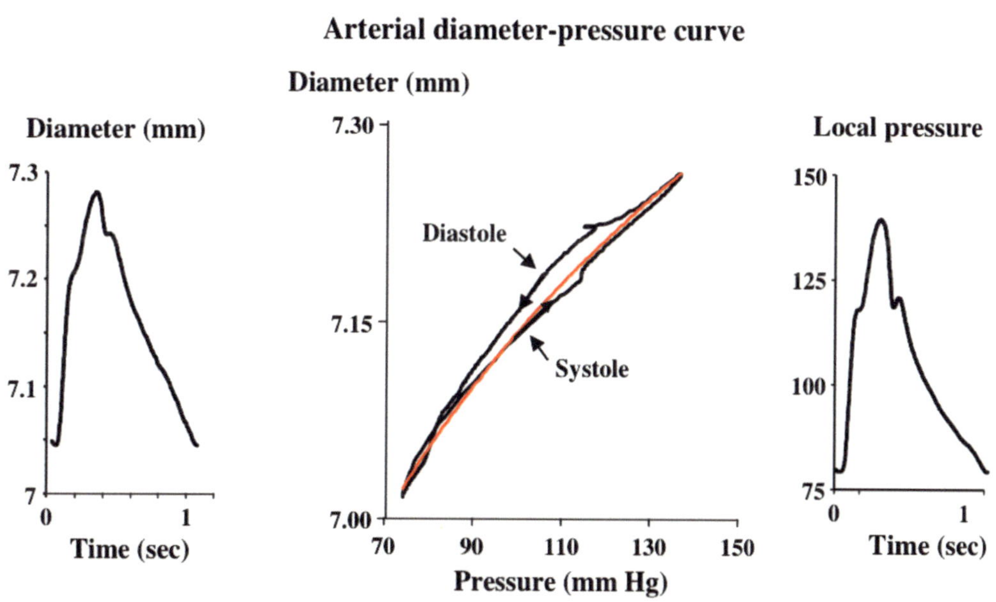

Fig. 5. Diameter-pressure curve (middle) derived from the diameter (left) and local pressure (right) of the common carotid artery. Differences in systole and diastole represent the energy dissipation due to viscous properties of the arterial wall. The red line is the averaged pressure-diameter curve. Reprinted and modified with permission (London & Pannier, 2010)

3.2.2 Calculations of local arterial stiffness

The elasticity of the arterial wall can be gauged by understanding the stress/strain relationship. While stress is the force producing deformation, strain is the resulting deformation incurred as a percentage change in length (Cavalcante et al., 2011). Strain therefore is dimensionless, and the stress/strain ratio is known as the elastic modulus, or Young's modulus (O'Rourke et al., 2002). In an artery, assuming the segment is a cylindrical tube with a circular luminal cross-section (Pannier et al., 2002; Reneman et al., 2005), compliance is considered the absolute change in volume (strain) due to a change in pressure (stress). Distensibility takes into account the initial dimensions of the artery, and is considered the relative change in volume for a given pressure. The equations are as follows:

$$\text{Compliance} = \frac{\Delta \text{CSA}}{\text{PP}} = \frac{\Pi r^2 - \Pi r^2}{\text{PP}} = \frac{\Pi\left(\frac{d\max}{2}\right)^2 - \Pi\left(\frac{d\min}{2}\right)^2}{\text{PP}} \tag{1}$$

$$\text{Distensibility} = \frac{\Pi\left(\frac{d\max}{2}\right)^2 - \Pi\left(\frac{d\min}{2}\right)^2}{\Pi\left(\frac{d\min}{2}\right)^2 \times \text{PP}} \tag{2}$$

where dmax is the maximum systolic diameter, dmin is the minimum diastolic diameter, and PP is the carotid pulse pressure. Compliance and distensibility can both be estimated as a change in radius, diameter, flow, or cross sectional area for a given change in pulse pressure, measured at the same site (Nichols & O'Rourke, 2005). The resistance to deformation is known as stiffness, which in turn is the reciprocal of compliance.

Local arterial stiffness of the central arteries is directly determined, as denoted from a change in pressure producing a given change in volume (Laurent et al., 2006) (Figure 6). In the large elastic arteries (i.e. the carotid artery or aorta) the relationship between lumen cross sectional area and change in pressure is linear (Meinders & Hoeks, 2004) and the error from this assumption is quite small (Reneman et al., 2005). In stiffer peripheral muscular arteries this error can be large (Reneman et al., 2005), therefore direct measures done at the carotid artery and aorta for determining local stiffness have been extensively explored.

Young's modulus, or the incremental elastic modulus (E_{inc}), outlined in equation [3], has been used extensively (Nichols & O'Rourke, 2005). It estimates the elastic properties of the arterial wall by taking into account it's thickness. Current measuring techniques unfortunately cannot differentiate the load bearing section of the wall (media/adventitia) from the non-load bearing portion (intima). Intima-media thickness (IMT) is used as a surrogate for wall thickness, as the adventitia is indistinguishable from surrounding structures with ultrasound imaging techniques. The assumptions are that the IMT is load bearing, and that the arterial wall is homogeneous (Adji et al., 2011; O'Rourke et al., 2002). Thus caution should be exercised in using Young's modulus as current measurements can be imprecise and unrealistic (O'Rourke et al., 2002).

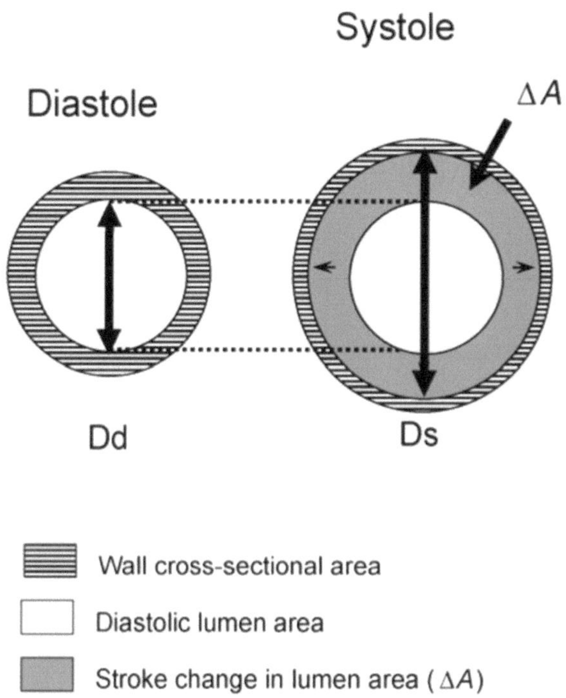

Fig. 6. Measurement of local arterial stiffness: change in luminal cross sectional area (ΔA) for a given change in pressure (diastole to systole). Reprinted and modified with permission (Laurent et al., 2006)

$$E_{inc} = \frac{3\left(\dfrac{1+\Pi\left(\frac{d\min}{2}\right)^2}{\Pi\left(\frac{de}{2}\right)^2 - \Pi\left(\frac{di}{2}\right)^2}\right)}{\dfrac{CSA}{\Pi\left(\frac{d\min}{2}\right)^2 \times PP}} \tag{3}$$

where de is the external diameter and di is the internal diameter, measured in diastole.

Peterson's elastic modulus (Peterson et al., 1960), outlined in equation [4], is different from Young's elastic modulus. It assumes a linear stress strain relationship, is inversely related to arterial distensibility, and needs to be specified at a given blood pressure (Cheng et al., 2002). In turn, an equation that provides an index of arterial compliance independent of distending pressure is the β stiffness index (Hirai et al., 1989), outlined in equation [5], where SBP is systolic blood pressure, and DBP is diastolic blood pressure.

$$\text{Peterson} = \frac{\Pi\left(\frac{d\min}{2}\right)^2 \times PP}{\Pi\left(\frac{d\max}{2}\right)^2 - \Pi\left(\frac{d\min}{2}\right)^2} \quad (4)$$

$$\beta = \frac{\ln\left(\frac{SBP}{DBP}\right)}{\left(\frac{d\max - d\min}{d\min}\right)} \quad (5)$$

3.2.3 Measurement of local arterial stiffness with ultrasound and tonometry

Ultrasound is a common tool used in the non-invasive assessment of the elastic properties of the arterial wall. Many devices have been developed to determine vascular diameters and IMT. These include echo tracking software (Hoeks et al., 1990; Tardy et al., 1991), which use radiofrequency signals to obtain a high precision image, as well as B-mode ultrasound equipped with a high-resolution linear array transducer (Currie et al., 2010; Nualnim et al., 2011; Redheuil et al., 2010; Tanaka et al., 2000) in combination with various edge detection and image analysis software. Both methods have been shown to have high agreement for assessing vessel diameter (A. S. Kelly et al., 2004). Measurement of IMT using non-invasive ultrasound systems is also an important tool and is used as a surrogate measure for wall thickness in measures of elasticity of the arterial wall such as Young's modulus. IMT is also often used as an indicator for cardiovascular disease (O'Leary et al., 1999) and has been employed in clinical studies (Molinari et al., 2010; Simon et al., 2002).

Most commonly, B-mode ultrasound images are collected at a minimum of 10 frames/sec with a 7.5-11 MHz linear array transducer positioned longitudinally to the common carotid artery with collection ~1-2 cm below the bifurcation of the external and internal carotid arteries. Analysis of time points associated with the maximal diameter in systole and the minimum diameter in diastole are selected and diameters are determined by measurement of the far wall from the interface of the lumen and intima to the near wall interface of the adventitia and media (Tanaka et al., 2000). Imaging of media-adventitia interface of the near wall is used, as the intima-lumen interface can be difficult to obtain. Determination of arterial diameters can be made manually using calipers, or with edge-detection software. Most edge-detection software determines the arterial diameter by identifying the arterial wall within a selected region of interest, based on the contrasting intensity of brightness between the arterial wall boundary and the lumen (Currie et al., 2010; Peters et al., 2011). Measurements are made at numerous points within the region of interest (typically ≥100 points), thereby increasing the precision of the measurement. Other software uses the radiofrequency signals generated from the tissue echo reflections to detect boundaries in tissue density. The radiofrequency detection has the added advantage of not being dependent on the post-processing of the B-mode images but is less commonly available (Woodman et al., 2001).

Local arterial measures also require measurement of local blood pressure. Applanation tonometry has been shown to produce near-identical pulse waveforms as those performed invasively (R. Kelly et al., 1989). Applanation tonometry uses a probe that incorporates a high fidelity strain gauge transducer which records continuous pressure waveforms in an artery. It is placed over the greatest area of pulsation, and requires support from solid structures (bone, bone plus ligaments) to flatten the artery slightly to produce a consistent and reproducible signal (R. Kelly et al., 1989). Based on the assumption that diastolic and mean blood pressure are constant through the arterial tree (Nichols & O'Rourke, 2005), Kelly and Fitchett developed a system of approximation of local arterial pressure using a tonometer (R. Kelly & Fitchett, 1992), which has been shown to provide the highest accuracy compared to invasive methods (Van Bortel et al., 2001). As baseline levels acquired by the tonometer are subject to hold down pressure, diastolic and mean blood pressures are equated to brachial blood pressures. Local systolic blood pressure is then determined by the extrapolation of the maximal tonometer signal and calibrated pressures, due to the amplification in systolic blood pressure (Nichols & O'Rourke, 2005). An example of this is provided in Figure 7. Ideally carotid artery pressures should be calibrated to concurrent brachial blood pressures measured continuously using various automated oscillometric blood pressure devices (Ex. Finometer (Finapres Medical Systems B.V.; Amsterdam, The Netherlands), Nexfin (BMEYE; Amsterdam, The Netherlands), CMB-700 (Colin Medical Instruments; San Antonio, TX, USA)), which correct to brachial blood pressure from either finger or radial artery waveforms. When this is not possible, carotid artery pressures can

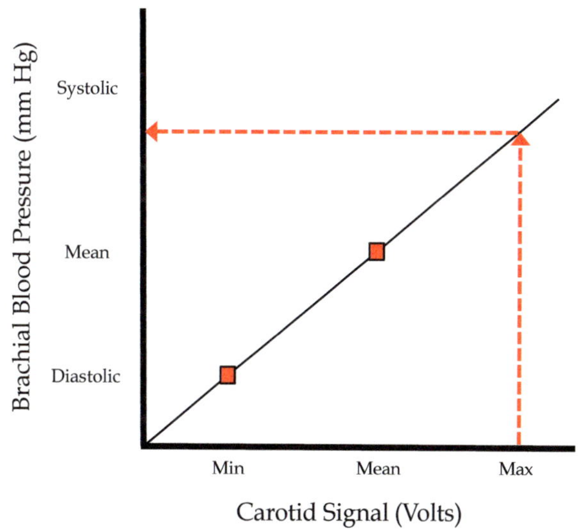

Fig. 7. Approximation of carotid systolic pressure. Minimum and mean carotid artery tonometry values are equated to the diastolic and mean brachial artery blood pressures (red squares), and the equation of the line connecting the points is generated. The pressure (y-axis) at which the maximum carotid artery tonometry value intersects with this line is identified as the predicted carotid artery systolic blood pressure.

also be calibrated to discrete brachial blood pressures collected using a manual sphygmomanometer or an automated oscillometric device. It should be mentioned that previous investigations (Barenbrock et al., 2002; Dijk et al., 2005; Tsivgoulis et al., 2006) have used brachial pulse pressures in the calculation of arterial stiffness measurements when the collection of localized pulse pressure is not available; however, this is not recommended.

Common carotid artery diameter and simultaneous carotid artery blood pressures are collected for 10 cardiac cycles (Currie et al., 2010) in the supine position following at least 10 minutes of quiet rest. Assessments should be performed in a temperature-controlled room, at the same time of day (for repeated measures), and individuals should abstain from caffeine, food consumption, and smoking for at least 3 hours, and alcohol consumption for at least 10 hours prior to testing (Laurent et al., 2006). Section 4 will discuss the association between local measures of carotid artery stiffness and disease; however; it has been suggested that local measures of arterial stiffness be used in mechanistic studies in pathophysiology, pharmacology, and therapeutics, rather than epidemiological studies moving forward (Laurent et al., 2006).

3.2.4 Validity, reliability, and reproducibility of local arterial measurements

Carotid measurements have been validated in clinical studies (Boutouyrie et al., 1999), as both ultrasound imaging for detection of lumen diameter and IMT (Gamble et al., 1994; Hoeks et al., 1990; Hoeks et al., 1997; A. S. Kelly et al., 2004) and use of applanation tonometry (R. Kelly et al., 1989) has been shown to be accurate and reproducible. Between visit coefficient of variation for distensibility measures using B-mode ultrasound imaging techniques is approximately 10% (Kanters et al., 1998; Liang et al., 1998), whereas IMT measures have a coefficient of variation of 2.6-2.8% (Currie et al., 2010; Liang et al., 1998).

3.2.5 Limitations of local arterial measurements

There are several limitations when measuring local arterial stiffness. Applanation of an artery requires a firm background surface to flatten the artery and low levels of subcutaneous fat to avoid dampening of the pulse (Reneman et al., 2005), therefore acquiring a pulse can be an issue in obese individuals. Local stiffness measures using ultrasound are also less sensitive than MRI measures of age-related ascending aortic stiffness in individuals free of cardiovascular disease (Redheuil et al., 2010). However, ultrasound is still a highly accessible clinical tool, and its use for determination of stiffness in the carotid artery is an accepted technique in the assessment of central artery stiffening. Finally, the predictive capacity of carotid stiffness measures for vascular events in patients with manifest arterial disease has been shown to be limited (Dijk et al., 2005). Although, brachial pressures were used in this study as a surrogate of local carotid pressure, therefore caution should be used when considering this result (see Figure 7).

3.3 Regional arterial stiffness and measurement

Regional arterial stiffness can be assessed using pulse wave velocity (PWV), which is commonly defined as the speed of the arterial pulse wave throughout the vasculature (O'Rourke et al., 2002). As previously described, ventricular ejection produces an incident pressure wave, which moves away from the heart and towards the peripheral vasculature at a finite speed. The assessment of how fast the incident wave travels, or its PWV, can provide information about the stiffness of different arterial segments. The faster the PWV, the stiffer the artery, which is addressed by the Moens-Korteweg equation (O'Rourke, 2006):

$$PWV = \sqrt{\frac{Eh}{2Rp}} \tag{6}$$

where E represents the intrinsic elastic properties of the vessel (Young's modulus in the circumferential direction), p is the blood density, and (h/2R) is the ratio of arterial wall thickness to vessel diameter. However, PWV can be determined practically and non-invasively using a variety of pulse detection tools including continuous wave or pulsed wave Doppler ultrasound.

3.3.1 Measurement of regional arterial stiffness

The assessment of PWV involves recording pulse waves at two different arterial sites, for a minimum of 10-15 seconds, to ensure measurement across at least one respiratory cycle (Van Bortel et al., 2002). Traditionally PWV is separated into central and peripheral measurements to account for differences in vascular composition of different portions of the vascular tree. Central PWV, also referred to as aortic PWV, provides an index of stiffness of the large elastic arteries, and is commonly measured as the PWV between the carotid and femoral arterial sites. Peripheral pulse wave velocity provides an index of stiffness of the medium sized muscular arteries, and can be separated into upper limb and lower limb measures. Upper limb assessments typically involve pulse detection at the carotid and brachial or radial arterial sites, where as lower limb PWV can be measured from the femoral artery to either the dorsalis pedis or posterior tibial arterial sites. Doppler ultrasound can be used to collect blood velocity signals at any of the sites listed above. However, aortic PWV can also be determined by collecting blood velocity signals at the suprasternal notch (root of the left subclavian artery), and the umbilicus (near the bifurcation of the abdominal aorta) (Lehmann et al., 1998).

3.3.2 Calculations of regional arterial stiffness

PWV is calculated using the following equation:

$$PWV = \frac{D}{\Delta t} \tag{7}$$

where D is the distance between measurement sites, and Δt is the pulse transit time.

Distance is measured along the surface of the body with anthropometric measuring tape, using specific anatomical landmarks. Central PWV measurements can be made using one of the following pathways: 1) total distance between carotid (carotid artery site to sternal notch) and femoral (sternal notch to inferior border of the umbilicus + inferior border of the umbilicus to the femoral artery site) arterial sites, 2) subtracting the distance of the carotid artery site from the total distance, or 3) subtracting the distance of the carotid artery site from the femoral artery site, which has recently been shown to have the best agreement with invasive measures (Weber et al., 2009). When standardization between distance measurement pathways is needed, central distance values can be converted to the total distance between carotid and femoral arterial sites (The Reference Values for Arterial Stiffness' Collaboration, 2010). PWV can then be multiplied by 0.8 to correct for the overestimation (The Reference Values for Arterial Stiffness' Collaboration, 2010). For upper limb PWV, the distance between the carotid artery site to the sternal notch is subtracted from the distance between the sternal notch and the upper limb site (brachial or radial artery site), which is measured when the arm is abducted 90 degrees. Lower limb measurements are made from the femoral artery site along the leg to either the dorsalis pedis or posterior tibial artery site.

The pulse transit time is determined as the time delay between the arrival of the pulse wave at the two arterial sites, and is calculated using the following equation:

$$\Delta t = T_2 - T_1 \tag{8}$$

where T_2 is the pulse arrival time at the distal site, and T_1 is the pulse arrival time at the proximal site. Time at each site can be determined online or offline. Online analysis uses the ECG trace and manual calipers to determine the time at the R-spike and at the arrival of the blood velocity waveform, which is commonly identified as the foot of the waveform. By subtracting the two values, you can determine time for that arterial site (either T_1 or T_2). To perform offline analysis, the raw audio signal from the color wave or pulsed wave Doppler ultrasound is outsourced to an external data collection system. The most reliable techniques include identifying, 1) the intersecting point between the tangent to the initial systolic upstroke of the blood velocity signal, and the horizontal line through the minimum point, and 2) the second derivative of the blood velocity signal, where the arrival of the waveform is identified as the maximum value (Figure 8) (Chiu et al., 1991). However, identification of the arrival of the pulse wave using derivatives has been criticized, since the shape of the waveform changes with heart rate fluctuations (Nichols & O'Rourke, 2005), altering where the peak of the derivative identifies. The arrival of the waveform can also be identified based on the phase velocity theory, which suggests the foot of the waveform is primarily composed of frequencies between 5 and 30 Hz, near the 30 Hz value (McDonald, 1968; Munakata et al., 2003). By filtering out the lower and higher frequencies from the signal using a band-pass filter (<5Hz, >30Hz), the foot of the waveform can be identified as the minimum value of the filtered signal. Unlike the derivative method, fluctuations in heart rate do not influence analysis since the frequencies are unaffected (Nichols & O'Rourke, 2005). When blood velocity signals are collected simultaneously using more than one Doppler probe, time at each site can easily be identified using the maximum or minimum value. When signals are collected sequentially, time at each site is determined using an ECG trace, similar to the online analysis.

3.3.3 Additional devices for the assessment of regional arterial stiffness

The assessment of PWV using Doppler ultrasound has been shown to be valid and reliable (Jiang et al., 2008; Sutton-Tyrrell et al., 2001). However, there are several other techniques available for the detection of the pulse wave in the determination of PWV including applanation tonometry (as previously described), photoplethysmographic sensors, and magnetic resonance imaging (MRI). Photoplethysmographic sensors contain an infrared emitting diode (peak wavelength 880nm), and a phototransistor detector. The infrared light is either absorbed by the blood and vascular tissue, scattered by other tissues, or reflected back to the detector. The arterial waveform in generated based on how much infrared light is reflected back to the detector (Loukogeorgakis et al., 2002). Flow measurements can also be made using MRI. This technique is capable of providing accurate PWV assessments since distance can be measured along the anatomical segment (Mohiaddin et al., 1993).

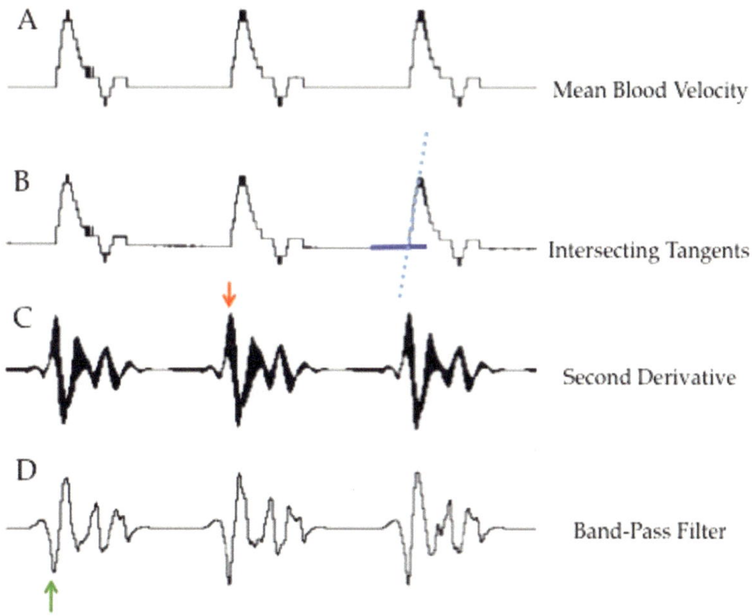

Fig. 8. Various analysis methods for identifying pulse transit time. The arrival of the mean blood velocity waveform (A) is identified with a red arrow. The intersecting tangent (B) analysis locates the point of intersection between the tangent to the initial systolic upstroke of the signal (dotted line), and the horizontal line through the minimum point (closed line). Pulse arrival can also be identified as the maximum value of the second derivative (C), or the minimum value of the band-pass filter (D).

3.3.4 Limitations of regional arterial stiffness measurements

PWV does have its limitations. The measurement of distance along the surface of the body is not a true anatomical representative of the arterial segment and therefore can introduce error into the PWV calculation. Pulse wave measurements at the two arterial sites should be collected simultaneously; however, equipment limitations may not permit this. While the collection of sequential measurements is sufficient, caution should be exercised when interpreting results. While MRI assessments of PWV are not subjective to these limitations, the technique is not that widely used given the lack of available equipment and high cost per use.

3.3.5 Local versus regional assessment of arterial stiffness

Aortic stiffness measures (via carotid-femoral PWV) and local carotid measures of distensibility have been compared (Paini et al., 2006). Strong correlations exist between the two measures in healthy subjects, but decrease with an increasing number of comorbidities (hypertension; hypertension and type 2 diabetes), as the aorta stiffens disproportionately to the carotid artery with age and other cardiovascular risk factors (Paini et al., 2006). Stiffness measures at the carotid artery, therefore, seem to provide a strong estimation for aortic stiffness in less diseased individuals, but aortic and carotid stiffness measures should not be used synonymously in higher risk populations.

4. Arterial stiffness in health and disease

Indices of arterial stiffness provide a non-invasive assessment of the health of the vasculature, and can provide relevant information about an individual's future risk of morbidity and mortality. While arterial stiffening is primarily attributed to modifications to the intrinsic structure of the vessel, several lifestyle factors can transiently augment or attenuate arterial stiffness. Caffeine consumption (Mahmud & Feely, 2001), smoking (Mahmud & Feely, 2003), and resistance exercise (DeVan et al., 2005) have been shown to temporarily increase arterial stiffness, whereas alcohol consumption (Mahmud & Feely, 2002), food consumption (Ahuja et al., 2009), and aerobic exercise (Kingwell et al., 1997) transiently decrease arterial stiffness. Chronic exposure to these factors, however, can lead to more permanent changes in arterial stiffness. Elevated resting arterial stiffness is observed in habitual smokers and individuals who consume excess caffeine and alcohol. Conversely, individuals who are habitually active, or who undergo an exercise training program are capable of attenuating or reversing age associated increases in arterial stiffness (Tanaka et al., 2000). Resting arterial stiffness is also affected by time of day, with larger arterial diameters and lower blood pressures reported at night (Kool et al., 1992).

Arterial stiffness increases naturally with age (O'Rourke & Hashimoto, 2007), and the rate of arterial stiffening is often associated with lifestyle factors (discussed above) and disease. Arterial stiffness is present in individuals with congenital diseases such as Marfan syndrome (Hirata et al., 1991), congenital heart diseases including coarctation of the aorta (de Divitiis et al., 2001) and tetralogy of Fallot (Cheung et al., 2006), as well as non-congenital conditions including but not limited to Kawasaki disease (Senzaki et al., 2005) and end-stage renal disease (Blacher et al., 1999). Traditional risk factors for cardiovascular disease are associated with increased arterial stiffening in adults, including obesity (Danias et al., 2003), type 2 diabetes (Henry et al., 2003), hypertension (Ting et al., 1986), and hypercholesterolemia (Wilkinson et al., 2002). Additionally, the presence of atherosclerosis is associated with arterial stiffening at various sites within the vascular tree (van Popele et al., 2001; van Popele et al., 2006). Not surprisingly, elevated arterial stiffness is present in individuals with cardiovascular diseases including coronary artery disease (Weber et al., 2004), heart failure (Kawaguchi et al., 2003), and stroke (Mattace-Raso et al., 2006).

Adolescents and children with cardiovascular disease risk factors including familial hypercholesterolemia (Aggoun et al., 2000), obesity (Tounian et al., 2001), and type 1 diabetes (Heilman et al., 2009) demonstrate greater arterial stiffness than their age and gender matched peers. While these studies are cross-sectional in design, and provide no information about their future outcomes, the research suggests children and adolescents with impaired arterial compliance are at a greater risk for disease development in adulthood.

Several investigations have examined the association between indices of arterial stiffness and future risk of cardiovascular morbidity and mortality and all-cause mortality. Aortic (carotid to femoral) PWV is considered the non-invasive gold standard measure of arterial stiffness. In apparently healthy men and women, higher aortic PWV ($\geq$ 11.8 m/s) is associated with a 48% increased risk of first major cardiovascular disease event including myocardial infarction, unstable angina, heart failure and/or stroke (Mitchell et al., 2010). According to a meta-analysis on aortic PWV, an increase of 1 m/s corresponds to an age, gender, and risk factor adjusted risk increase of 15% for cardiovascular and all-cause mortality (Vlachopoulos et al., 2010). This systematic review included a variety of populations and measurement techniques and therefore provides a comprehensive examination of the risk associated with elevated aortic stiffness. However, there are numerous other studies demonstrating increased risk of mortality in clinical populations with elevated aortic PWV including but not limited to end-stage renal disease (Blacher et al., 1999), hypertension (Laurent et al., 2001), and type 2 diabetes (Cruickshank et al., 2002).

The literature on the relationship between other indices of arterial stiffness and future risk of morbidity and mortality is not as well defined. Some investigations demonstrate no association between decreased carotid artery compliance and distensibility and future risk (Leone et al., 2008; van Dijk et al., 2001), whereas other studies demonstrate elevated risk in individuals with carotid artery stiffness (Barenbrock et al., 2002; Tsivgoulis et al., 2006). Additionally, not all of these investigations used local carotid pulse pressure in the calculation of arterial stiffness; therefore the findings should be interpreted with caution.

5. Future directions and conclusions

Efforts have recently been made to establish reference values of arterial stiffness for carotid-femoral PWV (The Reference Values for Arterial Stiffness' Collaboration, 2010). This is an important first step in understanding the baseline changes that occur with arterial stiffness in the healthy person as they age. Furthering these attempts will continue to elucidate the role of stiffness in aging, and will significantly contribute to understanding the role of stiffness in disease. Furthermore, even though stiffness measures have been shown to be strong prognostic indicators for the occurrence of cardiovascular events, work has yet to be done to show if the reduction or attenuation of arterial stiffness is associated with a reduction of cardiovascular events, independent of other risk factors (Laurent & Boutouyrie, 2007). Indeed, more immediate changes such as reductions in blood pressure, hyperglycemia, and lipids do show reductions in cardiovascular risk scores. However, improvements in the wall of the vessel (stiffness) may in fact suggest more long lasting reductions in cardiovascular risk, but this remains to be seen (Laurent & Boutouyrie, 2007).

Despite these future considerations, measurement of arterial stiffness is critical in understanding changes in the vascular tree, as its indices can be transiently and chronically altered by aging, disease, and lifestyle factors. Aortic PWV is considered the gold standard for non-invasive assessments of arterial stiffness, and can provide the most relevant information about an individual's future risk of cardiovascular morbidity and mortality, and all-cause mortality. Measurement of local arterial stiffness, while requiring more expertise and time, has also emerged as an important tool for the mechanistic study of vascular structure and function, especially in less diseased populations. In combination, these ultrasonic techniques provide a simple, comprehensive, and non-invasive approach to understand arterial structure and function. They should therefore be considered in the study of overall vascular health.

6. References

Adji, A., O'Rourke, M. F., & Namasivayam, M. (2011). Arterial stiffness, its assessment, prognostic value, and implications for treatment. *American Journal of Hypertension*, Vol. 24, No. 1 (Jan 2011), pp. 5-17. 1941-7225

Aggoun, Y., Bonnet, D., Sidi, D., Girardet, J. P., Brucker, E., Polak, M., Safar, M. E., & Levy, B. I. (2000). Arterial mechanical changes in children with familial hypercholesterolemia. *Arteriosclerosis, Thrombosis, and Vascular Biology*, Vol. 20, No. 9 (Sept 2000), pp. 2070-2075. 1524-4636

Ahuja, K. D., Robertson, I. K., & Ball, M. J. (2009). Acute effects of food on postprandial blood pressure and measures of arterial stiffness in healthy humans. *The American Journal of Clinical Nutrition*, Vol. 90, No. 2 (Aug 2009), pp. 298-303. 1938-3207

Armentano, R. L., Levenson, J., Barra, J. G., Fischer, E. I., Breitbart, G. J., Pichel, R. H., & Simon, A. (1991). Assessment of elastin and collagen contribution to aortic elasticity in conscious dogs. *American Journal of Physiology*, Vol. 260, No. 6 (Jun 1991), pp. H1870-1877. 0002-9513

Atkinson, J. (2008). Age-related medial elastocalcinosis in arteries: mechanisms, animal models, and physiological consequences. *Journal of Applied Physiology*, Vol. 105, No. 5 (Nov 2008), pp. 1643-1651. 8750-7587

Barenbrock, M., Kosch, M., Joster, E., Kisters, K., Rahn, K. H., & Hausberg, M. (2002). Reduced arterial distensibility is a predictor of cardiovascular disease in patients after renal transplantation. *Journal of Hypertension*, Vol. 20, No. 1 (Jan 2002), pp. 79-84. 0263-6352

Benetos, A., Laurent, S., Hoeks, A. P., Boutouyrie, P. H., & Safar, M. E. (1993). Arterial alterations with aging and high blood pressure. A noninvasive study of carotid and femoral arteries. *Arteriosclerosis, Thrombosis, and Vascular Biology*, Vol. 13, No. 1 (Jan 1993), pp. 90-97. 1049-8834

Blacher, J., Guerin, A. P., Pannier, B., Marchais, S. J., Safar, M. E., & London, G. M. (1999). Impact of aortic stiffness on survival in end-stage renal disease. *Circulation*, Vol. 99, No. 18 (May 1999), pp. 2434-2439. 1524-4539

Boutouyrie, P., Bussy, C., Lacolley, P., Girerd, X., Laloux, B., & Laurent, S. (1999). Association between local pulse pressure, mean blood pressure, and large-artery remodeling. *Circulation*, Vol. 100, No. 13 (Sept 1999), pp. 1387-1393. 1524-4539

Boutouyrie, P., Laurent, S., Benetos, A., Girerd, X. J., Hoeks, A. P., & Safar, M. E. (1992). Opposing effects of ageing on distal and proximal large arteries in hypertensives. *Journal of Hypertension Supplement*, Vol. 10, No. 6 (Aug 1992), pp. S87-91. 0952-1178

Cavalcante, J. L., Lima, J. A., Redheuil, A., & Al-Mallah, M. H. (2011). Aortic stiffness: current understanding and future directions. *Journal of the American College of Cardiology*, Vol. 57, No. 14 (Apr 2011), pp. 1511-1522. 1558-3597

Cheng, K. S., Baker, C. R., Hamilton, G., Hoeks, A. P., & Seifalian, A. M. (2002). Arterial elastic properties and cardiovascular risk/event. *European Journal of Vascular and Endovascular Surgery*, Vol. 24, No. 5 (Nov 2002), pp. 383-397. 1078-5884

Cheung, Y. F., Ou, X., & Wong, S. J. (2006). Central and peripheral arterial stiffness in patients after surgical repair of tetralogy of Fallot: implications for aortic root dilatation. *Heart*, Vol. 92, No. 12 (Dec 2006), pp. 1827-1830. 1468-201X

Chiu, Y. C., Arand, P. W., Shroff, S. G., Feldman, T., & Carroll, J. D. (1991). Determination of pulse wave velocities with computerized algorithms. *American Heart Journal*, Vol. 121, No. 5 (May 1991), pp. 1460-1470. 0002-8703

Cruickshank, K., Riste, L., Anderson, S. G., Wright, J. S., Dunn, G., & Gosling, R. G. (2002). Aortic pulse-wave velocity and its relationship to mortality in diabetes and glucose intolerance: an integrated index of vascular function? *Circulation*, Vol. 106, No. 16 (Oct 2002), pp. 2085-2090. 1524-4539

Currie, K. D., Proudfoot, N. A., Timmons, B. W., & MacDonald, M. J. (2010). Noninvasive measures of vascular health are reliable in preschool-aged children. *Applied Physiology, Nutrition, and Metabolism*, Vol. 35, No. 4 (Aug 2010), pp. 512-517. 1715-5312

Danias, P. G., Tritos, N. A., Stuber, M., Botnar, R. M., Kissinger, K. V., & Manning, W. J. (2003). Comparison of aortic elasticity determined by cardiovascular magnetic resonance imaging in obese versus lean adults. *American Journal of Cardiology*, Vol. 91, No. 2 (Jan 2003), pp. 195-199. 0002-9149

Davies, J. I., & Struthers, A. D. (2003). Pulse wave analysis and pulse wave velocity: a critical review of their strengths and weaknesses. *Journal of Hypertension*, Vol. 21, No. 3 (Mar 2003), pp. 463-472. 0263-6352

de Divitiis, M., Pilla, C., Kattenhorn, M., Zadinello, M., Donald, A., Leeson, P., Wallace, S., Redington, A., & Deanfield, J. E. (2001). Vascular dysfunction after repair of coarctation of the aorta: impact of early surgery. *Circulation*, Vol. 104, No. 12 (Sep 2001), pp. I165-170. 1524-4539

Dernellis, J., & Panaretou, M. (2005). Aortic stiffness is an independent predictor of progression to hypertension in nonhypertensive subjects. *Hypertension*, Vol. 45, No. 3 (Mar 2005), pp. 426-431. 1524-4563

DeVan, A. E., Anton, M. M., Cook, J. N., Neidre, D. B., Cortez-Cooper, M. Y., & Tanaka, H. (2005). Acute effects of resistance exercise on arterial compliance. *Journal of Applied Physiology*, Vol. 98, No. 6 (Jun 2005), pp. 2287-2291. 8750-7587

Dijk, J. M., Algra, A., van der Graaf, Y., Grobbee, D. E., & Bots, M. L. (2005). Carotid stiffness and the risk of new vascular events in patients with manifest cardiovascular disease. The SMART study. *European Heart Journal*, Vol. 26, No. 12 (Jun 2005), pp. 1213-1220. 0195-668X

Dobrin, P. B. (1999). Distribution of lamellar deformations: implications for properties of the arterial media. *Hypertension*, Vol. 33, No. 3 (Mar 1999), pp. 806-810. 0194-911X

Folkow, B. (1995). Hypertensive structural changes in systemic precapillary resistance vessels: how important are they for in vivo haemodynamics? *Journal of Hypertension*, Vol. 13, No. 12 (Dec 1995), pp. 1546-1559. 0263-6352

Gamble, G., Zorn, J., Sanders, G., MacMahon, S., & Sharpe, N. (1994). Estimation of arterial stiffness, compliance, and distensibility from M-mode ultrasound measurements of the common carotid artery. *Stroke*, Vol. 25, No. 1 (Jan 1994), pp. 11-16. 0039-2499

Harkness, M. L., Harkness, R. D., & McDonald, D. A. (1957). The collagen and elastin content of the arterial wall in the dog. *Proceedings of the Royal Society of London, Series B. Containing papers of a Biological character*, Vol. 146, No. 925 (Jun 1957), pp. 541-551. 0080-4649

Hayoz, D., Tardy, Y., Rutschmann, B., Mignot, J. P., Achakri, H., Feihl, F., Meister, J. J., Waeber, B., & Brunner, H. R. (1993). Spontaneous diameter oscillations of the radial artery in humans. *American Journal of Physiology*, Vol. 264, No. 6 (Jun 1993), pp. H2080-2084. 0002-9513

Heilman, K., Zilmer, M., Zilmer, K., Lintrop, M., Kampus, P., Kals, J., & Tillmann, V. (2009). Arterial stiffness, carotid artery intima-media thickness and plasma myeloperoxidase level in children with type 1 diabetes. *Diabetes Research and Clinical Practice*, Vol. 84, No. 2 (May 2009), pp. 168-173. 1872-8227

Henry, R. M., Kostense, P. J., Spijkerman, A. M., Dekker, J. M., Nijpels, G., Heine, R. J., Kamp, O., Westerhof, N., Bouter, L. M., & Stehouwer, C. D. (2003). Arterial stiffness increases with deteriorating glucose tolerance status: the Hoorn Study. *Circulation*, Vol. 107, No. 16 (Apr 2003), pp. 2089-2095. 1524-4539

Hirai, T., Sasayama, S., Kawasaki, T., & Yagi, S. (1989). Stiffness of systemic arteries in patients with myocardial infarction. A noninvasive method to predict severity of coronary atherosclerosis. *Circulation*, Vol. 80, No. 1 (Jul 1989), pp. 78-86. 0009-7322

Hirata, K., Triposkiadis, F., Sparks, E., Bowen, J., Wooley, C. F., & Boudoulas, H. (1991). The Marfan syndrome: abnormal aortic elastic properties. *Journal of the American College of Cardiology*, Vol. 18, No. 1 (Jul 1991), pp. 57-63. 0735-1097

Hoeks, A. P., Brands, P. J., Smeets, F. A., & Reneman, R. S. (1990). Assessment of the distensibility of superficial arteries. *Ultrasound in Medicine & Biology*, Vol. 16, No. 2 1990), pp. 121-128. 0301-5629

Hoeks, A. P., Willekes, C., Boutouyrie, P., Brands, P. J., Willigers, J. M., & Reneman, R. S. (1997). Automated detection of local artery wall thickness based on M-line signal processing. *Ultrasound in Medicine & Biology*, Vol. 23, No. 7 (1997), pp. 1017-1023. 0301-5629

Jiang, B., Liu, B., McNeill, K. L., & Chowienczyk, P. J. (2008). Measurement of pulse wave velocity using pulse wave Doppler ultrasound: comparison with arterial tonometry. *Ultrasound in Medicine & Biology*, Vol. 34, No. 3 (Mar 2008), pp. 509-512. 0301-5629

Kanters, S. D., Elgersma, O. E., Banga, J. D., van Leeuwen, M. S., & Algra, A. (1998). Reproducibility of measurements of intima-media thickness and distensibility in the common carotid artery. *European Journal of Vascular & Endovascular Surgery*, Vol. 16, No. 1 (Jul 1998), pp. 28-35. 1078-5884

Kawaguchi, M., Hay, I., Fetics, B., & Kass, D. A. (2003). Combined ventricular systolic and arterial stiffening in patients with heart failure and preserved ejection fraction: implications for systolic and diastolic reserve limitations. *Circulation*, Vol. 107, No. 5 (Feb 2003), pp. 714-720. 1524-4539

Kelly, A. S., Kaiser, D. R., Dengel, D. R., & Bank, A. J. (2004). Comparison of B-mode and echo tracking methods of assessing flow-mediated dilation. *Ultrasound in Medicine & Biology*, Vol. 30, No. 11 (Nov 2004), pp. 1447-1449. 0301-5629

Kelly, R., & Fitchett, D. (1992). Noninvasive determination of aortic input impedance and external left ventricular power output: a validation and repeatability study of a new technique. *Journal of the American College of Cardiology*, Vol. 20, No. 4 (Oct 1992), pp. 952-963. 0735-1097

Kelly, R., Hayward, C., Avolio, A., & O'Rourke, M. (1989). Noninvasive determination of age-related changes in the human arterial pulse. *Circulation*, Vol. 80, No. 6 (Dec 1989), pp. 1652-1659. 0009-7322

Kingwell, B. A., Berry, K. L., Cameron, J. D., Jennings, G. L., & Dart, A. M. (1997). Arterial compliance increases after moderate-intensity cycling. *Am J Physiol*, Vol. 273, No. 5 (Nov 1997), pp. H2186-2191. 0002-9513

Kool, M. J., Struijker-Boudier, H. A., Wijnen, J. A., Hoeks, A. P., & van Bortel, L. M. (1992). Effects of diurnal variability and exercise training on properties of large arteries. *Journal of Hypertension Supplement*, Vol. 10, No. 6 (Aug 1992), pp. S49-52. 0952-1178

Lanne, T., Sonesson, B., Bergqvist, D., Bengtsson, H., & Gustafsson, D. (1992). Diameter and compliance in the male human abdominal aorta: influence of age and aortic aneurysm. *European Journal of Vascular Surgery*, Vol. 6, No. 2 (Mar 1992), pp. 178-184. 0950-821X

Laurent, S., & Boutouyrie, P. (2007). Recent advances in arterial stiffness and wave reflection in human hypertension. *Hypertension*, Vol. 49, No. 6 (Jun 2007), pp. 1202-1206. 1524-4563

Laurent, S., Boutouyrie, P., Asmar, R., Gautier, I., Laloux, B., Guize, L., Ducimetiere, P., & Benetos, A. (2001). Aortic stiffness is an independent predictor of all-cause and cardiovascular mortality in hypertensive patients. *Hypertension*, Vol. 37, No. 5 (May 2001), pp. 1236-1241. 1524-4563

Laurent, S., Boutouyrie, P., & Lacolley, P. (2005). Structural and genetic bases of arterial stiffness. *Hypertension*, Vol. 45, No. 6 (Jun 2005), pp. 1050-1055. 1524-4563

Laurent, S., Cockcroft, J., Van Bortel, L., Boutouyrie, P., Giannattasio, C., Hayoz, D., Pannier, B., Vlachopoulos, C., Wilkinson, I., & Struijker-Boudier, H. (2006). Expert consensus document on arterial stiffness: methodological issues and clinical applications. *European Heart Journal*, Vol. 27, No. 21 (Nov 2006), pp. 2588-2605. 0195-668X

Learoyd, B. M., & Taylor, M. G. (1966). Alterations with age in the viscoelastic properties of human arterial walls. *Circulation Research*, Vol. 18, No. 3 (Mar 1966), pp. 278-292. 0009-7330

Lee, H. Y., & Oh, B. H. (2010). Aging and arterial stiffness. *Circulation Journal*, Vol. 74, No. 11 (Nov 2010), pp. 2257-2262. 1347-4820

Lehmann, E. D., Hopkins, K. D., Rawesh, A., Joseph, R. C., Kongola, K., Coppack, S. W., & Gosling, R. G. (1998). Relation between number of cardiovascular risk factors/events and noninvasive Doppler ultrasound assessments of aortic compliance. *Hypertension*, Vol. 32, No. 3 (Sept 1998), pp. 565-569. 0194-911X

Leone, N., Ducimetiere, P., Gariepy, J., Courbon, D., Tzourio, C., Dartigues, J. F., Ritchie, K., Alperovitch, A., Amouyel, P., Safar, M. E., & Zureik, M. (2008). Distension of the carotid artery and risk of coronary events: the three-city study. *Arteriosclerosis, Thrombosis, and Vascular Biology*, Vol. 28, No. 7 (Jul 2008), pp. 1392-1397. 1524-4636

Levy, D., & Brink, S. (2005). *A Change of Heart: How the People of Framingham, Massachusetts, Helped Unravel the Mysteries of Cardiovascular Disease* (1st edition), Knopf, 0375412751, New York

Liang, Y. L., Teede, H., Kotsopoulos, D., Shiel, L., Cameron, J. D., Dart, A. M., & McGrath, B. P. (1998). Non-invasive measurements of arterial structure and function:

repeatability, interrelationships and trial sample size. *Clinical Science (London)*, Vol. 95, No. 6 (Dec 1998), pp. 669-679. 0143-5221

London, G. M., & Pannier, B. (2010). Arterial functions: how to interpret the complex physiology. *Nephrology, Dialysis, Transplantation*, Vol. 25, No. 12 (Dec 2010), pp. 3815-3823. 1460-2385

Loukogeorgakis, S., Dawson, R., Phillips, N., Martyn, C. N., & Greenwald, S. E. (2002). Validation of a device to measure arterial pulse wave velocity by a photoplethysmographic method. *Physiological Measurements*, Vol. 23, No. 3 (Aug 2002), pp. 581-596. 0967-3334

Mahmud, A., & Feely, J. (2001). Acute effect of caffeine on arterial stiffness and aortic pressure waveform. *Hypertension*, Vol. 38, No. 2 (Aug 2001), pp. 227-231. 1524-4563

Mahmud, A., & Feely, J. (2002). Divergent effect of acute and chronic alcohol on arterial stiffness. *American Journal of Hypertension*, Vol. 15, No. 3 (Mar 2002), pp. 240-243. 0895-7061

Mahmud, A., & Feely, J. (2003). Effect of smoking on arterial stiffness and pulse pressure amplification. *Hypertension*, Vol. 41, No. 1 (Jan 2003), pp. 183-187. 1524-4563

Mattace-Raso, F. U., van der Cammen, T. J., Hofman, A., van Popele, N. M., Bos, M. L., Schalekamp, M. A., Asmar, R., Reneman, R. S., Hoeks, A. P., Breteler, M. M., & Witteman, J. C. (2006). Arterial stiffness and risk of coronary heart disease and stroke: the Rotterdam Study. *Circulation*, Vol. 113, No. 5 (Feb 2006), pp. 657-663. 1524-4539

McDonald, D. A. (1968). Regional pulse-wave velocity in the arterial tree. *Journal of Applied Physiology*, Vol. 24, No. 1 (Jan 1968), pp. 73-78. 0021-8987

McEniery, C. M., Spratt, M., Munnery, M., Yarnell, J., Lowe, G. D., Rumley, A., Gallacher, J., Ben-Shlomo, Y., Cockcroft, J. R., & Wilkinson, I. B. (2010). An analysis of prospective risk factors for aortic stiffness in men: 20-year follow-up from the Caerphilly prospective study. *Hypertension*, Vol. 56, No. 1 (Jul 2010), pp. 36-43. 1524-4563

Meinders, J. M., & Hoeks, A. P. (2004). Simultaneous assessment of diameter and pressure waveforms in the carotid artery. *Ultrasound in Medicine & Biology*, Vol. 30, No. 2 (Feb 2004), pp. 147-154. 0301-5629

Mitchell, G. F., Hwang, S. J., Vasan, R. S., Larson, M. G., Pencina, M. J., Hamburg, N. M., Vita, J. A., Levy, D., & Benjamin, E. J. (2010). Arterial stiffness and cardiovascular events: the Framingham Heart Study. *Circulation*, Vol. 121, No. 4 (Feb 2010), pp. 505-511. 1524-4539

Mohiaddin, R. H., Firmin, D. N., & Longmore, D. B. (1993). Age-related changes of human aortic flow wave velocity measured noninvasively by magnetic resonance imaging. *Journal of Applied Physiology*, Vol. 74, No. 1 (Jan 1993), pp. 492-497. 8750-7587

Molinari, F., Zeng, G., & Suri, J. S. (2010). A state of the art review on intima-media thickness (IMT) measurement and wall segmentation techniques for carotid ultrasound. *Computer Methods and Programs in Biomedicine*, Vol. 100, No. 3 (Dec 2010), pp. 201-221. 1872-7565

Munakata, M., Ito, N., Nunokawa, T., & Yoshinaga, K. (2003). Utility of automated brachial ankle pulse wave velocity measurements in hypertensive patients. *American Journal of Hypertension*, Vol. 16, No. 8 (Aug 2003), pp. 653-657. 0895-7061

Naghavi, M. (2009). *Asymptomatic Atherosclerosis* (1st edition), Humana Press, 9781603271783, New York

Naidu, M. U., Reddy, B. M., Yashmaina, S., Patnaik, A. N., & Rani, P. U. (2005). Validity and reproducibility of arterial pulse wave velocity measurement using new device with oscillometric technique: a pilot study. *Biomedical Engineering Online*, Vol. 4, No. (2005), pp. 49. 1475-925X

Najjar, S. S., Scuteri, A., & Lakatta, E. G. (2005). Arterial aging: is it an immutable cardiovascular risk factor? *Hypertension*, Vol. 46, No. 3 (Sept 2005), pp. 454-462. 1524-4563

Nichols, W. W., & O'Rourke, M. F. (2005). *McDonald's Blood Flow in Arteries: Theoretical, Experimental and Clinical Principles* (5th edition), Hodder Arnold, 0340809418, London

Nualnim, N., Barnes, J. N., Tarumi, T., Renzi, C. P., & Tanaka, H. (2011). Comparison of central artery elasticity in swimmers, runners, and the sedentary. *American Journal of Cardiology*, Vol. 107, No. 5 (Mar 2011), pp. 783-787. 1879-1913

O'Leary, D. H., Polak, J. F., Kronmal, R. A., Manolio, T. A., Burke, G. L., & Wolfson, S. K., Jr. (1999). Carotid-artery intima and media thickness as a risk factor for myocardial infarction and stroke in older adults. Cardiovascular Health Study Collaborative Research Group. *New England Journal of Medicine*, Vol. 340, No. 1 (Jan 1999), pp. 14-22. 0028-4793

O'Rourke, M. F. (2006). Principles and definitions of arterial stiffness, wave reflections and pulse pressure amplification, In: *Arterial Stiffness in Hypertension*, Safar, M. E. & O'Rourke, M. F., pp. 3-20, Elsevier, Amsterdam

O'Rourke, M. F., & Hashimoto, J. (2007). Mechanical factors in arterial aging: a clinical perspective. *Journal of the American College of Cardiology*, Vol. 50, No. 1 (Jul 2007), pp. 1-13. 1558-3597

O'Rourke, M. F., & Safar, M. E. (2005). Relationship between aortic stiffening and microvascular disease in brain and kidney: cause and logic of therapy. *Hypertension*, Vol. 46, No. 1 (Jul 2005), pp. 200-204. 1524-4563

O'Rourke, M. F., Staessen, J. A., Vlachopoulos, C., Duprez, D., & Plante, G. E. (2002). Clinical applications of arterial stiffness; definitions and reference values. *American Journal of Hypertension*, Vol. 15, No. 5 (May 2002), pp. 426-444. 0895-7061

Paini, A., Boutouyrie, P., Calvet, D., Tropeano, A. I., Laloux, B., & Laurent, S. (2006). Carotid and aortic stiffness: determinants of discrepancies. *Hypertension*, Vol. 47, No. 3 (Mar 2006), pp. 371-376. 1524-4563

Pannier, B. M., Avolio, A. P., Hoeks, A., Mancia, G., & Takazawa, K. (2002). Methods and devices for measuring arterial compliance in humans. *American Journal of Hypertension*, Vol. 15, No. 8 (Aug 2002), pp. 743-753. 0895-7061

Papaioannou, T. G., Stamatelopoulos, K. S., Gialafos, E., Vlachopoulos, C., Karatzis, E., Nanas, J., & Lekakis, J. (2004). Monitoring of arterial stiffness indices by applanation tonometry and pulse wave analysis: reproducibility at low blood pressures. *Journal of Clinical Monitoring and Computing*, Vol. 18, No. 2 (Apr 2004), pp. 137-144. 1387-1307

Peters, S. A., den Ruijter, H. M., Palmer, M. K., Grobbee, D. E., Crouse, J. R., 3rd, O'Leary, D. H., Evans, G. W., Raichlen, J. S., Lind, L., & Bots, M. L. (2011). Manual or semi-automated edge detection of the maximal far wall common carotid intima-media thickness: a direct comparison. *Journal of Internal Medicine*, Vol. No. (Jul 2011), pp. 1365-2796

Peterson, L. H., Jensen, R. E., & Parnell, J. (1960). Mechanical Properties of Arteries in Vivo. *Circulation Research*, Vol. 8, No. 3 (May 1960), pp. 622-639.

Redheuil, A., Yu, W. C., Wu, C. O., Mousseaux, E., de Cesare, A., Yan, R., Kachenoura, N., Bluemke, D., & Lima, J. A. (2010). Reduced ascending aortic strain and distensibility: earliest manifestations of vascular aging in humans. *Hypertension*, Vol. 55, No. 2 (Feb 2010), pp. 319-326. 1524-4563

Reneman, R. S., Meinders, J. M., & Hoeks, A. P. (2005). Non-invasive ultrasound in arterial wall dynamics in humans: what have we learned and what remains to be solved. *European Heart Journal*, Vol. 26, No. 10 (May 2005), pp. 960-966. 0195-668X

Roman, M. J., Devereux, R. B., Schwartz, J. E., Lockshin, M. D., Paget, S. A., Davis, A., Crow, M. K., Sammaritano, L., Levine, D. M., Shankar, B. A., Moeller, E., & Salmon, J. E. (2005). Arterial stiffness in chronic inflammatory diseases. *Hypertension*, Vol. 46, No. 1 (Jul 2005), pp. 194-199. 1524-4563

Saito, M., Okayama, H., Nishimura, K., Ogimoto, A., Ohtsuka, T., Inoue, K., Hiasa, G., Sumimoto, T., & Higaki, J. (2008). Possible link between large artery stiffness and coronary flow velocity reserve. *Heart*, Vol. 94, No. 6 (Jun 2008), pp. e20. 1468-201X

Senzaki, H., Chen, C. H., Ishido, H., Masutani, S., Matsunaga, T., Taketazu, M., Kobayashi, T., Sasaki, N., Kyo, S., & Yokote, Y. (2005). Arterial hemodynamics in patients after Kawasaki disease. *Circulation*, Vol. 111, No. 16 (Apr 2005), pp. 2119-2125. 1524-4539

Simon, A., Gariepy, J., Chironi, G., Megnien, J. L., & Levenson, J. (2002). Intima-media thickness: a new tool for diagnosis and treatment of cardiovascular risk. *Journal of Hypertension*, Vol. 20, No. 2 (Feb 2002), pp. 159-169. 0263-6352

Sutton-Tyrrell, K., Mackey, R. H., Holubkov, R., Vaitkevicius, P. V., Spurgeon, H. A., & Lakatta, E. G. (2001). Measurement variation of aortic pulse wave velocity in the elderly. *American Journal of Hypertension*, Vol. 14, No. 5 (May 2001), pp. 463-468. 0895-7061

Taddei, S., Virdis, A., Ghiadoni, L., Salvetti, G., Bernini, G., Magagna, A., & Salvetti, A. (2001). Age-related reduction of NO availability and oxidative stress in humans. *Hypertension*, Vol. 38, No. 2 (Aug 2001), pp. 274-279. 1524-4563

Tanaka, H., Dinenno, F. A., Monahan, K. D., Clevenger, C. M., DeSouza, C. A., & Seals, D. R. (2000). Aging, habitual exercise, and dynamic arterial compliance. *Circulation*, Vol. 102, No. 11 (Sept 2000), pp. 1270-1275. 1524-4539

Tardy, Y., Meister, J. J., Perret, F., Brunner, H. R., & Arditi, M. (1991). Non-invasive estimate of the mechanical properties of peripheral arteries from ultrasonic and photoplethysmographic measurements. *Clinical Physics and Physiological Measurement*, Vol. 12, No. 1 (Feb 1991), pp. 39-54. 0143-0815

The Reference Values for Arterial Stiffness' Collaboration. (2010). Determinants of pulse wave velocity in healthy people and in the presence of cardiovascular risk factors: 'establishing normal and reference values'. *European Heart Journal*, Vol. 31, No. 19 (Oct 2010), pp. 2338-2350. 1522-9645

Ting, C. T., Brin, K. P., Lin, S. J., Wang, S. P., Chang, M. S., Chiang, B. N., & Yin, F. C. (1986). Arterial hemodynamics in human hypertension. *The Journal of Clinical Investigations*, Vol. 78, No. 6 (Dec 1986), pp. 1462-1471. 0021-9738

Tounian, P., Aggoun, Y., Dubern, B., Varille, V., Guy-Grand, B., Sidi, D., Girardet, J. P., & Bonnet, D. (2001). Presence of increased stiffness of the common carotid artery and endothelial dysfunction in severely obese children: a prospective study. *Lancet*, Vol. 358, No. 9291 (Oct 2001), pp. 1400-1404. 0140-6736

Tsivgoulis, G., Vemmos, K., Papamichael, C., Spengos, K., Daffertshofer, M., Cimboneriu, A., Zis, V., Lekakis, J., Zakopoulos, N., & Mavrikakis, M. (2006). Common carotid arterial stiffness and the risk of ischaemic stroke. *European Journal of Neurology*, Vol. 13, No. 5 (May 2006), pp. 475-481. 1351-5101

Van Bortel, L. M., Balkestein, E. J., van der Heijden-Spek, J. J., Vanmolkot, F. H., Staessen, J. A., Kragten, J. A., Vredeveld, J. W., Safar, M. E., Struijker Boudier, H. A., & Hoeks, A. P. (2001). Non-invasive assessment of local arterial pulse pressure: comparison of applanation tonometry and echo-tracking. *Journal of Hypertension*, Vol. 19, No. 6 (Jun 2001), pp. 1037-1044. 0263-6352

Van Bortel, L. M., Duprez, D., Starmans-Kool, M. J., Safar, M. E., Giannattasio, C., Cockcroft, J., Kaiser, D. R., & Thuillez, C. (2002). Clinical applications of arterial stiffness, Task Force III: recommendations for user procedures. *American Journal of Hypertension*, Vol. 15, No. 5 (May 2002), pp. 445-452. 0895-7061

van Dijk, R. A., Dekker, J. M., Nijpels, G., Heine, R. J., Bouter, L. M., & Stehouwer, C. D. (2001). Brachial artery pulse pressure and common carotid artery diameter: mutually independent associations with mortality in subjects with a recent history of impaired glucose tolerance. *European Journal of Clinical Investigations*, Vol. 31, No. 9 (Sept 2001), pp. 756-763. 0014-2972

van Popele, N. M., Grobbee, D. E., Bots, M. L., Asmar, R., Topouchian, J., Reneman, R. S., Hoeks, A. P., van der Kuip, D. A., Hofman, A., & Witteman, J. C. (2001). Association Between Arterial Stiffness and Atherosclerosis: The Rotterdam Study. *Stroke*, Vol. 32, No. 2 (2001), pp. 454-460.

van Popele, N. M., Mattace-Raso, F. U., Vliegenthart, R., Grobbee, D. E., Asmar, R., van der Kuip, D. A., Hofman, A., de Feijter, P. J., Oudkerk, M., & Witteman, J. C. (2006). Aortic stiffness is associated with atherosclerosis of the coronary arteries in older adults: the Rotterdam Study. *Journal of Hypertension*, Vol. 24, No. 12 (2006), pp. 2371-2376.

Vlachopoulos, C., Aznaouridis, K., & Stefanadis, C. (2010). Prediction of cardiovascular events and all-cause mortality with arterial stiffness: a systematic review and meta-analysis. *Journal of the American College of Cardiology*, Vol. 55, No. 13 (Mar 2010), pp. 1318-1327. 1558-3597

Vlachopoulos, C., Dima, I., Aznaouridis, K., Vasiliadou, C., Ioakeimidis, N., Aggeli, C., Toutouza, M., & Stefanadis, C. (2005). Acute systemic inflammation increases arterial stiffness and decreases wave reflections in healthy individuals. *Circulation*, Vol. 112, No. 14 (Oct 2005), pp. 2193-2200. 1524-4539

Weber, T., Ammer, M., Rammer, M., Adji, A., O'Rourke, M. F., Wassertheurer, S., Rosenkranz, S., & Eber, B. (2009). Noninvasive determination of carotid-femoral pulse wave velocity depends critically on assessment of travel distance: a comparison with invasive measurement. *Journal of Hypertension*, Vol. 27, No. 8 (Aug 2009), pp. 1624-1630. 1473-5598

Weber, T., Auer, J., O'Rourke, M. F., Kvas, E., Lassnig, E., Berent, R., & Eber, B. (2004). Arterial stiffness, wave reflections, and the risk of coronary artery disease. *Circulation*, Vol. 109, No. 2 (Jan 2004), pp. 184-189. 1524-4539

Widlansky, M. E., Gokce, N., Keaney, J. F., Jr., & Vita, J. A. (2003). The clinical implications of endothelial dysfunction. *Journal of the American College of Cardiology*, Vol. 42, No. 7 (Oct 2003), pp. 1149-1160. 0735-1097

Wilkinson, I. B., Mohammad, N. H., Tyrrell, S., Hall, I. R., Webb, D. J., Paul, V. E., Levy, T., & Cockcroft, J. R. (2002). Heart rate dependency of pulse pressure amplification and arterial stiffness. *American Journal of Hypertension*, Vol. 15, No. 1 (Jan 2002), pp. 24-30. 0895-7061

Wilkinson, I. B., Prasad, K., Hall, I. R., Thomas, A., MacCallum, H., Webb, D. J., Frenneaux, M. P., & Cockcroft, J. R. (2002). Increased central pulse pressure and augmentation index in subjects with hypercholesterolemia. *Journal of the American College of Cardiology*, Vol. 39, No. 6 (Mar 2002), pp. 1005-1011. 0735-1097

Woodman, R. J., Playford, D. A., Watts, G. F., Cheetham, C., Reed, C., Taylor, R. R., Puddey, I. B., Beilin, L. J., Burke, V., Mori, T. A., & Green, D. (2001). Improved analysis of brachial artery ultrasound using a novel edge-detection software system. *Journal of Applied Physiology*, Vol. 91, No. 2 (Aug 2001), pp. 929-937. 8750-7587

Zieman, S. J., Melenovsky, V., & Kass, D. A. (2005). Mechanisms, pathophysiology, and therapy of arterial stiffness. *Arteriosclerosis, Thrombosis, and Vascular Biology*, Vol. 25, No. 5 (May 2005), pp. 932-943. 1524-4636

7

The Role of Ultrasonography in the Assessment of Arterial Baroreflex Function

Yu-Chieh Tzeng
Cardiovascular Systems Laboratory
University of Otago
New Zealand

1. Introduction

Cardiovascular disease is the leading cause of mortality in the developed world [1]. Experimental research indicates that in addition to traditional risk factors such as hypertension and dyslipidemia, dysfunction of the autonomic nervous system is also a powerful independent risk factor for death from cardiovascular disease. Although not yet routinely assessed in clinical practice, depressed baroreflex function increases the risk of death following myocardial infarction [2], in chronic heart failure [3], and recent trials also clearly indicate an increased risk for both ischemic and hemorrhagic stroke [4, 5]. In the context of these morbid epidemiological correlations, it is not difficult to justify the need for a better understanding of the mechanisms and factors involved in normal human baroreflex regulation.

Ultrasonography has played a vital role over the past decades not only in clinical medicine but also in advancing our understanding of fundamental biological processes. This proposition is certainly true for human cardiovascular research, where the non-invasive nature of ultrasonography has enabled physiologists and clinicians to study regulatory mechanisms that could otherwise only be examined in animal models under sedation or anaesthesia. The aim of this chapter is to review the pivotal role that ultrasonography has played in advancing our understanding of human baroreflex function. The chapter will begin with an overview of the human baroreflex in section 2 with particular emphasis on cardio-vagal regulation of the heart, and vascular sympathetic regulation of peripheral vascular resistance. Section 3 will introduce the technical application of ultrasonography in baroreflex research with emphasis on the use of B-mode imaging in the evaluation of the mechanical and neural components of the baroreflex arc. Important practical, analytical, and physiological considerations will be discussed. Finally, the literature will be reviewed in section 4 to illustrate how the practical application of vascular ultrasound imaging has lead to deeper insights into the workings of the human baroreflex not otherwise possible.

2. Physiology of the baroreflex

The arterial baroreflex is critical to both short and long term regulation of blood pressure. The sensory components of this reflex comprise of stretch sensitive nerve endings situated in vessel walls of some arteries, particularly in the carotid sinus and the aortic arch that respond to changes in vascular distention pressure by altering afferent discharge activity in the carotid sinus nerve (a branch of the glossopharyngeal nerve) and the aortic nerves.

Afferent baroreceptor inputs project to regions of the nucleus tractus solitarius, which extends almost over the entire length of the medulla and is the exclusive first relay station and integration area for afferent baroreceptor information [6]. Numerous inter-connections exist between the nucleus tractus solitarius and other structures important in the baroreflex, including the hypothalamus, amygdala, parabrachial nuclei, subfornical organ, cerebellum, and rostral ventrolateral medulla [7]. However, the precise central interneuronal connections that drive parasympathetic and sympathetic motoneurons, and the locations of vagal-cardiac motoneurons have not been located in humans. In animals they are found in variable locations, including the nucleus ambigus in the cat [8], and dorsal motor nucleus of the vagus in dogs and monkeys [9]. Sympathetic pre-ganglionic motoneurons are located in the intermediolateral column of the spinal cord [10]. Irrespective of the precise central neuronal connections mediating the baroreflex, it is clear that the end effector response to arterial baroreflex stimulation is an increase in efferent vagal activity, and a decrease in efferent sympathetic activity [11].

The efferent limbs of the baroreflex can be functionally considered as consisting of a cardiac component and a vascular component. The cardiac baroreflex refers to the prompt adjustment of heart rate, stroke volume (and therefore cardiac output) in response to changes in blood pressure. These responses are mediated primarily via the vagus nerve because they are markedly attenuated following surgical vagotomy and muscarinic cholinergic [12]. In healthy humans at rest, and during exercise, the cardiac baroreflex can respond rapidly with cardiac period intervals beginning to adjust within 0.5 sec following baroreceptor loading with neck suction [13]. Although maximal responses increase with advancing age, in the young, they generally takes place within 3-4 seconds following baroreceptor loading, and 2-3 sec following baroreceptor unloading respectively in the young [14]. Reflex alterations in heart rate can also arise due to the action of the sympathetic nervous system. Increased sympathetic activity can increase heart rate via the release of noradrenalin in postganglionic nerve terminals, or the release of adrenaline into the systemic circulation from the adrenal medulla. It is important to recognize that whereas the chronotropic response of the heart to baroreflex stimulation is dominated by vagal activity (via the release of acetylcholine), the inotropic responses to baroreflex stimulation responsible for changes in stroke volume are mediated via the sympathetic nervous systems.

In contrast, the vascular baroreflex refers to regulation of peripheral vascular smooth muscle tone. The major site of vascular resistance is thought to reside in the arterioles and capillaries, which in the systemic circulation are densely innervated with post-ganglionic sympathetic fibers. Although sympathetic regulation of venous tone is not a key determinant of peripheral vascular resistance, venous constriction influences blood volume distribution. The reaction times of the vascular sympathetic baroreflex are slower compared to cardiac responses. Even though changes in sympathetic nerve activity can occur with latencies of ~200ms after changes of afferent nervous activity to the central nervous system, the lag times associated with sympathetic neurovascular transduction at the level of the neuromuscular junction are substantially longer such that the first changes in end organ response are seen only after 2-3 seconds. The maintenance of blood pressure therefore requires the effective regulation and integration of both the cardiac and vascular baroreflex arc.

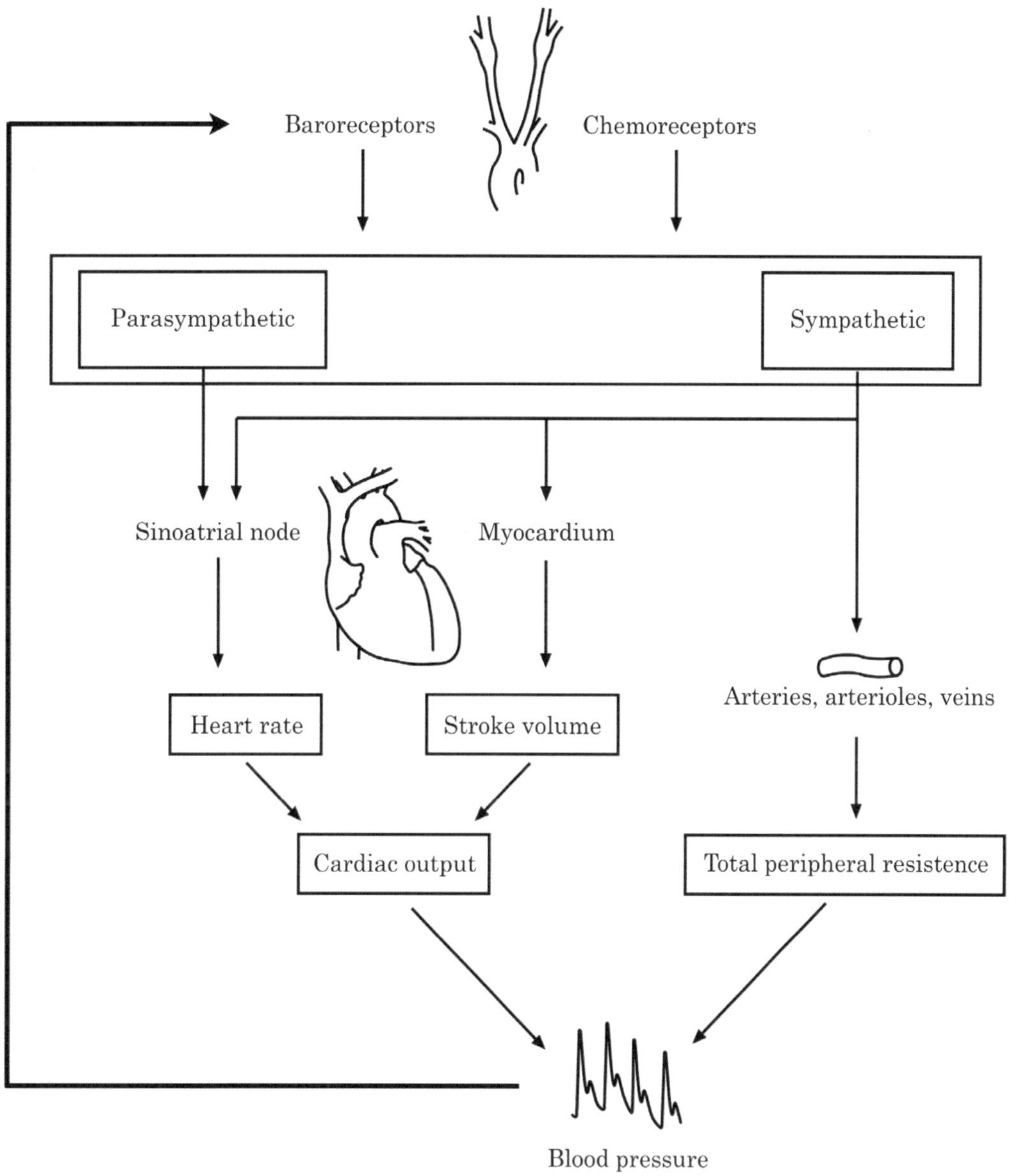

Fig. 1. Schematic showing the major mechanistic pathways involved with short-term systemic blood pressure control. Note that in vivo the baroreflex arc is a closed-loop system.

3. Assessment of the mechanical and neural components of the cardiac baroreflex

3.1 Overview

Baroreflex gain has traditionally been quantified as the relation between changes in arterial blood pressure and cardiac period (R-R intervals), heart rate, or sympathetic nerve activity. This analysis assumes that blood pressure is the input that drives reflex autonomic changes. However, baroreceptors respond to mechanical deformation and not the pressure *per se*. Therefore, the transduction of blood pressure into barosensory stretch, and the consequent transduction of barosensory stretch into efferent parasympathetic and sympathetic neural outflow are critical steps that determine the integrated baroreflex response. The major contribution of vascular ultrasound imaging to baroreflex research has been the enabling of these critical components of the integrated baroreflex arc to be studied separately and non-invasively in humans through the use of B and M-mode imaging processes [15].

In principal, the imaging analysis can be combined with any baroreflex assessment technique provided adequate ultrasound images can be obtained. In practice, however, apart from the modified Oxford method, the approach has only been successfully applied in subjects performing the Valsalva maneuver [16] and under steady state resting conditions using linear transfer function analysis [17]. Therefore, considering the relative novelty of the approach, and the fact that no method can be considered the gold standard, investigators wishing to undertake this form of analysis should choose their approach based on their unique experimental requirements, and an understanding of the analytical and theoretical shortcomings of each method. In this section, methods that are *technically* suitable for this form of analysis from an imaging perspective will be presented in context of some of these considerations. Beyond the scope are methods that do not permit the accurate acquisition of carotid images (e.g. neck suction/pressure, dynamic squat-stand maneuvers) and techniques based on highly controversial physiological assumptions (e.g. spontaneous sequence method, high frequency transfer function gain) [18, 19].

3.2 Carotid ultrasound scanning protocol

The assessment begins with the identification of wall boundaries, which appear as parallel echogenic lines separated by a hypoechonic space in longitudinal B-mode image (figure 2). Although the internal carotid, bulb, and common carotid arteries can all be imaged (figure 3), the latter generally yields the best image quality because the vessel course is parallel to the surface of the skin and is positioned at right angles to the ultrasound beam. The first echo along the far wall corresponds to the lumen-intima interface whilst the second and normally brighter echo corresponds to the media-adventitia interface. The echolucent zone in between corresponds to the media. It is important to recognize that interfaces may be difficult to discern when the near and far walls of the vessels are curvilinear and not at right angels to the ultrasound beam. Therefore, within the carotid bulb where the walls flare and dilate, or along the proximal internal carotid where the walls do not lie in parallel, only short segments of wall may be seen on a single frame. For these reasons, vascular distention waveforms are generally acquired 1-2cm of the bifurcation even though baroreceptor density is greatest at the carotid bulb. Other causes for the loss of wall interface that are unrelated to scanning technique include the presence of atherosclerotic plaques or the presence of fat in the arterial wall.

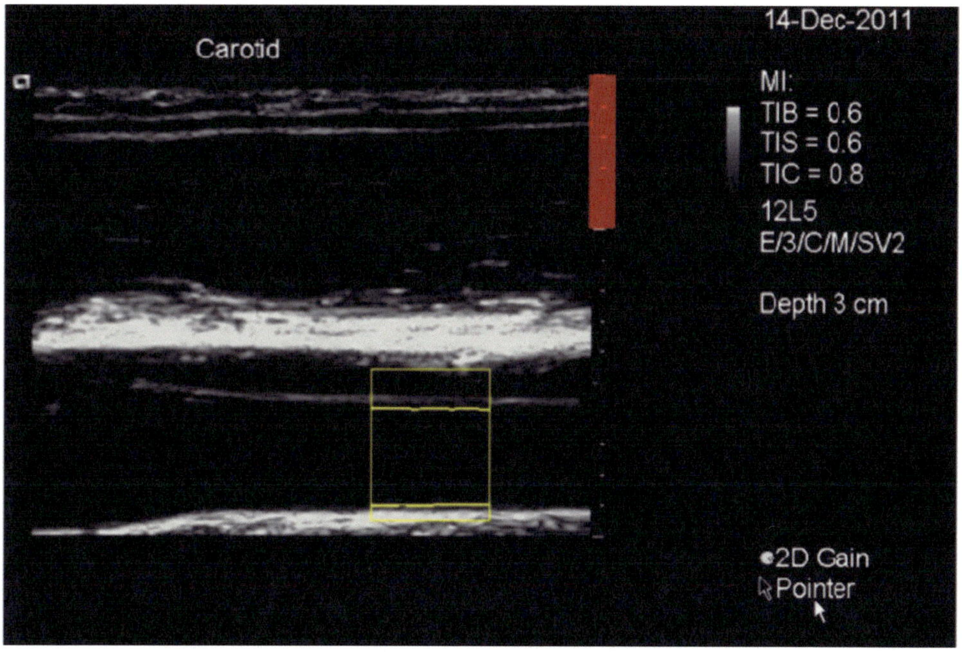

Fig. 2. Sample screen shot showing the custom edge tracking of the carotid luminal diameter.

Studies are conducted using linear array probes (7.5-13 Mhz) with the subjects head tilted ~45° away from the side of the study to capture a longitudinal section of the common carotid artery ~1 cm proximal to the bifurcation. This usually requires an initial cursory scan to orient the sonographer to the subject's carotid anatomy to establish the site of the bifurcation and to differentiate between the internal and the external the external carotid artery. Upon identifying the distance common carotid immediately proximal to the bulb, the probe should be manipulated to optimize the view of the arterial wall such that the lumen-intima and media-adventitia interfaces over a 1-cm length can be clearly displayed. Images should be captured as close to a 45 degrees angle as possible and both the near and far walls should be clearly visible for robust analysis.

The continuous digital video screen shot of the optimized B-mode images are then recorded and saved for offline analysis using custom written edge-tracking software (figure 2). The region of interest is calibrated for length, and using a pixel-density algorithm the vessel walls are tracked and diameter measured at 30 Hz resolution for the entire video that encompassed the Oxford trial. In contrast to methods originally described by Hunt et al., where hardware limitations meant that image sets could only be acquired on approximately every other cardiac cycle, our technique enables the carotid diameter data to be acquired for every cardiac cycle throughout the duration of the baroreflex test (~3 minutes). High resolution tracking of carotid distension waveforms can also be obtained using a number of commercially available systems that employ interlaced M-mode and B-mode imaging, such as the ART.Lab system (Esaote, Maastrict) or the QFM-21 (Haedco, Japan). However, the use of A-mode imaging with the QFM-21 limits the utility of this device given there is no visual feedback in B-mode to guide the accurate placement of the probe relative to the length of the carotid artery.

Method	Strength	Weaknesses
Modified Oxford method	Partial open loop analysis of baroreflex gain Not confounded by differences in respiration rate Enables the assessment of baroreflex hysteresis Evaluate cardiac baroreflex gain as well as the neural arc of the smpathetic baroreflex	Invasive procedure require venous cannulation Potential influence of drugs on vascular transduction Does not permit evaluation of sympathetic neurovascular transduction given the use of vasoactive drugs Subjectivity of analysis
Valsalva manuever	Non-invasive Non-pharmacological Partial open loop analysis of baroreflex gain Enables the assessment of baroreflex hysteresis Evaluate both cardiac and symaptethic baroreflex function	Need for subject compliance Poor consistency across subjects
Spectral methods	Non-invasive Non-pharmacological Does not permit assessment of baroreflex hysteresis Prone to confounding by changes in respiration	Liable to confounding by non-baroreflex mediated fluctuations in vagal outflow (e.g. respiration) Controversial physiological assumptions Closed-loop analysis

Table 1. Comparison of methods for the assessment of baroreflex function

3.3 Overview of techniques and data analysis

The following overview summaries the data analysis that is involved in the quantification of integrated, mechanical and neural baroreflex gains. Only methods involving general linear regression and linear transfer function analysis will be outlined. Higher order mathematical models of baroreflex function fall outside the scope of this chapter.

The modified Oxford method

In 1969 Smyth et al., proposed a method for assessing arterial baroreflex gain that involved regressing reflex cardiac interval responses to systolic blood pressure changes induced with vasoactive drugs [20]. Commonly referred to as the 'Oxford method', this technique has become widely regarded as the gold standard measure of baroreflex function. Although the assessment was originally carried out using bolus injections of angiotensin, the method has undergone many incremental modifications since its introduction. These include, for example, the use of drugs with minimal direct cardiac chronotropic effects, and the administration of vasodilator and vasoconstriction drugs in sequence to enable the complete characterization of both the cardiac and sympathetic baroreflex function (modified 'Oxford method').

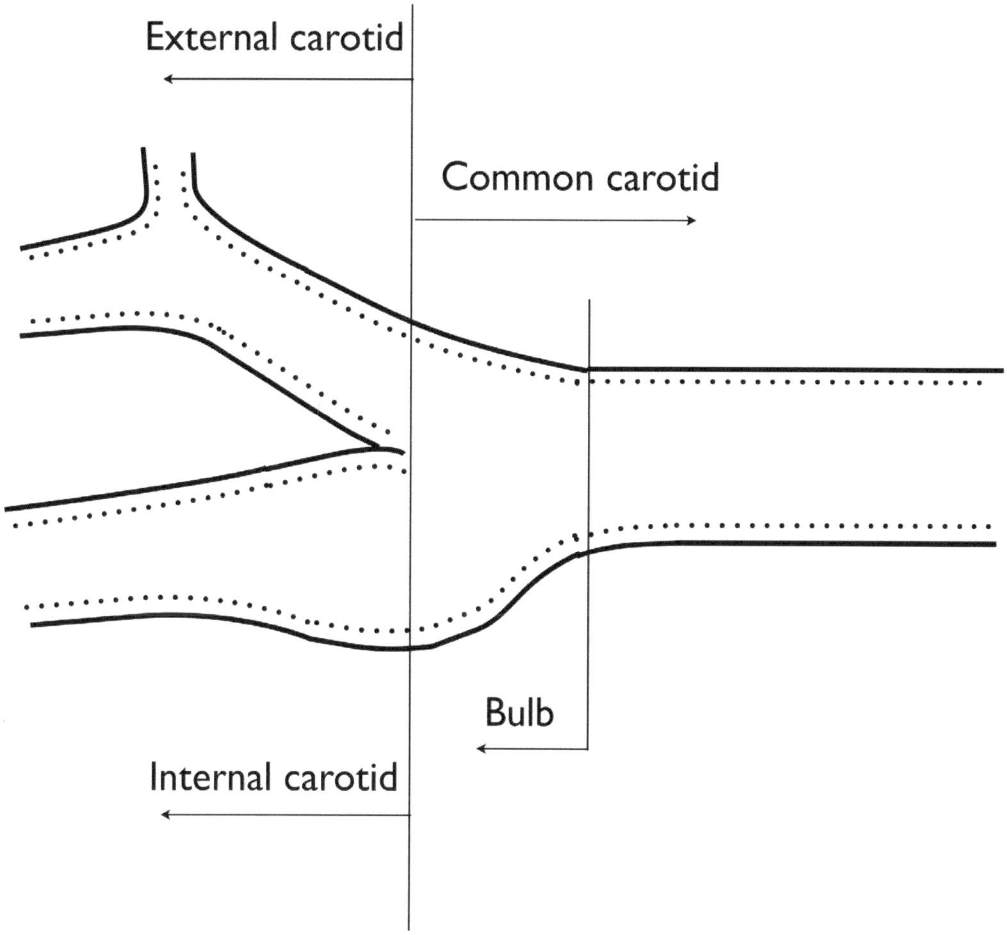

Fig. 3. Schematic showing the common, internal and external carotid arteries. The carotid bulb can be recognized in most subjects as the site where common carotid dilates slightly and the vessel walls flare out such that they're no longer parallel to each other. The elliptically shaped bulb is geometrically complex in the longitudinal view and therefore can be difficult to image in its entirety within a single frame. The external carotid artery lies anterior and medial to the internal carotid in 90% of subjects but is reversed in the remaining 10%. The internal carotid artery is generally larger than the external carotid, and has no braches as it ascends into the skull to supply the brain, whereas the external carotid has branches that supply the neck and face.

A key advantage of the method is that blood pressure can be perturbed across a wide range within a sufficiently short time frame to *clearly* engage the baroreflex. This is a critical consideration given the baroreflex is a closed-loop system (figure 1) and accurate quantification of input-output relations in theory requires the loop to be opened. Whilst the open-loop condition cannot be meet under the majority of human experimental settings, the active perturbation of blood pressure does allow the loop to be partial-opened to yield robust estimates of baroreflex gain [21]. The key objection to the Oxford method relates to the use of vaso-active agents, which may exert unquantifiable effects on baroreceptor transduction, cardiopulmonary afferent activity and sinus node activity. However, the practical significance of these concerns remains unclear. Other strengths and weaknesses of the method are summarized in Table 1.

Technically the modified Oxford method involves sequential intravenous bolus injections sodium nitroprusside (SNP) and phenylephrine hydrochloride (PE). Once recordings of hemodynamic measurements have begun, blood pressure should be carefully monitored and allowed to stabilize, after which the injection of SNP can be administered. This should be followed ~60 seconds later by the injection of PE. Recording can cease when systolic blood pressure began to plateau after the rise after the PE injection. Oxford trials, therefore, typically last 120 to 180 seconds. Doses given for SNP and PE are typically 150 and 200g, respectively, although this should be adjusted on an individual basis if an insufficient blood pressure perturbation is achieved (systolic blood pressure change <15 mm Hg). It is common practice to account for known baroreflex delays, which can be done by matching systolic blood pressure values to either the concurrent heartbeat for R-R intervals >800 ms or a 1 beat delay for shorter heart periods (typically between 500 and 800 ms). Due to baroreflex hysteresis, baroreflex sensitivities should be calculated separately for SNP and PE injections to identify the gain (or sensitivity) against falling and rising blood pressure.

Figure 4 shows a representative tracing of heart rate, carotid artery lumen diameter, and finger blood pressure during a modified Oxford baroreflex test sequence. For the assessment of cardio-vagal BRS, the pressure to R-R interval relation for falling pressures are examined at the onset of the systolic blood pressure decrease, which typically occur ~30 sec after the bolus injection of SNP, and ends when systolic blood pressure reached its nadir. For rising pressures, data selection begins at the nadir in systolic blood pressure and end when pressure peaks after the bolus injection of PE.

It is common for the identification and elimination of the saturation and threshold regions to be done via visual data inspection [22, 23]. However, mathematical modeling procedures can be applied for more objective analysis. For example, a piecewise linear regression can be applied to the raw data points to statistically identify breakpoints that occur at the upper and lower ends of the data set (Figure 5) [24, 25]. Other approaches for the objective identification of cardiac-vagal BRS have been reported in the literature including the use sigmoid [26], logistic [27] and elliptical functions [28].

Typically, an arbitrary threshold for the correlation coefficient of the linear segment is set at 0.6 to justify the use of a linear regression model. It is also conventional to account for respiratory-related fluctuations in R-R interval and systolic blood pressure by averaging R-R intervals or heart rate across 2 or 3 mm Hg bins. However, although data binning improves the correlation coefficients, neither respiratory rate [23] nor data binning [26] materially influence the magnitude of the gain estimates.

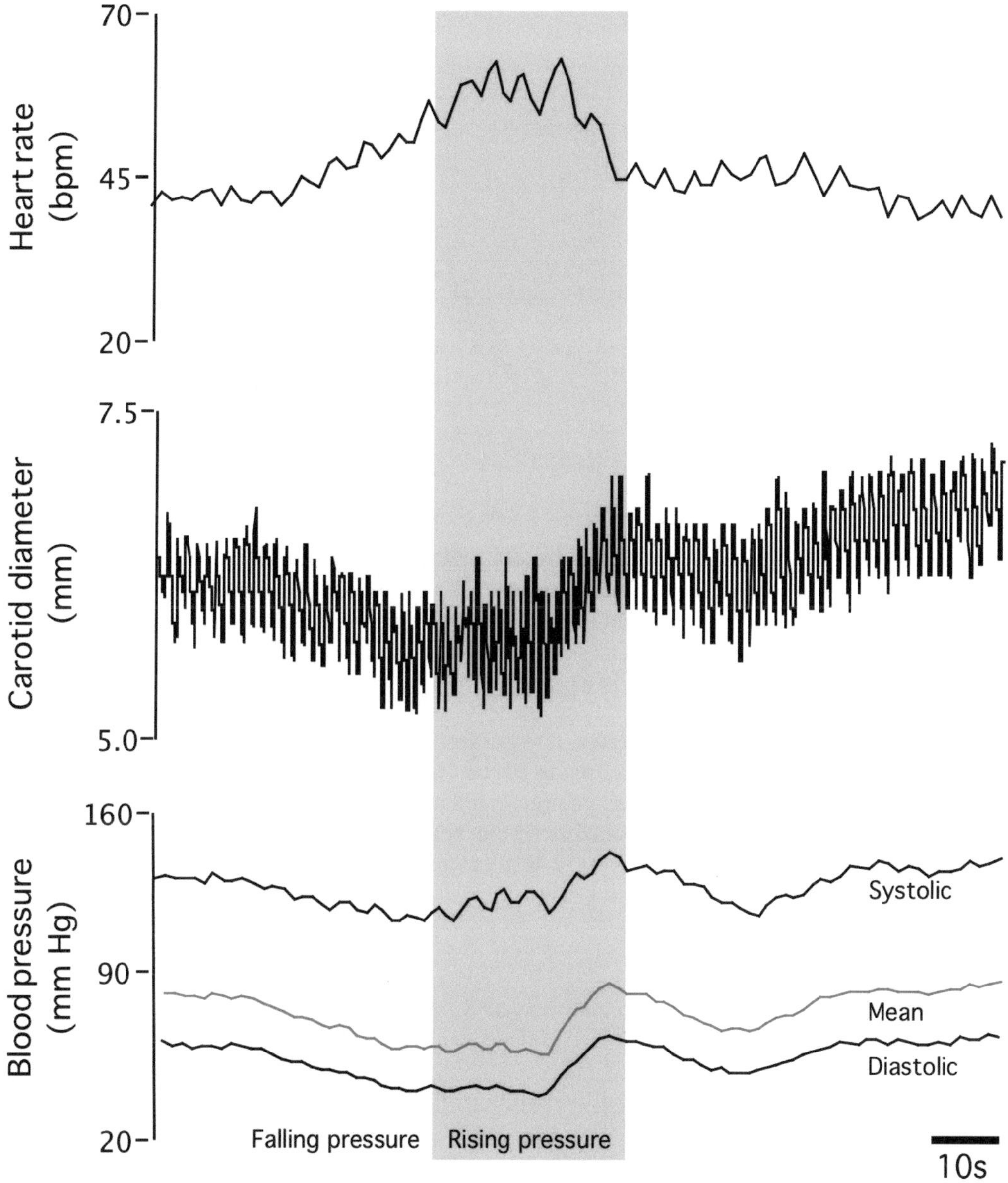

Fig. 4. Representative recording of a modified Oxford baroreflex test sequence. Intravenous bolus injections of sodium nitroprusside were followed ~60 s later by phenylephrine hydrochloride. The grey scale areas indicate the data segments typically taken for the determination of baroreflex gain.

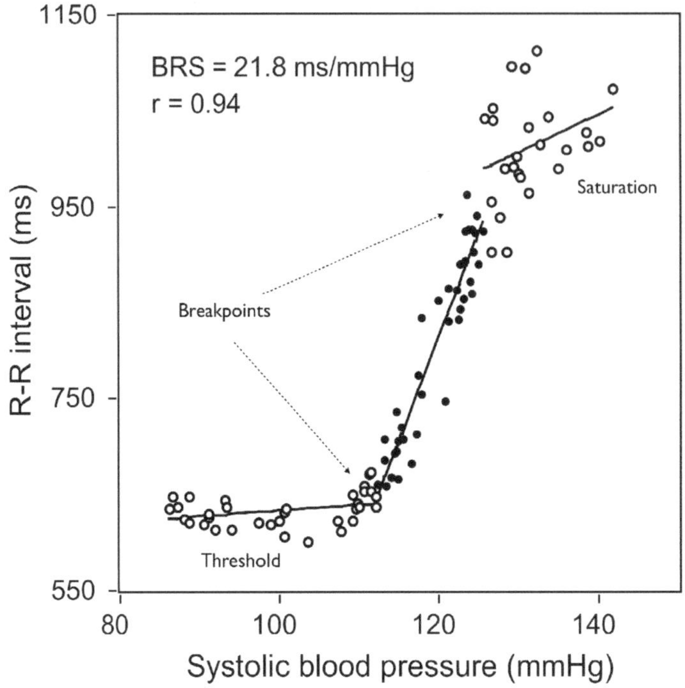

Fig. 5. Piecewise regression model for elimination of threshold and saturation regions of the integrated baroreflex response to rising pressures. Open circles (○) represent the threshold and saturation regions and the closed circles (•) represent the linear portion of the baroreflex gain. Arrows indicate breakpoints that separate the threshold, saturation, and linear region (Adapted from Taylor et al., 2011).

The gain of the mechanical and neural components can be calculated separately for both rising and falling pressures, with exclusion of the threshold and saturation regions as done for the assessment of integrated gain. For the mechanical component, systolic carotid lumen diameter measurements within a cardiac cycle should be plotted against systolic blood pressure, and for the neural component, R-R intervals or heart rate should be plotted against systolic carotid lumen diameter (figure 6).

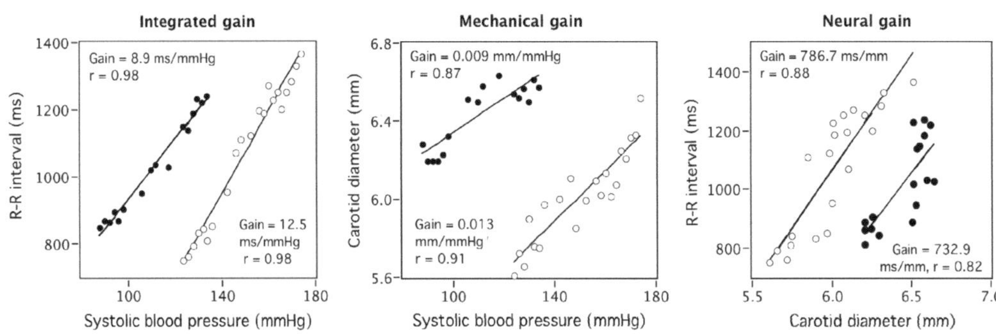

Fig. 6. Integrated, mechanical and neural gains for rising pressures in the morning (•) and afternoon (○) for one subject. (adapted from Taylor et a., 2011).

For assessment of integrated, mechanical, and neural components of the sympathetic baroreflex, simple linear regression procedures are generally applied but with few modifications. First, instead of systolic lumen diameters and systolic pressures, integrated and mechanical gains for the sympathetic arc are derived using diastolic lumen diameters and diastolic blood pressure. This is because diastolic pressure correlates more strongly to sympathetic activity, which in humans are generally recordings of muscle sympathetic nerve activity (MSNA) made in the peroneal nerve [29]. Second, sympathetic activity has a bursting pattern that rarely maintains a 1:1 relation with cardiac cycles even at low blood pressures where baroreflex-mediated sympatho-inhibition is low. Therefore, pharmacological baroreflex testing across a wide range of blood pressures invariably results in an over-representation of cardiac cycles with zero sympathetic activity. To account for this error, cardiac cycles can be weighted according to the presence or absence of observable sympathetic bursts. For example, cardiac cycles with zero's below the lowest pressure associated with a sympathetic burst are assigned a weight of 0 ('false' zero) whereas zeros above the highest pressure associated with a sympathetic burst were assigned a weight of 1 ('true' zero) [30]. Some groups employ data binning (e.g. across 3mmHg blood pressure increments) to reduce the statistical impact of inherent beat-to-beat variability in nerve activity [31], which are generally represented as total integrated sympathetic activity (i.e. the product of burst frequency and average burst area in arbitrary units).

The Valsalva maneuver

The Valsalva maneuver was first described by Antonia Maria Valsalva in the 17th century as a method for testing the patency of the Eustachian tube. However, the maneuver has gained subsequent acceptance as a means of stressing the baroreflex due to its well-characterized effects on cardiac output, venous return, and blood pressure. Essentially the maneuver involves forced expiration against a closed glottis, or a short tube to enhance expiratory resistance. Mouth pressure is measured and maintained at a constant level (e.g. 40 mmHg) for 15 seconds. Figure 7 shows the typical response in blood pressure and heart rate (MSNA not shown), which have been characterized into four phases. Phase one is the initial blood pressure rise and heart rate and MSNA reduction (via the baroreflex) due to a mild rise in stroke volume secondary to elevated intrathoracic pressure forcing blood out of the pulmonary circulation into the left atrium. The sustained elevation in introthoracic pressure

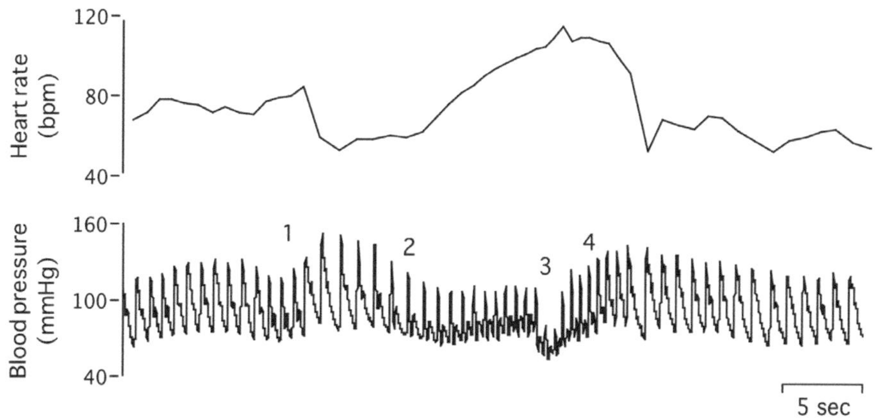

Fig. 7. Blood pressure and heart rate changes during the Valsalva manuver.

during phase two impedes venous return and consequently reduces cardiac output. This phase triggers a baroreflex mediated increase in heart rate and MSNA. Phase three commences with the pressure release and resumption of normal breathing. During this phase blood pressure decreases briefly as the external compression on the aorta is released and heart rate increases. This is followed by phase four as blood pressure starts to rise due to an increased in cardiac output secondary to a rapid increase in venous return, and the background of elevated sympathetic vascular resistance that occurred during phase two. During phase four, heart rate decreases and MSNA falls.

The regression approaches described for the modified Oxford method are also applicable to the Valsalva maneuver. In general, estimates of cardia-vagal baroreflex gain can be determined from both phase two or four of the response. However, satisfactory sympathetic baroreflex slopes may only be obtainable during phase two, given the relative paucity of sympathetic bursts during phase four [32].

Transfer function analysis

Integrated, neural, and mechanical baroreflex gains can be quantified using transfer-function analysis of spontaneously occurring low frequency (0.14-0.15 Hz) blood pressure, carotid lumen diameter, R-R interval, and normalized MSNA fluctuations. The data processing typically begins with interpolation (e.g. linear, spline) and re-sampling (1-4 Hz) of beat-to-beat systolic pressure, carotid lumen diameter, and R-R intervals to provide equidistant time series that are required for Fourier analysis. Due to noise inherent in finite data series, its common to apply the Welch averaging technique to minimize data variance in exchange for reduced frequency resolution. Welch averaging involves the subdivision of the entire data epoch into successive overlapping segments of equal lengths. The data within each window should be de-trended and passed through a Hanning window before spectral analysis. The frequency-domain transforms can be computed with a fast Fourier transformation algorithm. The transfer function H (*f*) between the two signals was calculated as:

$$H(f) = Sxy(f)/Sxx(f)$$

where $S_{xx}(f)$ is the autospectrum of input signal and $S_{xy}(f)$ is the cross-spectrum between the two signals. The transfer function gain $|H(f)|$ and phase spectrum $|\Phi(f)|$ were obtained from the real part $H_R(f)$ and imaginary part $H_I(f)$ of the complex transfer function:

$$|H(f)| = \{[HR(f)]2 + [HI(f)]2\}$$

$$\Phi(f) = \tan\text{-}1[HI(f)/HR(f)]$$

The squared coherence function MSC (f) was estimated as:

$$MSC(f) = |Sxy(f)|2/[Sxx(f)Syy(f)],$$

where $S_{yy}(f)$ is the autospectrum of changes in output signal. Given that transfer function analysis is a linear methodology that is yields only valid gain estimates if the cross-spectral coherence is sufficiently high. This threshold is conventionally set at 0.5 although lower thresholds have been applied.

According to this approach, the integrated cardiac baroreflex gain corresponds to the average systolic pressure to R-R interval transfer function gain within the low frequency range (0.04-0.15) [33]. The mechanical component is the average transfer function gain between systolic blood pressure and systolic carotid diameter fluctuations whereas the neural gain is the average systolic carotid diameter to R-R interval transfer function gain within the same frequency range. In theory the transduction of carotid diameter fluctuations to changes in MSNA can also be assessed although details of these transfer function characteristics in humans have not yet been reported in the literature.

The major advantage of the spontaneous spectral approach is that the assessment can be made non-invasively without the use of drugs or special provocation maneuvers (the procedure becomes invasive if MSNA recordings are made). However, there are important potential shortcomings with this technique. First, because input and output relationships between the various haemodynamics parameters are assessed under spontaneous conditions, the derived transfer function parameters reflect close-loop relations that may not accurately reflex open-loop gains [34]. Furthermore, the technique is highly liable to confounding from respiratory influences. For example, fluctuations in R-R intervals associated with respiratory activity (respiratory sinus arrhythmia) can merge, accentuate, and confound the magnitude of low frequency fluctuations if breathing rate falls within the low frequency range (i.e.<0.15Hz) [23]. Such respiratory influences need to be carefully controlled for and may be minimized with the use of pace respiration.

4. New insights into baroreflex physiology gain through the application of vascular ultrasound

The technical advances described in section 3 offer the potential for more detailed understanding of mechanisms underlying changes in baroreflex function not previously attainable in health and disease [35]. The following is a summary of new insights into baroreflex physiology that have been gained with the aid of ultrasonography.

4.1 Baroreflex hysteresis

It is well recognised that cardiac baroreflex function exhibits hysteresis; baroreflex responses are greater for rising vs. falling blood pressures. Hysteresis is an intrinsic feature to the cardiac baroreflex, and is observable with both pharmacologically induced changes in blood pressure (Pickering et al. 1972; Bonyhay et al. 1997; Rudas et al. 1999) and direct neck pressure stimulation (Eckberg & Sleight, 1992). This pattern of hysteresis has classically been attributed solely to the visoelastic properties of barosensory vessels such that, for a given blood pressure, vessel diameters are greater if the pressure was on the ascent. However, Studinger et al., showed that hysteresis derives not only from barosensory vessel mechanics, but also from complex interactions with neural resetting which often offset the changes in mechanical gain [24]. These findings further reinforce the concept that the integrated baroreflex gain derives from the combined influences of mechanical transduction of pressure into baroreceptor stretch, and neural transduction of baroreceptor stretch into vagal outflow.

4.2 Baroreflex changes with aerobic exercise

Although baroreflex impairment is a strong predictor of adverse cardiac and cerebrovascular outcomes, very few interventions have been shown to successful ameliorate the decline in baroreflex function associated with aging and cardiovascular disease. Some data suggest that aerobic exercise training may enhance cardiac baroreflex function although the mechanisms underpinning these changes are poorly understood. Using the valsalva technique, Komine et al., showed that in young men who had engaged in regular running exercise for ~80 min/day, 5 days/week for 6-7 years showed increases in arterial baroreflex gain through changes in the neural component of the baroreflex arc and not through alterations in carotid artery compliance [16]. Similarly, Deley showed that among previously sedentary elderly men and women, participation in a regular aerobic training program involving treadmill, elliptical training, and bicycle exercise at 70-80% heart rate reserve for six months enhanced baroreflex gain by 26%. The improvement in baroreflex gain was directly related to the amount of exercise performed and was derived primarily from changes in the neural component [36].

4.3 Effects of posture

Baroreflex function testing is generally conducted in the supine position. However, there are many activities in day-to-day living that produce physiological challenges and that have been associated with changes in baroreflex function, such as the assumption of an upright posture.[37] The risk of vasovagal syncope is greatly increased in the morning,[38] which may be associated with insufficient baroreflex function to maintain adequate blood pressure during orthostatic stress.[39] A number of studies have been performed to investigate the effects of orthostatic stress on integrated baroreflex function. The current consensus is that orthostatic stress augments vascular sympathetic gainand reduces cardio-vagal.[37, 40] Saeed et al., have provided further insight by showing that the differences in observed integrated BRS primarily arise from reduced mechanical transduction. These studies suggest that the propensity to orthostatic intolerance may be greater in those with structural vascular disease that affect the mechanical transduction properties of the integrated baroreflex arc.[41]

4.4 Stress response and baroreceptor function

Greater blood pressor responses to mental stress have been associated with greater risk of cardiovascular events, including the development of hypertension, stroke, coronary artery disease (CAD). Although blunting of baroreceptor function may underpin the exaggerated pressure responses associated with mental stress, the mechanisms underpinning the baroreceptor dysfunction are poorly understood. Deley et al., recently studied the mechanical and neural component of the baroreflex among healthy individuals and patients with documented coronary artery disease during the performance of a mental arithmetic and speaking task [42]. However, whilst patients with CAD showed exaggerated heart rate and blood pressure responses to the tasks, there were no differences in integrated, mechanical or neural baroreflex gains between healthy and CAD patients, which suggests that the augmented pressure response does not result from generalised baroreflex dysfunction.

4.5 Post exercise depression of baroreflex function

A single bout of moderate to high intensity exercise is associated with a period of post-exercise hypotension. Although the underlying cause of the hypotension remains unclear, studies have shown that following exercise in borderline hypertensive and young healthy subjects the integrated cardiac baroreflex gain changes dynamically. This change is characterised by an initial reduction [43] or no change [44] shortly after exercise (10-30 minutes), followed by elevation above baseline levels 40-55 minutes post exercise cessation. However, although these results clearly indicate that cardiac baroreflex function is altered during the post-exercise period, details regarding the sites and mechanisms underlying the changes remain entirely unknown.

Recently we examined for the first time the changes in cardiac baroreflex function before and at 10, 30, and 60 minutes after 40 minutes of cycling at 60% estimated maximal oxygen consumption.[45] We found that following aerobic exercise baroreflex gain is reduced and hysteresis manifests. The reduction in baroreflex gain to falling blood pressure is mediated by decreased mechanical and neural gains, whereas the decreased baroreflex gain to rising blood pressure is mediated by a reduced mechanical gain only. These findings indicate that impaired neural transduction of the cardiac baroreflex plays an important role in transient autonomic dysfunction after exercise that account for the increased propensity for syncope in the period immediately post exercise.

4.6 Diurnal variations in baroreflex function

We applied the technique to further understand the mechanisms underlying circadian variation in blood pressure, which exhibit a characteristic 'morning surge' following waking that has been linked to higher incidence of cardiac and cerebrovascular events [46]. We have shown that 1) the morning rise in blood pressure is related to overall reductions in integrated baroreflex gain, 2) that for falling pressures the lower integrated gain in the morning was caused by reduced neural gain compared with the afternoon, and 3) for rising pressures the lower integrated gain in the morning was caused by reduced mechanical gain compared with the afternoon [25]. These unique findings hold the prospect of guiding the development of future treatment strategies aimed at lowering cardio- and cerebrovascular events that occur more frequently in the morning. For example, given increases in blood pressure such as those that occur in the morning, may predispose to cerebral haemorrhage [47], hypertensive patients may benefit most from clinical interventions that focus augmenting the mechanical component by enhancing vascular properties. Conversely, individuals suffering from orthostatic intolerance, for which the risk is also greatest in the morning [48], may benefit from interventions aimed at enhancing the neural component [49].

5. References

[1] Grundy SM, D'Agostino Sr RB, Mosca L, Burke GL, Wilson PW, Rader DJ, Cleeman JI, Roccella EJ, Cutler JA, Friedman LM. Cardiovascular risk assessment based on us cohort studies: Findings from a national heart, lung, and blood institute workshop. *Circulation.* 2001;104:491-496.

[2] La Rovere MT, Pinna GD, Hohnloser SH, Marcus FI, Mortara A, Nohara R, Bigger JT, Jr., Camm AJ, Schwartz PJ. Baroreflex sensitivity and heart rate variability in the

identification of patients at risk for life-threatening arrhythmias: Implications for clinical trials. *Circulation.* 2001;103:2072-2077.
[3] La Rovere MT, Pinna GD, Maestri R, Robbi E, Caporotondi A, Guazzotti G, Sleight P, Febo O. Prognostic implications of baroreflex sensitivity in heart failure patients in the beta-blocking era. *J Am Coll Cardiol.* 2009;53:193-199.
[4] Sykora M, Diedler J, Rupp A, Turcani P, Rocco A, Steiner T. Impaired baroreflex sensitivity predicts outcome of acute intracerebral hemorrhage. *Crit Care Med.* 2008;36:3074-3079.
[5] Sykora M, Diedler J, Turcani P, Hacke W, Steiner T. Baroreflex: A new therapeutic target in human stroke? *Stroke.* 2009
[6] Jordan D, Spyer KM. Brainstem integration of cardiovascular and pulmonary afferent activity. *Prog Brain Res.* 1986;67:295-314.
[7] Scharf SM, Pinsky MR, Magder S. Heart-lung interactions. In: Scharf sm, pinsky mr, magder s, editors, respiratory-circulatory interactions in health and disease. Marcel dekker, new york, basel. 2001:1-7.
[8] Nosaka S, Yamamoto T, Yasunaga K. Localization of vagal cardioinhibitory preganglionic neurons with rat brain stem. *J Comp Neurol.* 1979;186:79-92.
[9] Gunn CG, Sevelius G, Puiggari J, Myers FK. Vagal cardiomotor mechanisms in the hindbrain of the dog and cat. *Am J Physiol.* 1968;214:258-262.
[10] Calaresu FR, Faiers AA, Mogenson GJ. Central neural regulation of heart and blood vessels in mammals. *Prog Neurobiol.* 1975;5:1-35.
[11] Fritsch JM, Smith ML, Simmons DT, Eckberg DL. Differential baroreflex modulation of human vagal and sympathetic activity. *Am J Physiol.* 1991;260:R635-641.
[12] Casadei B, Meyer TE, Coats AJ, Conway J, Sleight P. Baroreflex control of stroke volume in man: An effect mediated by the vagus. *J Physiol.* 1992;448:539-550.
[13] Eckberg DL, Kifle YT, Roberts VL. Phase relationship between normal human respiration and baroreflex responsiveness. *J Physiol.* 1980;304:489-502.
[14] Fisher JP, Kim A, Young CN, Ogoh S, Raven PB, Secher NH, Fadel PJ. Influence of ageing on carotid baroreflex peak response latency in humans. *J Physiol.* 2009;587:5427-5439.
[15] Hunt BE, Fahy L, Farquhar WB, Taylor JA. Quantification of mechanical and neural components of vagal baroreflex in humans. *Hypertension.* 2001;37:1362-1368.
[16] Komine H, Sugawara J, Hayashi K, Yoshizawa M, Yokoi T. Regular endurance exercise in young men increases arterial baroreflex sensitivity through neural alteration of baroreflex arc. *J Appl Physiol.* 2009;106:1499-1505.
[17] Saeed M, Link MS, Mahapatra S, Mouded M, Tzeng D, Jung V, Contreras R, Swygman C, Homoud M, Estes NA, 3rd, Wang PJ. Analysis of intracardiac electrograms showing monomorphic ventricular tachycardia in patients with implantable cardioverter-defibrillators. *Am J Cardiol.* 2000;85:580-587.
[18] Eckberg DL. Point:Counterpoint: Respiratory sinus arrhythmia is due to a central mechanism vs. Respiratory sinus arrhythmia is due to the baroreflex mechanism. *J Appl Physiol.* 2009;106:1740-1742.
[19] Karemaker JM. Counterpoint: Respiratory sinus arrhythmia is due to the baroreflex mechanism. *J Appl Physiol.* 2009;106:1742-1743.

[20] Smyth HS, Sleight P, Pickering GW. Reflex regulation of arterial pressure during sleep in man. A quantitative method of assessing baroreflex sensitivity. *Circ Res.* 1969;24:109-121.
[21] Diaz T, Taylor JA. Probing the arterial baroreflex: Is there a 'spontaneous' baroreflex? *Clin Auton Res.* 2006;16:256-261.
[22] Lipman RD, Salisbury JK, Taylor JA. Spontaneous indices are inconsistent with arterial baroreflex gain. *Hypertension.* 2003;42:481-487.
[23] Tzeng YC, Sin PY, Lucas SJ, Ainslie PN. Respiratory modulation of cardiovagal baroreflex sensitivity. *J Appl Physiol.* 2009;107:718-724.
[24] Studinger P, Goldstein R, Taylor JA. Mechanical and neural contributions to hysteresis in the cardiac vagal limb of the arterial baroreflex. *J Physiol.* 2007;583:1041-1048.
[25] Taylor CE, Atkinson G, Willie CK, Jones H, Ainslie PN, Tzeng YC. Diurinal variation in the mechanical and neural component of the baroreflex. *Hypertension.* 2011;Under review
[26] Hunt BE, Farquhar WB. Nonlinearities and asymmetries of the human cardiovagal baroreflex. *Am J Physiol Regul Integr Comp Physiol.* 2005;288:R1339-1346.
[27] Leitch JW, Newling R, Nyman E, Cox K, Dear K. Limited utility of the phenylephrine-nitroprusside sigmoid curve method of measuring baroreflex function after myocardial infarction. *J Cardiovasc Risk.* 1997;4:179-184.
[28] Ler AS, Cohen MA, Taylor JA. A planar elliptical model of cardio-vagal hysteresis. *Physiol Meas.* 2010;31:857-873.
[29] Vallbo AB, Hagbarth KE, Torebjork HE, Wallin BG. Somatosensory, proprioceptive, and sympathetic activity in human peripheral nerves. *Physiol Rev.* 1979;59:919-957.
[30] Studinger P, Goldstein R, Taylor JA. Age- and fitness-related alterations in vascular sympathetic control. *J Physiol.* 2009;587:2049-2057.
[31] Hart EC, Joyner MJ, Wallin BG, Karlsson T, Curry TB, Charkoudian N. Baroreflex control of muscle sympathetic nerve activity: A nonpharmacological measure of baroreflex sensitivity. *Am J Physiol Heart Circ Physiol.* 2010;298:H816-822.
[32] Kamiya A, Iwase S, Kitazawa H, Mano T, Vinogradova OL, Kharchenko IB. Baroreflex control of muscle sympathetic nerve activity after 120 days of 6 degrees head-down bed rest. *Am J Physiol Regul Integr Comp Physiol.* 2000;278:R445-452.
[33] Electrophysiology TFotESoCatNASoPa. Heart rate variability: Standards of measurement, physiological interpretation and clinical use. *Circulation.* 1996;93:1043-1065.
[34] Kamiya A, Kawada T, Shimizu S, Sugimachi M. Closed-loop spontaneous baroreflex transfer function is inappropriate for system identification of neural arc but partly accurate for peripheral arc: Predictability analysis. *J Physiol.* 2011;589:1769-1790.
[35] Halliwill JR, Taylor JA, Hartwig TD, Eckberg DL. Augmented baroreflex heart rate gain after moderate-intensity, dynamic exercise. *Am J Physiol.* 1996;270:R420-426.
[36] Deley G, Picard G, Taylor JA. Arterial baroreflex control of cardiac vagal outflow in older individuals can be enhanced by aerobic exercise training. *Hypertension.* 2009;53:826-832.
[37] O'Leary DD, Kimmerly DS, Cechetto AD, Shoemaker JK. Differential effect of head-up tilt on cardiovagal and sympathetic baroreflex sensitivity in humans. *Exp Physiol.* 2003;88:769-774.

[38] Mineda Y, Sumiyoshi M, Tokano T, Yasuda M, Nakazato K, Nakazato Y, Nakata Y, Yamaguchi H. Circadian variation of vasovagal syncope. *J Cardiovasc Electrophysiol.* 2000;11:1078-1080.

[39] Cooper VL, Hainsworth R. Effects of head-up tilting on baroreceptor control in subjects with different tolerances to orthostatic stress. *Clin Sci (Lond).* 2002;103:221-226.

[40] Taylor JA, Eckberg DL. Fundamental relations between short-term rr interval and arterial pressure oscillations in humans. *Circulation.* 1996;93:1527-1532.

[41] Saeed NP, Reneman RS, Hoeks AP. Contribution of vascular and neural segments to baroreflex sensitivity in response to postural stress. *J Vasc Res.* 2009;46:469-477.

[42] Deley G, Lipman RD, Kannam JP, Bartolini C, Taylor JA. Stress responses and baroreflex function in coronary disease. *J Appl Physiol.* 2009;106:576-581.

[43] Somers VK, Conway J, LeWinter M, Sleight P. The role of baroreflex sensitivity in post-exercise hypotension. *J Hypertens Suppl.* 1985;3:S129-130.

[44] Halliwill JR, Taylor JA, Eckberg DL. Impaired sympathetic vascular regulation in humans after acute dynamic exercise. *J Physiol.* 1996;495 (Pt 1):279-288.

[45] Willie CK, Ainslie PN, Taylor CE, Jones H, Sin PY, Tzeng YC. Neuromechanical features of the cardiac baroreflex after exercise. *Hypertension.* 2011;57:927-933.

[46] Elliott WJ. Circadian variation in the timing of stroke onset: A meta-analysis. *Stroke.* 1998;29:992-996.

[47] Muller JE, Tofler GH, Willich SN, Stone PH. Circadian variation of cardiovascular disease and sympathetic activity. *J Cardiovasc Pharmacol.* 1987;10 Suppl 2:S104-109; discussion S110-101.

[48] Lewis NC, Atkinson G, Lucas SJ, Grant EJ, Jones H, Tzeng YC, Horsman H, Ainslie PN. Diurnal variation in time to presyncope and associated circulatory changes during a controlled orthostatic challenge. *Am J Physiol Regul Integr Comp Physiol.* 2010;299:R55-61.

[49] Thomas KN, Burgess KR, Basnyat R, Lucas SJ, Cotter JD, Fan JL, Peebles KC, Lucas RA, Ainslie PN. Initial orthostatic hypotension at high altitude. *High Alt Med Biol.* 2010;11:163-167.

8

Detection of Intracardiac and Intrapulmonary Shunts at Rest and During Exercise Using Saline Contrast Echocardiography

Andrew T. Lovering and Randall D. Goodman
University of Oregon, Oregon Heart & Vascular Institute, USA

1. Introduction

Ultrasound has become a valuable tool for making non-invasive physiological measurements that are clinically important, one of which is detection of anatomic shunts using saline contrast echocardiography. Right-to-left intrapulmonary and intracardiac shunts are clinically relevant for two reasons. First, they allow deoxygenated blood to mix with oxygenated blood, thereby reducing the overall efficiency of pulmonary gas exchange. Thus, the opening of either intrapulmonary or intracardiac shunts at rest and/or during exercise may play a role in determining pulmonary gas exchange efficiency (Sun *et al.*, 2002; Stickland & Lovering, 2006; Lovering *et al.*, 2011). The opening of these shunts may also explain why some people with pulmonary diseases such as chronic obstructive pulmonary disease (COPD) desaturate so profoundly during even mild exercise (Miller *et al.*, 1984; Dansky *et al.*, 1992). The second reason that these pathways are clinically relevant is that anatomic right-to-left shunts may allow for thrombi to bypass the pulmonary capillary filter. Indeed, a patent foramen ovale and pulmonary arteriovenous malformations are associated with increased risk for neurological sequelae such as migraines, transient ischemic attacks and stroke (Movsowitz *et al.*, 1992; Petty *et al.*, 1997; De Castro *et al.*, 2000; Lamy *et al.*, 2002).

Where there is a right-to-left shunt it is likely that there may also be a left-to-right shunt following the same path but during a different phase of the cardiac and/or respiratory cycle. Left-to-right shunts are clinically relevant because they can result in right heart volume overload and irreversible pulmonary hypertension (Mulder, 2010). Thus, evidence of right heart chamber enlargement or right-to-left shunt by saline contrast echocardiography is sufficient reason for further investigation to rule out significant left-to-right shunting.

This chapter will focus on the ultrasound measurements used for detecting anatomic right-to-left shunts at rest, during exercise and during pharmacological-induced stress in both clinical and research settings. We also include a section on recent findings from our lab and others using saline contrast to detect right-to-left shunts in healthy human subjects and subjects with COPD.

2. Right-to-left intrapulmonary and intracardiac shunt

Intracardiac shunts include patent foramen ovale (PFO), atrial septal defects (ASD) and ventricular septal defects (VSD). It is generally accepted that 25 to 30% of the general population has a probe-patent foramen ovale (Hagen *et al.*, 1984). Interestingly, recent estimates of the prevalence of PFO using saline contrast echocardiography suggest a slightly higher prevalence of approximately 40% (Woods *et al.*, 2010; Elliott *et al.*, 2011b). The association of PFO with neurological sequelae such as migraine, transient ischemic attack and stroke make these pathways highly clinically relevant (Homma *et al.*, 1997; Petty *et al.*, 1997; De Castro *et al.*, 2000; Lamy *et al.*, 2002; Carpenter *et al.*, 2010).

It has been documented for over 70 years that anatomic right-to-left intrapulmonary shunts exist in normal human lungs. The studies that established the existence of these pathways used solid, large diameter microspheres to prove that there are large diameter pathways that bypass pulmonary capillaries (von Hayek, 1940; Tobin & Zariquiey, 1950; Tobin, 1966). More recent studies by our group have used microspheres to demonstrate the existence of large diameter (>25 to 50 μm) intrapulmonary arteriovenous anastomoses in isolated, ventilated and perfused healthy human and baboon lungs under physiologic conditions (Lovering *et al.*, 2007).

Intrapulmonary right-to-left pathways can be pulmonary arteriovenous malformations (PAVMs), grossly distended capillaries or arteriovenous anastomoses. The prevalence of PAVMs and grossly distended capillaries that result from rare diseases such as hepatopulmonary syndrome and hemorrhagic hereditary telangiectasia is considered to be very small, on the order of 1 in 50,000 (Khurshid & Downie, 2002; Liu *et al.*, 2010). However, we have found that greater than 95% of healthy humans have intrapulmonary arteriovenous anastomoses that are closed at rest but open up during exercise (Stickland & Lovering, 2006; Lovering *et al.*, 2010). Furthermore, the existence of these pathways in baboon lungs suggests that they may not be evolutionary disadvantageous since humans, gorillas and chimpanzees diverged from the old world monkeys (baboons, macaques, etc.) approximately 25 to 30 million years ago (Purvis, 1995; Goodman *et al.*, 1998; Stewart & Disotell, 1998). Although there is a high prevalence of these pathways in healthy humans, a significant impact on physiologic processes has not yet been proven.

3. Echocardiography for the detection of anatomic right-to-left shunt at rest

Saline contrast echocardiography is a proven non-invasive technique for the detection of right-to-left shunts at rest. This technique is used in both clinical and research settings, although certified ultrasonographers are typically required to obtain images of diagnostic quality. We strongly suggest that all recommendations by the American Society for Echocardiography for performance, interpretation and application of saline contrast echocardiography be followed accordingly (Waggoner *et al.*, 2001; Mulvagh *et al.*, 2008).

3.1 Theory

Echocardiography used as a technique for the detection of right-to-left shunts assumes that intravenously-infused saline contrast bubbles are filtered out by the pulmonary capillaries or collapse before reaching the left side of the heart (Yang, 1971; Yang *et al.*, 1971a, b; Meltzer *et al.*, 1980a; Meltzer *et al.*, 1980b; Meltzer *et al.*, 1981; Bommer *et al.*, 1984; Woods & Patel, 2006). Thus, large diameter bubbles do not reach the left side of the heart unless they travel through large diameter pathways such as pulmonary arteriovenous malformations (PAVMs) or a PFO. Saline contrast echocardiography is therefore considered to be the most sensitive test for detection of intracardiac shunts (Belkin *et al.*, 1994). With a prevalence of 30 to 40%, it is difficult to argue the existence of a PFO if intravenously injected saline contrast bubbles appear in the left heart. Alternatively, saline contrast echocardiography as a technique for intrapulmonary right-to-left shunts remains less well established, despite the fact that it is more sensitive than pulmonary angiography for detection of even the smallest right-to-left intrapulmonary shunts (Cottin *et al.*, 2004; van Gent *et al.*, 2009).

3.2 Equipment, instrumentation & technique

Subjects are instrumented with an intravenous catheter (i.v.) in a peripheral vein for the introduction of the contrast agent, which is normally air and sterile saline. Typically, 0.5-1 ml of air and 4-10 ml of saline are used to manually agitate between two syringes connected by stopcocks for a total injection volume of 10 ml (Otto, 2004; Feigenbaum, 2005; Woods *et al.*, 2010). In a research setting, equal success has been achieved in detecting right-to-left shunts via intrapulmonary arteriovenous anastomoses using 0.5-1 ml of air and 3-5 ml of saline, for a total injection volume of 5 ml (Stickland & Lovering, 2006; Laurie *et al.*, 2010; Lovering *et al.*, 2010; Elliott *et al.*, 2011a). The agitated saline mix solution should be injected as a bolus, forcibly by hand. Simultaneously, a well-trained sonographer should be acquiring a four chamber apical view of the heart. For superior image quality, the resting subject should be positioned in the left lateral decubitus position so that the heart moves anteriorly and laterally within the chest cavity. If necessary, the left arm should be folded upwards behind the head to expand the ribcage. A mattress cutout/drop-down is beneficial when the subject must be rolled steeply onto their left side to reduce lung artifact during inspiration. The echocardiograph should be preset to digitally acquire a 20-beat loop and the sonographer should employ settings that achieve high resolution without compromising penetration. The focal zone should be set near the base of the heart.

Technique and timing are important for a successful agitated saline contrast echocardiogram with a Valsalva maneuver. The subject should be instructed in the Valsalva maneuver and it is often helpful if they practice it a few times prior to contrast injection. The sonographer should position the patient and locate the best apical imaging window. The patient is asked to inhale a small breath, stop breathing, tighten the stomach muscles and sustain this effort for a minimum of ten seconds. The sonographer should move the imaging plane (typically inferiorly and medially) with the heart during the maneuver and then follow the heart back to the original window upon release of the maneuver. During the maneuver, a second caregiver forcibly agitates the saline mixture by plunging it back and forth between two syringes. When the 10 second maneuver is nearly completed, the contrast is quickly injected. Image acquisition should commence the moment contrast is injected. Immediately following injection, the subject is instructed to release the Valsalva maneuver and take small breaths. Upon release of Valsalva a rush of contrast will quickly opacify the right heart. Additional injections are performed if initial findings are equivocal.

Transesophageal echocardiography (TEE) provides image resolution that is superior to transthoracic echocardiography (TTE). Saline contrast injections are a routine element of every TEE and intracardiac shunt pathways are often easily identified as contrast passes through them. Patient sedation can prevent adequate Valsalva maneuvers during TEE so right-to-left shunts across a patent foramen ovale may go undetected (Fisher *et al.*, 1995).

3.3 Differentiating between intrapulmonary and intracardiac shunt

Once the agitated saline contrast mix is injected as a bolus, forcibly by hand, timing becomes critical in differentiating between intrapulmonary and intracardiac right-to-left shunts. After the appearance of saline contrast on the right side of the heart, timing of the appearance of saline contrast bubbles on the left heart will determine whether an intrapulmonary or intracardiac shunt is suspected. In general, if bubbles appear on the left side of the heart in ≤ 3 heart beats, then an intracardiac shunt is suspected, e.g. patent foramen ovale, atrial septal defect (Meltzer *et al.*, 1980a; Woods & Patel, 2006). If an intracardiac shunt is suspected, then a second contrast injection should be performed upon the subject's release of a Valsalva maneuver (Woods & Patel, 2006). Performing and releasing the Valsalva maneuver transiently elevates right heart pressure, which reverses the pressure gradient between the atria, creating conditions favorable for right-sided contrast to move to the left side of the heart across the intracardiac shunt. The second injection should confirm the presence of an intracardiac shunt if there is increased contrast and/or if the contrast bubbles continue to appear in the left heart in ≤ 3 heartbeats. Alternatively, if saline contrast bubbles appear in the left heart in > 3 heartbeats after their appearance in the right heart, then an intrapulmonary shunt is suspected, e.g., pulmonary arteriovenous malformation, pulmonary arteriovenous anastomoses (Nanthakumar *et al.*, 2001; Lee *et al.*, 2003; van Gent *et al.*, 2009; Elliott *et al.*, 2011a). The different types of intracardiac and intrapulmonary shunts are outlined in detail below.

3.3.1 Intracardiac shunts

The most common intracardiac shunt pathway is the PFO. Unlike ASDs, a PFO is a feature of normal cardiac development. Although the foramen is no longer patent in the majority of adults, a PFO is detectible in 25 to 40% of the general population (Hagen *et al.*, 1984; Woods *et al.*, 2010; Elliott *et al.*, 2011b). A PFO typically has the echocardiographic appearance of a valve-like flap of tissue covering the foramen ovale in the middle portion of the interatrial septum. This flap can be seen opening intermittently into the left atrium whenever right atrial pressure exceeds left atrial pressure. If fusion of the flap provides a nearly complete seal, the remaining orifice is shaped more like a narrow slit or tunnel. Standard TTE views for visualizing a PFO include the parasternal short-axis view at the level of the aortic valve, the right parasternal bicaval view and the subcostal bicaval view. The atrial septum is best imaged by TEE and a small PFO may only be visualized using this technique. However, saline contrast TTE during the release of a Valsalva maneuver has been found to be even more sensitive than TEE for revealing a PFO (Lam *et al.*, 2010; Gonzalez-Alujas *et al.*, 2011). To achieve the highest sensitivity for intracardiac right-to-left shunting, one should always coordinate contrast injection with the release of a Valsalva maneuver.

Right-to-left shunting may also occur through an ASD. The most common type is a secundum ASD. Unlike a PFO, a secundum ASD typically has the appearance of a hole with defined edges. Similar to a PFO, a secundum defect is located in the middle of the interatrial septum and may be quite small and difficult to visualize. It is best viewed using the same imaging planes one would use to view a PFO, and might only be detected by a saline contrast injection. Three-dimensional imaging, either TTE or TEE, is a useful method of examining the true shape and area of the defect. It is important to differentiate between a PFO and an ASD because an ASD is less likely to restrict left-to-right shunting and therefore may present a greater risk of right heart volume overload and associated sequelae.

An ostium primum ASD results from the incomplete fusion of the inferior and superior endocardial cushions and therefore is located in the inferior portion of the interatrial septum. An ostium primum ASD may exist in isolation and may be referred to as a partial AV canal. Commonly it is paired with an inlet ventricular septal defect, in which case it bears the name atrioventricular septal defect (AVSD) or complete AV canal. A distinguishing feature of AVSD is that both atrioventricular valves share the same annulus and valve plane. This valvular alignment is visible by TTE in the apical four-chamber view. This is easily distinguishable from normal heart alignment because the normal tricuspid valve plane is displaced towards the apex relative to the mitral valve plane.

A defect adjoining the atria near the junction of the superior or inferior vena cava with the right atrium is a sinus venosus ASD. It most often involves the superior and posterior portion of the interatrial septum and is commonly associated with partial anomalous pulmonary venous return. It can be difficult to detect using standard TTE views but is readily visible by TEE in the bicaval view. An effort should be made to rule out sinus venosus ASD if a substantial and early right-to-left shunt is detected by saline contrast injection without evidence of defects in the secundum or primum septum.

The absence of separation between the roof of the coronary sinus and the floor of the left atrium (coronary sinus defect) has often been categorized as an atrial septal defect because it effectively provides a shunt pathway between the atria via the coronary sinus. This defect is sometimes associated with a common thoracic venous abnormality known as persistent left superior vena cava (PLSVC). A PLSVC provides venous return from the left upper extremity (or both if the right SVC is absent) into the right atrium via the coronary sinus resulting in coronary sinus dilatation. For direct visualization of a coronary sinus defect, TEE is superior to TTE. However, a customized saline contrast TTE can uncover both PLSVC and coronary sinus defect with one injection. Whenever a dilated coronary sinus is detected (usually an incidental finding), a PLSVC and/or coronary sinus defect should be suspected as the cause and a saline contrast injection should be performed (Goyal *et al.*, 2008). The sonographer images the heart using an inferiorly tilted apical four-chamber view to reveal coronary sinus drainage into the right atrium. Once contrast appears within the coronary sinus, the sonographer quickly tilts the scanhead anteriorly to the standard apical four-chamber view. If a PLSVC is present, contrast will be seen in the coronary sinus before it reaches the right atrium. If both a PLSVC and a coronary sinus defect are present, contrast will appear within the left atrium and right atrium simultaneously. If contrast appears within the left atrium shortly following opacification of the right atrium, a PFO is likely but a coronary sinus defect is effectively ruled-out.

Saline contrast echocardiography should not be used to rule out suspected small ventricular septal defects (VSD). Shunting through a small VSD is primarily systolic, left-to-right, and because of the high-pressure gradient they are readily apparent by color flow Doppler on the right ventricular side of the septum. If a small VSD is suspected by 2D imaging, but there is no high-velocity systolic color jet on the right side of the septum and right ventricular systolic pressure is normal, VSD has been effectively ruled out.

3.3.2 Intrapulmonary shunts

As listed above, the interrogator should count the number of cardiac cycles between right atrial opacification and the arrival of contrast in the left atrium. If the delay is > 3 cardiac cycles, the passage of microbubbles followed a transpulmonary pathway. Intrapulmonary pathways include pulmonary arteriovenous malformations (PAVMs) and intrapulmonary arteriovenous anastomoses. Although PAVMs are considered to be rare, and associated with diseases states, more recent work suggests a prevalence of ~20% in the general population (Woods *et al.*, 2010; Elliott *et al.*, 2011b). Whether or not these pathways detected by Woods and colleagues are truly PAVMS or intrapulmonary arteriovenous anastomoses is unknown. Preliminary findings from our lab suggest that they are the latter (Elliott *et al.*, 2011b), however further research into this area is needed.

Clinically, subjects lay in the supine position for ultrasound imaging. In a research setting, subjects can be in a supine, upright or reclined position, however interpretation of the echocardiograms should take into account body positioning during ultrasound imaging. Specifically, there are data suggesting that intrapulmonary arteriovenous anastomoses are patent in the supine position, but not in the upright position (Stickland *et al.*, 2004; Elliott *et al.*, 2011b). Also, Tobin & Zariquiey demonstrated that intrapulmonary arteriovenous anastomoses 20 to 500 μm in functional diameter are located in the apex of the human lung (Tobin & Zariquiey, 1950). Together, these data support the idea that perfusion of the apices of the lung may open these vessels. Thus, if the goal is to identify the presence of intrapulmonary right-to-left shunts, then subjects should be screened in the supine position. When subjects are in the reclined position, it is recommended that they be rotated 45 degrees on their left side to allow for optimal imaging conditions.

In summary, the chance to detect either an intracardiac or an intrapulmonary right-to-left shunt in healthy human subjects at rest is approximately 60% (40% PFO + 20% intrapulmonary). In subjects with a PFO, it is not possible to unequivocally detect intrapulmonary right-to-left shunts. The reason for this is that bubbles may cross over the inter-atrial septum at any time during echocardiographic imaging. Thus, if bubbles appear in the left ventricle after 10 heartbeats in subjects with a PFO, there is no way to determine if those bubbles crossed the atrium via an intracardiac or intrapulmonary shunt pathway.

3.4 Semi-quantification of right-to-left shunt

There are numerous scoring methods used in both clinical and research settings for *semi-quantification* of right-to-left shunt with saline contrast bubbles (Barzilai *et al.*, 1991; Lovering *et al.*, 2008b; La Gerche *et al.*, 2010; Laurie *et al.*, 2010). These scoring methods take into account the density and spatial distribution of saline contrast bubbles in the left heart. As such, a score of 0 typically represents no saline contrast bubbles, while increasing numbers indicate increasing amounts of saline contrast (Figure 1). Better anatomic approaches to quantification of right-to-left shunts use radiolabeled albumin macroaggregates in conjunction with nuclear medicine imaging (Whyte *et al.*, 1992; Lovering *et al.*, 2009b), but this topic is beyond the scope of the current chapter.

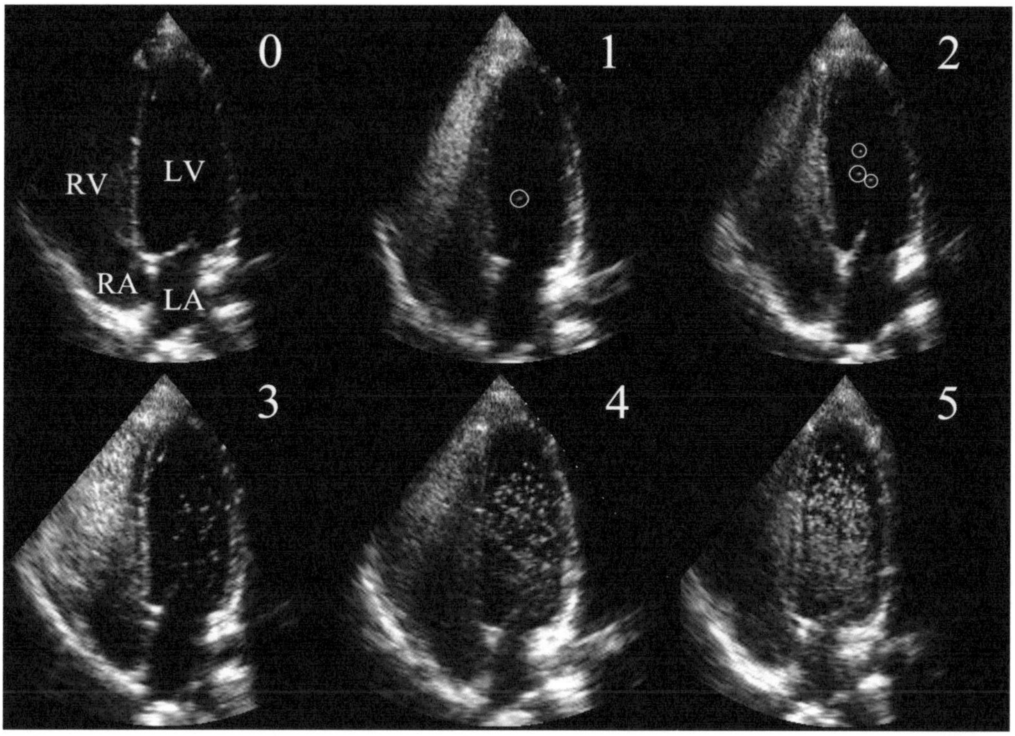

Fig. 1. Representative echocardiograms of bubble scores. Scores are assigned based on both the density and spatial distribution of microbubbles in the left ventricle from the frame with the largest amount of contrast. A score of 0 = 0 microbubbles; 1 = 1 - 3 microbubbles; 2 = 4 - 12 microbubbles; 3 = more than 12 microbubbles in a bolus; 4 = more than 12 microbubbles heterogeneously distributed throughout the left ventricle; 5 = more than 12 microbubbles homogeneously distributed throughout the left ventricle. Scores 1 and 2 have bubbles circled for clarity. RA, LA = right & left atrium; RV, LV = right & left ventricle.

4. Echocardiography for the detection of anatomic right-to-left shunt during exercise & stress

Stress echocardiography is a proven non-invasive technique frequently used to test for flow-limiting coronary artery disease in patients with symptoms of angina. Less commonly, it is used in combination with Doppler techniques to evaluate the effect of stress on valvular lesions and outflow tract obstruction. Saline contrast is also useful during exercise to enhance the Doppler signal or to assess the effect of exercise on right-to-left shunting. Performing echocardiography on an individual during exercise is a challenge to the skill of the sonographer. Obtaining images of diagnostic quality is made more difficult by respiratory artifact, motion of the patient, exaggerated cardiac motion, and tachycardia. It is recommended that only experienced sonographers be selected for the performance of these tests. Furthermore, we strongly suggest that all recommendations by the American Society for Echocardiography for performance, interpretation and application of stress echocardiography be followed accordingly (Pellikka *et al.*, 2007).

4.1 Technical considerations for echocardiographic measurements during exercise

The ultrasound equipment required for saline contrast echocardiography during exercise are the same as those listed above for resting imaging. Continuous 12-lead electrocardiography is often performed during exercise testing. Depending upon the locations of the imaging windows in an individual during rest and exercise, some of the precordial EKG leads may need to be relocated to allow for echocardiographic imaging. This varies significantly between individuals, but the leads most likely to be affected are V2, V4 and V5. If they must be moved, V2 can be moved to a higher rib space and V4 and V5 can be moved to a lower rib space to accommodate echocardiographic imaging (Figure 2).

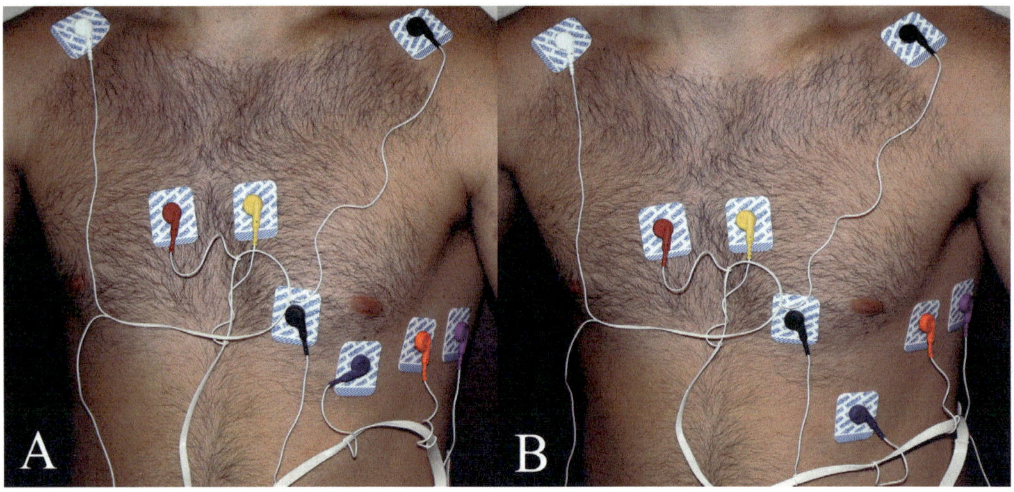

Fig. 2. Placement of 12 lead electrodes for use with ultrasound imaging during exercise. A) normal configuration, B) adaptive configuration example.

4.2 Treadmill versus cycle ergometer exercise:

Most stress echocardiograms are performed using a treadmill and three minute stages of increasing workload. Treadmill exercise has the advantage in that it allows most patients to achieve their target heart rate (85% of the age-predicted maximum) on a treadmill. However, it bears the significant disadvantage that echocardiographic images cannot be acquired during exercise. Images must be acquired immediately following exercise during the recovery phase on an exam table, and for this reason, transient exercise-induced cardiac abnormalities, and right-to-left shunting, can be missed.

Supine and/or recumbent cycle ergometers are popular in many clinical settings because echocardiographic imaging can be performed during exercise (Stickland *et al.*, 2004). The cycling apparatus is built into an exam table so that an individual is able to exercise while lying in the supine or recumbent position. These tables normally include the capacity to be tilted sideward and are equipped with a drop-down section to expose the apical imaging window. These features permit high quality imaging during various levels of exercise. The primary disadvantage of supine cycle stress is that some patients find it difficult to exercise well in that position and are consequently unable to achieve the target heart rate.

We have considerable experience successfully performing diagnostic contrast-enhanced spectral Doppler studies during exercise and evaluations of right-to-left shunting during exercise on subjects in the forward-leaning upright bike arrangement, or "Aerobar" position (Lovering *et al.*, 2008b; Elliott *et al.*, 2011a) (Figure 3). The "Aerobar" position has several advantages: One, subjects are able to lean forward resting their forearms on bars that allow them to maintain a relatively still upper body during exercise. Two, the apex of the heart falls forward in this position allowing for superior image quality during exercise. Three, this is a more comfortable and more natural position for exercise than the supine bike, so the likelihood of achieving the target heart rate is greater than in supine exercise. Four, evaluation of global and regional left and right ventricular wall motion may also be successfully performed during exercise in this position. A disadvantage is that it can be difficult to image a patient during exercise in this position if they have abdominal obesity. To date, similar results have been found when comparing right-to-left shunt during recumbent and upright exercise (Stickland *et al.*, 2004; La Gerche *et al.*, 2010; Elliott *et al.*, 2011a). There are no published data examining intrapulmonary shunting during supine exercise. We would suggest that body positioning be taken into consideration when making these measurements in the supine position during exercise given the fact that previous work has shown differences in patency of intrapulmonary arteriovenous anastomoses at rest (see **3.3.2 Intrapulmonary Shunts** above). Thus it seems appropriate to use the cycle ergometer-testing paradigm that best suits the investigator needs.

4.3 Non-exercise stress modalities

In addition to cycle ergometer exercise, pharmacologic-induced stress can be used in lieu of "true exercise." Pharmacological stress echocardiography allows for better image quality than any of the competing exercise modalities because the patient is lying still in a position best suited for imaging while the heart is stressed chemically. The most common protocol calls for continuous infusion of dobutamine that increases in three to five minute stages with atropine injections performed during the later stages if necessary to reach the target heart rate (Pellikka *et al.*, 2007). Pharmacological stress echocardiography is the preferred method when a patient is physically unable to exercise or when valvular lesions or outflow tract obstructions need to be assessed. The disadvantage of pharmacological stress is that it is not true exercise. Additionally, many patients do not tolerate the drugs well.

5. Recent research advancements using echocardiography in healthy humans & patient populations

5.1 Research using echocardiography in healthy humans during exercise

Work by our group and others have focused on detection of intrapulmonary and intracardiac shunting at rest and during exercise using saline contrast echocardiography. Succinylated gelatin has been used to detect patent intrapulmonary arteriovenous anastomoses (La Gerche *et al.*, 2010) but there are no data suggesting that this contrast agent is superior to using air and saline alone. Given the fact that additives may increase the risk of adverse reactions in research subjects, the use of saline and air seems to be the best choice (Bommer *et al.*, 1984; Mulvagh *et al.*, 2008). Commercially available contrast agents contain microbubbles small enough to transit pulmonary capillaries and opacify the left ventricle. By design these agents opacify all four cardiac chambers preventing the viewer from detecting an intracardiac shunt. They are also specifically contraindicated for use when there is a known or suspected intracardiac shunt (Mulvagh *et al.*, 2008).

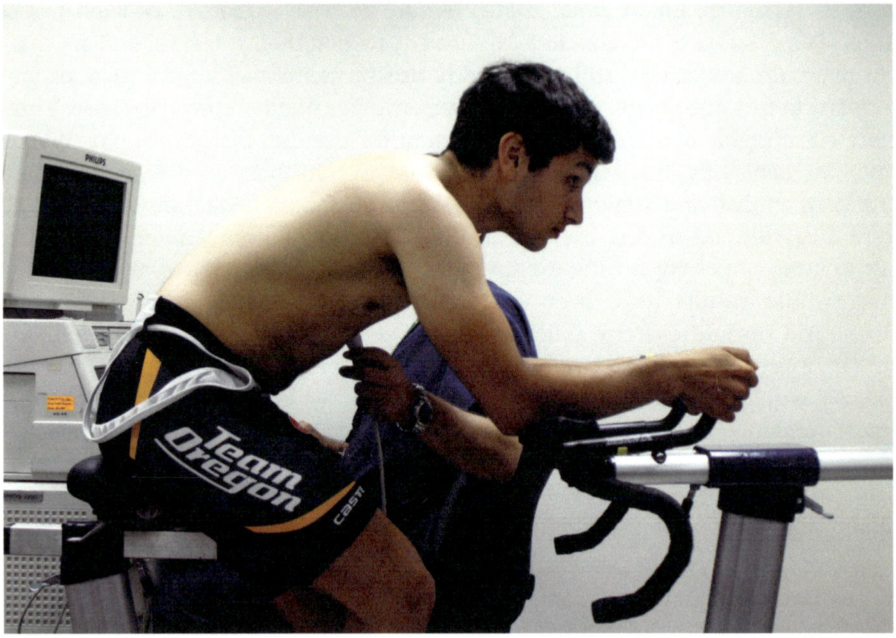

Fig. 3. Subject in the "aerobar" position. Note aerobars on the cycle ergometer with subject in the forward leaning position.

It has been demonstrated that exercise opens intrapulmonary arteriovenous anastomoses that were closed at rest in healthy humans (Eldridge *et al.*, 2004; Stickland *et al.*, 2004; La Gerche *et al.*, 2010; Elliott *et al.*, 2011a). Furthermore, increasing exercise intensity increases the amount of saline contrast that is detected in the left ventricle, which is indicative of increased intrapulmonary shunting (Stickland *et al.*, 2004). It has been suggested that blood flowing through intrapulmonary arteriovenous anastomoses is acting as a "true" shunt (Stickland & Lovering, 2006; Lovering *et al.*, 2009a), however the physiologic role of these vessels remains highly controversial and as of yet, unproven (Hopkins *et al.*, 2009).

The effect of inspired oxygen concentration is another intervention that has been shown to have a modulatory effect on the patency of intrapulmonary arteriovenous anastomoses. We have demonstrated that breathing hyperoxic gas closes intrapulmonary arteriovenous anastomoses at rest and during exercise (Elliott *et al.*, 2011a). This may play a role in detecting intrapulmonary arteriovenous anastomoses at rest in patients with lung disease or healthy human subjects (Elliott *et al.*, 2011b). Conversely, we have also demonstrated that breathing hypoxic gas mixtures will open intrapulmonary arteriovenous anastomoses in healthy humans at rest and will increase the degree of shunting during exercise compared to exercise in normoxia (Lovering *et al.*, 2008a; Elliott *et al.*, 2011a) (Figure 4). Since arterial hypoxemia is associated with patent intrapulmonary arteriovenous anastomoses in healthy humans, this may have an effect on patient populations with arterial hypoxemia (see below).

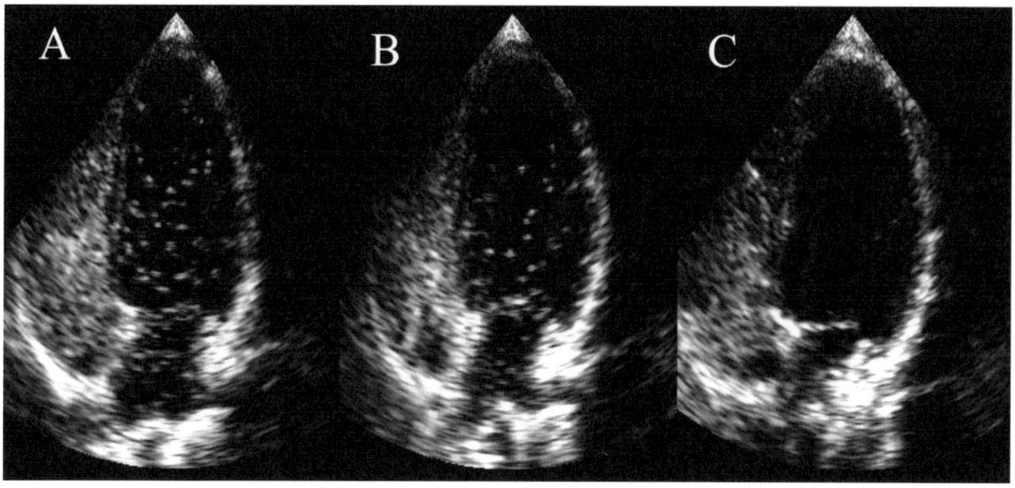

Fig. 4. Echocardiograms during exercise in hypoxia (A), normoxia (B) and hyperoxia (C). Note left side contrast is greatest in hypoxia (A) but is absent during in hyperoxia (C).

Of note, it has been argued that changing inspired oxygen tension may affect the external partial pressure environment (i.e. PO_2 of the blood) such that breathing hyperoxia may shorten the lifespan of saline contrast bubbles whereas hypoxia may lengthen the life span of saline contrast bubbles (Van Liew & Vann, 2010). Although this argument follows mathematical modeling and theoretical calculations, when this question was directly addressed *in vivo* using various inspired gases and saline contrast bubbles made of 100% carbon dioxide, 100% nitrogen, 100% helium, 100% room air or 100% oxygen, it was found that there was no effect on either the bubble score or the sensitivity of the technique (Elliott *et al.*, 2011a). Thus, any effect on inspired oxygen tension is likely a direct effect on the pulmonary vasculature rather than an effect on *in vivo* gas bubble dynamics. These data are further supported by the fact that ventilating dogs with low and high oxygen mixtures results in increased and decreased intrapulmonary shunt fractions, respectively (Niden & Aviado, 1956). In these studies the authors detected right-to-left shunting using solid microspheres (60 to 420 μm in diameter), which clearly would not be affected by altered *in vivo* external partial pressure environments.

5.2 Research using echocardiography in patients with lung disease at rest

Special considerations are suggested when examining certain patient populations. For example, patients with chronic obstructive pulmonary disease (COPD) who also have arterial hypoxemia are likely to have patent intrapulmonary right-to-left shunts at rest (Miller *et al.*, 1984; Dansky *et al.*, 1992). Preliminary work in our lab using saline contrast echocardiography has detected these pathways in subjects with COPD who do not have a PFO (Figure 5). Interestingly, administration of supplemental oxygen to these subjects with COPD closes intrapulmonary pathways suggesting that they are actively regulated.

Other diseases associated with arterial hypoxemia such as hepatopulmonary syndrome and hereditary hemorrhagic telangiectasia are known to have arteriovenous malformations that will allow for the transpulmonary passage of saline contrast bubbles under resting conditions (Woods & Patel, 2006). Thus, patients with underlying lung diseases and arterial hypoxemia, may desaturate further as a result of the opening of hypoxia-induced intrapulmonary arteriovenous anastomoses. It is unknown whether or not hyperoxia would close intrapulmonary arteriovenous anastomoses in these patients, but data from healthy humans suggests that it would be possible (Lovering *et al.*, 2008b; Elliott *et al.*, 2011a).

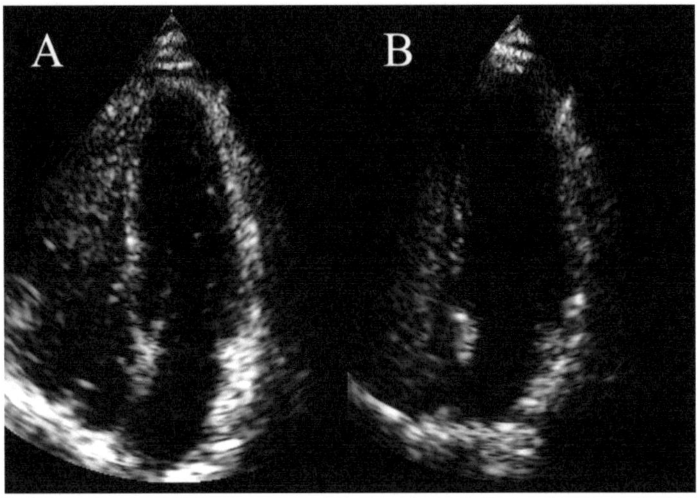

Fig. 5. Intrapulmonary arteriovenous anastomoses in COPD subjects. A) left side contrast in subject at rest with arterial saturation of 94%, B) absence of left side contrast in the same subject breathing 100% O_2 with a saturation of 100%.

6. Conclusion

In conclusion, saline contrast echocardiography is a non-invasive technique that can be used to detect right-to-left shunts in healthy humans and in various patient populations. Timing of the appearance of saline contrast bubbles in the left heart can be used to differentiate intracardiac shunts (e.g. PFOs) from intrapulmonary shunts (e.g. PAVMs) in subjects who do not have both. Special considerations should be taken with the interpretation of the echocardiograms depending on the subject's body positioning, the fraction of inspired oxygen the subject is breathing and the disease status of the patient.

7. Acknowledgement

We thank Kara M. Beasley, BS for assistance with preparation of figures. Andrew Lovering thanks John Hokanson, MD for introducing him to saline contrast echocardiography. Financial support: Oregon Health & Science University Medical Research Foundation Grant, American Lung Association in Oregon Research Grant, University of Oregon/Peace Health Oregon Region Translational Research Award, American Physiological Society's Giles F. Filley Memorial Award for Excellence in Respiratory Physiology & Medicine.

8. References

Barzilai B, Waggoner AD, Spessert C, Picus D & Goodenberger D. (1991). Two-dimensional contrast echocardiography in the detection and follow-up of congenital pulmonary arteriovenous malformations. *Am J Cardiol* 68, 1507-1510.

Belkin RN, Pollack BD, Ruggiero ML, Alas LL & Tatini U. (1994). Comparison of transesophageal and transthoracic echocardiography with contrast and color flow Doppler in the detection of patent foramen ovale. *American heart journal* 128, 520-525.

Bommer WJ, Shah PM, Allen H, Meltzer R & Kisslo J. (1984). The safety of contrast echocardiography: report of the Committee on Contrast Echocardiography for the American Society of Echocardiography. *J Am CollCardiol* 3, 6-13.

Carpenter DA, Ford AL & Lee JM. (2010). Patent foramen ovale and stroke: Should PFOs be closed in otherwise cryptogenic stroke? *Curr Atheroscler Rep* 12, 251-258.

Cottin V, Plauchu H, Bayle JY, Barthelet M, Revel D & Cordier JF. (2004). Pulmonary arteriovenous malformations in patients with hereditary hemorrhagic telangiectasia. *American journal of respiratory and critical care medicine* 169, 994-1000.

Dansky HM, Schwinger ME & Cohen MV. (1992). Using contrast material-enhanced echocardiography to identify abnormal pulmonary arteriovenous connections in patients with hypoxemia. *Chest* 102, 1690-1692.

De Castro S, Cartoni D, Fiorelli M, Rasura M, Anzini A, Zanette EM, Beccia M, Colonnese C, Fedele F, Fieschi C & Pandian NG. (2000). Morphological and functional characteristics of patent foramen ovale and their embolic implications. *Stroke; a journal of cerebral circulation* 31, 2407-2413.

Eldridge MW, Dempsey JA, Haverkamp HC, Lovering AT & Hokanson JS. (2004). Exercise-induced intrapulmonary arteriovenous shunting in healthy humans. *J Appl Physiol* 97, 797-805.

Elliott JE, Choi Y, Laurie SS, Yang X, Gladstone IM & Lovering AT. (2011a). Effect of initial gas bubble composition on detection of inducible intrapulmonary arteriovenous shunt during exercise in normoxia, hypoxia, or hyperoxia. *Journal of Appl Physiol* 110, 35-45.

Elliott JE, Nigam SM, Lauire SS, Yang X, Beasley KM, Goodman RD, Gladstone IM & Lovering AT. (2011b). Pulmonary arteriovenous malformations or intrapulmonary arteriovenous anastomoses in healthy humans at rest. Unpublished Observations.

Feigenbaum H. (2005). *Feigenbaum's Echocardiography*. Lippincott Williams & Wilkins, Philadelphia.

Fisher DC, Fisher EA, Budd JH, Rosen SE & Goldman ME. (1995). The incidence of patent foramen ovale in 1,000 consecutive patients. A contrast transesophageal echocardiography study. *Chest* 107, 1504-1509.

Gonzalez-Alujas T, Evangelista A, Santamarina E, Rubiera M, Gomez-Bosch Z, Rodriguez-Palomares JF, Avegliano G, Molina C, Alvarez-Sabin J & Garcia-Dorado D. (2011). Diagnosis and quantification of patent foramen ovale. Which is the reference technique? Simultaneous study with transcranial Doppler, transthoracic and transesophageal echocardiography. *Rev Esp Cardiol* 64, 133-139.

Goodman M, Porter CA, Czelusniak J, Page SL, Schneider H, Shoshani J, Gunnell G & Groves CP. (1998). Toward a phylogenetic classification of Primates based on DNA evidence complemented by fossil evidence. *MolPhylogenetEvol* 9, 585-598.

Goyal SK, Punnam SR, Verma G & Ruberg FL. (2008). Persistent left superior vena cava: a case report and review of literature. *Cardiovasc Ultrasound* 6, 50.

Hagen PT, Scholz DG & Edwards WD. (1984). Incidence and size of patent foramen ovale during the first 10 decades of life: an autopsy study of 965 normal hearts. *Mayo ClinProc* 59, 17-20.

Homma S, Di Tullio MR, Sacco RL, Sciacca RR, Smith C & Mohr JP. (1997). Surgical closure of patent foramen ovale in cryptogenic stroke patients. *Stroke* 28, 2376-2381.

Hopkins SR, Olfert IM & Wagner PD. (2009). Last Word on Point:Counterpoint: Exercise-induced intrapulmonary shunting is imaginary vs. real. *J Appl Physiol* 107, 1002.

Khurshid I & Downie GH. (2002). Pulmonary arteriovenous malformation. *Postgrad Med J* 78, 191-197.

La Gerche A, Macisaac AI, Burns AT, Mooney DJ, Inder WJ, Voigt JU, Heidbuchel H & Prior DL. (2010). Pulmonary transit of agitated contrast is associated with enhanced pulmonary vascular reserve and right ventricular function during exercise. *J Appl Physiol.*

Lam YY, Yu CM, Zhang Q, Yan BP & Yip GW. (2010). Enhanced detection of patent foramen ovale by systematic transthoracic saline contrast echocardiography. *International journal of cardiology.*

Lamy C, Giannesini C, Zuber M, Arquizan C, Meder JF, Trystram D, Coste J & Mas JL. (2002). Clinical and imaging findings in cryptogenic stroke patients with and without patent foramen ovale: the PFO-ASA Study. Atrial Septal Aneurysm. *Stroke* 33, 706-711.

Laurie SS, Yang X, Elliott JE, Beasley KM & Lovering AT. (2010). Hypoxia-induced intrapulmonary arteriovenous shunting at rest in healthy humans. *J Appl Physiol* 109, 1072-1079.

Lee WL, Graham AF, Pugash RA, Hutchison SJ, Grande P, Hyland RH & Faughnan ME. (2003). Contrast echocardiography remains positive after treatment of pulmonary arteriovenous malformations. *Chest* 123, 351-358.

Liu FY, Wang MQ, Fan QS, Duan F, Wang ZJ & Song P. (2010). Endovascular embolization of pulmonary arteriovenous malformations. *Chin Med J (Engl)* 123, 23-28.

Lovering AT, Eldridge MW & Stickland MK. (2009a). Counterpoint: Exercise-induced intrapulmonary shunting is real. *J Appl Physiol* 107, 994-997.

Lovering AT, Elliott JE, Beasley KM & Laurie SS. (2010). Pulmonary pathways and mechanisms regulating transpulmonary shunting into the general circulation: An update. *Injury* 41S2, S16-S23.

Lovering AT, Haverkamp HC, Romer LM, Hokanson JS & Eldridge MW. (2009b). Transpulmonary passage of 99mTc macroaggregated albumin in healthy humans at rest and during maximal exercise. *J Appl Physiol* 106, 1986-1992.

Lovering AT, Romer LM, Haverkamp HC, Pegelow DF, Hokanson JS & Eldridge MW. (2008a). Intrapulmonary shunting and pulmonary gas exchange during normoxic and hypoxic exercise in healthy humans. *J ApplPhysiol* 104, 1418-1425.

Lovering AT, Stickland MK, Amann M, Murphy JC, O'Brien MJ, Hokanson JS & Eldridge MW. (2008b). Hyperoxia prevents exercise-induced intrapulmonary arteriovenous shunt in healthy humans. *J Physiol* 586, 4559-4565.

Lovering AT, Stickland MK, Amann M, O'Brien MJ, Hokanson JS & Eldridge MW. (2011). Effect of a patent foramen ovale on pulmonary gas exchange efficiency at rest and during exercise. *Journal of applied physiology* 110, 1354-1361.

Lovering AT, Stickland MK, Kelso AJ & Eldridge MW. (2007). Direct demonstration of 25- and 50- μm arteriovenous pathways in healthy human and baboon lungs. *Am J Physiol Heart CircPhysiol* 292, H1777-H1781.

Meltzer RS, Sartorius OE, Lancee CT, Serruys PW, Verdouw PD, Essed CE & Roelandt J. (1981). Transmission of ultrasonic contrast through the lungs. *Ultrasound MedBiol* 7, 377-384.

Meltzer RS, Tickner EG & Popp RL. (1980a). Why do the lungs clear ultrasonic contrast? *Ultrasound Med Biol* 6, 263-269.

Meltzer RS, Tickner EG, Sahines TP & Popp RL. (1980b). The source of ultrasound contrast effect. *J ClinUltrasound* 8, 121-127.

Miller WC, Heard JG & Unger KM. (1984). Enlarged pulmonary arteriovenous vessels in COPD. Another possible mechanism of hypoxemia. *Chest* 86, 704-706.

Movsowitz C, Podolsky LA, Meyerowitz CB, Jacobs LE & Kotler MN. (1992). Patent foramen ovale: a nonfunctional embryological remnant or a potential cause of significant pathology? *J Am Soc Echocardiogr* 5, 259-270.

Mulder BJ. (2010). Changing demographics of pulmonary arterial hypertension in congenital heart disease. *Eur Respir Rev* 19, 308-313.

Mulvagh SL, Rakowski H, Vannan MA, Abdelmoneim SS, Becher H, Bierig SM, Burns PN, Castello R, Coon PD, Hagen ME, Jollis JG, Kimball TR, Kitzman DW, Kronzon I, Labovitz AJ, Lang RM, Mathew J, Moir WS, Nagueh SF, Pearlman AS, Perez JE, Porter TR, Rosenbloom J, Strachan GM, Thanigaraj S, Wei K, Woo A, Yu EH & Zoghbi WA. (2008). American Society of Echocardiography Consensus Statement on the Clinical Applications of Ultrasonic Contrast Agents in Echocardiography. *Journal of the American Society of Echocardiography : official publication of the American Society of Echocardiography* 21, 1179-1201; quiz 1281.

Nanthakumar K, Graham AT, Robinson TI, Grande P, Pugash RA, Clarke JA, Hutchison SJ, Mandzia JL, Hyland RH & Faughnan ME. (2001). Contrast echocardiography for detection of pulmonary arteriovenous malformations. *Am Heart J* 141, 243-246.

Niden AH & Aviado DM, Jr. (1956). Effects of pulmonary embolism on the pulmonary circulation with special reference to arteriovenous shunts in the lung. *CircRes* 4, 67-73.

Otto C. (2004). *Textbook of Clinical Echocardiography*. Saunders, Philadelphia.

Pellikka PA, Nagueh SF, Elhendy AA, Kuehl CA & Sawada SG. (2007). American Society of Echocardiography recommendations for performance, interpretation, and application of stress echocardiography. *Journal of the American Society of Echocardiography : official publication of the American Society of Echocardiography* 20, 1021-1041.

Petty GW, Khandheria BK, Chu CP, Sicks JD & Whisnant JP. (1997). Patent foramen ovale in patients with cerebral infarction. A transesophageal echocardiographic study. *Arch Neurol* 54, 819-822.

Purvis A. (1995). A composite estimate of primate phylogeny. *PhilosTransRSocLond B BiolSci* 348, 405-421.

Stewart CB & Disotell TR. (1998). Primate evolution - in and out of Africa. *CurrBiol* 8, R582-R588.

Stickland MK & Lovering AT. (2006). Exercise-induced intrapulmonary arteriovenous shunting and pulmonary gas exchange. *ExercSport SciRev* 34, 99-106.

Stickland MK, Welsh RC, Haykowsky MJ, Petersen SR, Anderson WD, Taylor DA, Bouffard M & Jones RL. (2004). Intra-pulmonary shunt and pulmonary gas exchange during exercise in humans. *J Physiol* 561, 321-329.

Sun XG, Hansen JE, Oudiz RJ & Wasserman K. (2002). Gas exchange detection of exercise-induced right-to-left shunt in patients with primary pulmonary hypertension. *Circulation* 105, 54-60.

Tobin CE. (1966). Arteriovenous shunts in the peripheral pulmonary circulation in the human lung. *Thorax* 21, 197-204.

Tobin CE & Zariquiey MO. (1950). Arteriovenous shunts in the human lung. *Proc Soc Exp Biol Med* 75, 827-829.

van Gent MW, Post MC, Luermans JG, Snijder RJ, Westermann CJ, Plokker HW, Overtoom TT & Mager JJ. (2009). Screening for pulmonary arteriovenous malformations using transthoracic contrast echocardiography: a prospective study. *Eur Respir J* 33, 85-91.

Van Liew HD & Vann RD. (2010). Sonic echocardiography: what does it mean when there are no bubbles in the left ventricle? *J Appl Physiol* 110, 295; author reply 296-7.

von Hayek H. (1940). öber einen Kurzschlusskreislauf (arterio-venîse Anastomosen) in der menschlichen Lunge. *ZtschrfAnatuEntwklsg* 110, 412-422.

Waggoner AD, Ehler D, Adams D, Moos S, Rosenbloom J, Gresser C, Perez JE & Douglas PS. (2001). Guidelines for the cardiac sonographer in the performance of contrast echocardiography: recommendations of the American Society of Echocardiography Council on Cardiac Sonography. *Journal of the American Society of Echocardiography : official publication of the American Society of Echocardiography* 14, 417-420.

Whyte MK, Peters AM, Hughes JM, Henderson BL, Bellingan GJ, Jackson JE & Chilvers ER. (1992). Quantification of right to left shunt at rest and during exercise in patients with pulmonary arteriovenous malformations. *Thorax* 47, 790-796.

Woods TD, Harmann L, Purath T, Ramamurthy S, Subramanian S, Jackson S & Tarima S. (2010). Small and Moderate Size Right-to-Left Shunts Identified By Saline Contrast Echocardiography Are Normal and Unrelated To Migraine Headache. *Chest*.

Woods TD & Patel A. (2006). A critical review of patent foramen ovale detection using saline contrast echocardiography: when bubbles lie. *J Am SocEchocardiogr* 19, 215-222.

Yang WJ. (1971). Dynamics of gas bubbles in whole blood and plasma. *J Biomech* 4, 119-125.

Yang WJ, Echigo R, Wotton DR & Hwang JB. (1971a). Experimental studies of the dissolution of gas bubbles in whole blood and plasma. I. Stationary bubbles. *J Biomech* 4, 275-281.

Yang WJ, Echigo R, Wotton DR & Hwang JB. (1971b). Experimental studies of the dissolution of gas bubbles in whole blood and plasma. II. Moving bubbles or liquids. *J Biomech* 4, 283-288.

9

Ultrasonography of the Stomach

Laurence Trahair and Karen L. Jones
University of Adelaide, Discipline of Medicine, Royal Adelaide Hospital
Adelaide, South Australia,
Australia

1. Introduction

Ultrasound is a versatile imaging modality with the potential to provide much quantitative and qualitative information in both clinical and research settings. Ultrasound has the capacity to provide both anatomical and physiological information in real-time, and also offers images with high temporal and spatial resolution. Furthermore, ultrasound is relatively non-invasive and is not associated with a radiation burden to the patient. These advantages, as well as the capacity to provide this information in a simple, fast and pain free examination has meant that there has been a huge increase in the number of applications of ultrasound since its introduction in the early 1960s. It was not until the 1980s that ultrasonographic assessment of the stomach and its contents were explored, and, since that time, a number of new techniques have been developed which can provide more comprehensive information in a single ultrasonographic exam.

This chapter will describe a number of these techniques, specifically, ultrasound imaging of the fundus and antrum (including area and volume), 2D and 3D assessment of gastric emptying, measurement of antropyloroduoenal motility and transpyloric flow as well as gastric strain rate imaging. Within each of these sections both clinical and research applications will be discussed. Strengths and limitations of the techniques, as well as comparisons with other methodological or diagnostic techniques will also be addressed.

2. Scanning techniques

Generally, no specific patient preparation is necessary (Nylund *et al.*, 2009). Fasting for a period of time prior to the examination will minimise the fluid and air present in the stomach and small intestine, resulting in better quality images (Folvik *et al.*, 1999; Nylund *et al.*, 2009), this is, however, not strictly necessary. If air is present, the ultrasonographer can apply gentle pressure with the transducer to move the air away from the area being scanned (Tarjan *et al.*, 2000). Additionally, it is important to minimise respiration effects when scanning, and this can be achieved by taking images at a constant point throughout the respiration cycle, or by asking patients to hold their breath as images are acquired (Jones *et al.*, 1997).

The patient should be positioned comfortably, in a supine position; however, measurement of gastric emptying (with both 2D and 3D ultrasound) should be performed seated or semirecumbent position, to allow better visualisation of the entire stomach, and to reflect gastric emptying in a physiological situation (Hveem *et al.*, 1996; Gilja *et al.*, 1997a; Gilja *et al.*, 2005). Scanning should be performed with a 3.5 - 5 MHz transducer, allowing for complete visualisation of the area of interest (Nylund *et al.*, 2009).

The transducer should be placed on the surface of the skin in such a way as to acquire an image of the entirety of the region being examined, as this varies from individual to individual, and is easily modified throughout the exam. This location is normally in the region of the epigastrium, down to the subcostal margins, or over the umbilicus (Hveem *et al.*, 1996; Gilja *et al.*, 1997a; Gilja *et al.*, 2005).

The use of colour and power Doppler should be considered, as well as duplex ultrasonography. These can add additional anatomical information, particularly relating to the vasculature, which can be impossible to see with B-mode ultrasonography (Nylund *et al.*, 2009).

3. Imaging of the antrum

The way in which the stomach regulates the emptying of food to optimise digestion and absorption is complex. The function of the proximal stomach is generally recognised as a storage facility relaxing to accommodate food which is then passed down into the antrum where it is ground down into particles <1mm in size before emptying into the small intestine. Several techniques have been used to provide insights into the mechanisms regulating this process. Ultrasonographic imaging of the antrum can be used to provide information relating to the volume or area of the distal stomach both in the fasted state and postprandially, thereby providing information about distension of this region.

Imaging should ideally be performed with the subject seated, and the transducer positioned vertically to obtain a sagittal image of the antrum, with the superior mesenteric vein and the abdominal aorta in a longitudinal section (Hveem *et al.*, 1996) (Figure 1). Images should be taken at the end of inspiration to minimise the effects of the normal motion of the stomach which occurs with regular breathing (Jones *et al.*, 1997). The area of the antrum is defined by a region of interest drawn around the cross section of the antrum and is expressed in cm^2.

The use of ultrasound to assess the antrum is appealing in both the clinical and research setting due to the ease and simplicity with which it can be applied, especially in favour of other imaging modalities that are more expensive and time consuming.

The ability to assess gastric distension is of particular relevance in patients with diabetes mellitus and functional dyspepsia in whom the prevalence of upper gastrointestinal symptoms is substantial (Hausken & Berstad, 1992; Undeland *et al.*, 1996). Studies using 2D ultrasound have demonstrated in these patient populations that antral area is increased; both in the fasted and postprandial state (Hausken & Berstad, 1992; Undeland *et al.*, 1996).

The use of ultrasound to assess gastric distension can also be applied to evaluate mechanisms relating to appetite regulation. For example, in both healthy young (Jones *et al.*, 1997), and older (Sturm *et al.*, 2004) subjects, antral distension (as measured by antral area on a 2D ultrasound image) following a meal has been shown to correlate with perceptions of fullness and energy intake indicating the importance of antral distension in appetite regulation (Figure 2).

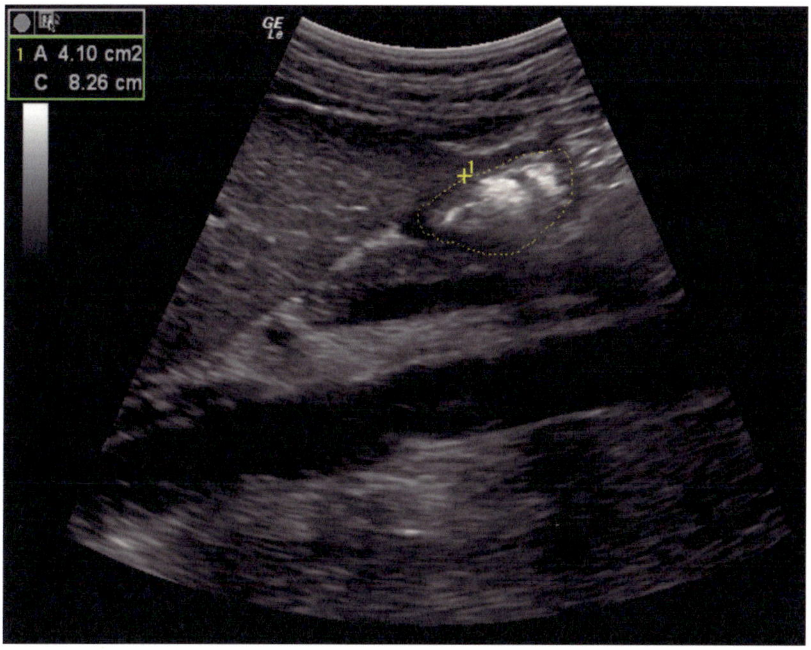

Fig. 1. 2D image of the antrum, with area calculation. The abdominal aorta and superior mesenteric vein are visible in the longitudinal section of the image.

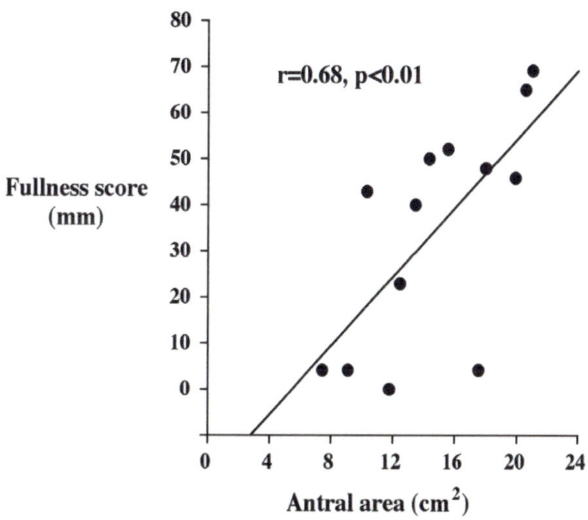

Fig. 2. Relationship between fullness score as measured by a visual questionnaire and antral area, measured by 2D ultrasound, 45 minutes after the consumption of a high-nutrient dextrose drink (75g dextrose dissolved in 350mL water) (n=14 healthy, young volunteers). (Am. J. Clin. Nutr. (1997;66:127-32), American Society for Nutrition).

Ultrasonographic assessment of the antrum has also been used pre-operatively to assess the likelihood of perioperative complications arising from the aspiration of gastric contents during surgery (Perlas *et al.*, 2009). Physicians acquiring a single image of the antrum were able to distinguish between a fasted and fed stomach 2 hours following the ingestion of either a solid or a liquid meal (Bouvet *et al.*, 2009).

4. Imaging of the proximal stomach

Ultrasonographic imaging of the proximal stomach was first described in 1995 (Gilja *et al.*, 1995). With the patient seated, leaning backwards slightly, the transducer is be placed on the epigastrium, by the left subcostal margin, and tilted cranially (Gilja *et al.*, 2007). Two images are acquired, the first being a sagittal slice of the proximal stomach, with the left renal pelvis in the longitudinal section of the image, using the left lobe of the liver and pancreas as anatomical landmarks. The area of the fundus is defined as a region from the top margin of the fundus to a point 7 cm downward, along the axis of the stomach (Gilja *et al.*, 1995). A second image, taken in the oblique plane can be acquired with the transducer in the same location. The top margin of the fundus should remain clearly visible in this image. The diameter of the fundus can be calculated on this image and is defined as the maximum diameter of the fundus kept within 7 cm along the axis of the proximal stomach (Gilja *et al.*, 1995). Proximal stomach volume can be derived using these measurements. In addition to measurements of diameter, area and volume, this ultrasound technique also enables the calculation of the initial emptying fractions of the proximal stomach, if imaging is performed soon after ingestion of a meal (Gilja *et al.*, 1995).

Imaging of the proximal stomach and estimation of fundic accommodation was traditionally performed with either a gastric barostat or scintigraphy. Currently, the 'gold standard' for assessment of proximal stomach accommodation is the use of a barostat device, a thin, plastic, inflatable balloon attached to an orogastric catheter, which, when positioned correctly and inflated in the proximal stomach, can measure gastric wall relaxation, and from this the tone of the muscle can be inferred (Azpiroz & Malagelada, 1987). Unlike ultrasonographic assessment, the barostat technique only measures the volume of a sealed balloon, therefore it offers no information about the size or true muscle tone of the stomach (Szarka & Camilleri, 2009). The barostat device can be uncomfortable, is highly invasive and has been shown to influence gastric motor patterns (Moragas *et al.*, 1993; Parys *et al.*, 1993). The barostat bag has also been shown to cause dilation of the antrum due to its placement, which may affect gastric emptying (Mundt *et al.*, 2002), an effect clearly overcome with ultrasound. Ultrasound enables the accommodation of the proximal stomach to be assessed with high inter- and intra-observer agreement (De Schepper *et al.*, 2004) with the added advantage of also assessing gastric emptying, antral motility and transpyloric flow, if desired, in a single examination (De Schepper *et al.*, 2004).

Scintigraphic single photon emission computed tomography (SPECT) scanning has the capacity to non-invasively provide information about gastric volume (Vasavid *et al.*, 2010), without interfering with gastric motor patterns. The technique requires intravenous administration of radioactive technetium pertechnetate which is taken up by the gastric mucosa to facilitate imaging. Gastric accommodation can be assessed using this technique in a reproducible fashion, however, there is evidence that SPECT is not very sensitive in detecting fundic relaxation when compared to the gastric barostat (van den Elzen *et al.*, 2003). Ultrasonographic imaging of the proximal stomach has similar advantages to that of imaging of the antrum, in that its cost, absence of radiation burden, accessibility and simplicity makes it more approachable than other imaging modalities. In addition, ultrasound imaging is performed in the sitting position, which is more reflective of the 'physiological' way one would be positioned when eating as opposed to SPECT, which requires the patient to be scanned in the supine position (De Schepper *et al.*, 2004; Hausken & Gilja, 2006).

While ultrasound has several advantages over the barostat technique, there remains some controversy as to whether measurements acquired by ultrasound, or even SPECT, can be compared directly to those acquired with a barostat device. The barostat, when inflated, can adjust to the changes in gastric pressure by adjusting the intrabag volume, therefore, changes in intrabag volume are said to reflect changes in muscle tone (Azpiroz & Malagelada, 1987). Ultrasound and scintintigraphic imaging methods, however, measure the physical size of the proximal stomach, which can only be used to infer movements of contraction and relaxation of the stomach (Hausken & Gilja, 2006). Whilst this information is not directly comparable, both changes in gastric volume, as well as the contraction and relaxation of the stomach provide valuable information about disordered motility (Hausken & Gilja, 2006).

Ultrasonographic imaging of the fundus has largely been used in the research setting while clinical applications of this type of imaging remain to be explored. Patients with functional dyspepsia and diabetes studied with ultrasound have demonstrated reduced proximal stomach accommodation (Gilja *et al.*, 1996b; Undeland *et al.*, 1998) when compared to healthy subjects. In patients with functional dyspepsia, glyceryl trinitrate (an exogenous donor of NO, a key neurotransmitter in mediating the relaxation of the smooth muscle of the stomach), administered sublingually has been shown to improve the accommodation of the proximal stomach, as measured by ultrasound, and reduce the postprandial symptoms associated with this condition (Gilja *et al.*, 1997b). In patients with reflux esophagitis, the area of the fundus has been shown to be significantly greater after a meal when compared to healthy controls, and these patients experienced greater epigastric fullness (Tefera *et al.*, 2001; Tefera *et al.*, 2002).

5. 2D assessment of gastric emptying

Scintigraphy is currently the 'gold standard' for clinical measurement of gastric emptying (Collins *et al.*, 1983; Collins *et al.*, 1991); however, it requires access to expensive equipment and carries a radiation burden to the patient and operator. Other techniques involve the use of an orogastric catheter, which is invasive and associated with a high degree of discomfort (Sheiner, 1975), or stable radioisotopes such as C^{14}-octanoic acid, which are not as readily available as ultrasound and requires specialised equipment to analyse (Vantrappen, 1994). Ultrasonography of the stomach has the ability to overcome these disadvantages. It provides an indirect measurement of gastric emptying by quantifying changes in antral area over time (Holt *et al.*, 1980; Bolondi *et al.*, 1985; Holt *et al.*, 1986).

The skills to acquire 2D ultrasound images are relatively easy to learn from an experienced operator. To optimise measurement, the subject should remain seated in approximately the same position for the duration of the examination, and ultrasound images of antral area should be taken at consistent times through the respiration cycle (Jones *et al.*, 1997). A variety of both liquid and semi-solid test meals, including low-nutrient beef soup, beans, pasta, orange juice and dextrose (Holt *et al.*, 1980; Bolondi *et al.*, 1985; Holt *et al.*, 1986; Brown *et al.*, 1993; Benini *et al.*, 1994; Hveem *et al.*, 1996) have been used to assess gastric emptying. The rate of gastric emptying, or gastric emptying half time (T50), defined as the time it takes for 50% of a given meal to empty from the stomach, can be calculated (Collins *et al.*, 1983) and the retention of a meal, expressed as a percentage of the total meal, at any given time, is defined as in equation (1) below.

$$\text{Retention } (\%) = \frac{AA(t) - AA(f)}{AA(max) - AA(f)} x100 \quad (1)$$

Where AA(t) is the antral area measured at any given time point, AA(f) is the fasting antral area and AA(max) is the maximum antral area recorded after drink ingestion (Hveem *et al.*, 1996).

Ultrasonographic assessment of gastric emptying has been validated against scintigraphy. Studies comparing emptying of a low nutrient beef soup (Holt *et al.*, 1986) and high nutrient dextrose drink (Hveem *et al.*, 1996; Jones *et al.*, 1997) demonstrate good correlation and agreement between techniques (Figure 3).

Studies using 2D ultrasonography in the research setting are particularly attractive as several measurements can be taken over a given time frame or in a single exam. Research studies have shown an overall delayed rate of gastric emptying in functional dyspepsia, with occasional, more rapid initial emptying (Lunding *et al.*, 2006) and an overall delayed rate of gastric emptying in patients with longstanding type 1 (Darwiche *et al.*, 1999) and type 2 (Bian *et al.*, 2011) diabetes.

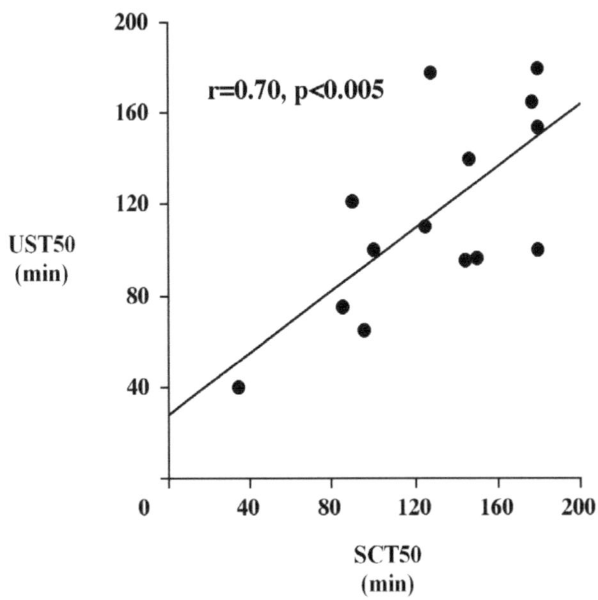

Fig. 3. Relationship between the gastric emptying half times (T50) of a high-nutrient dextrose drink (75g dextrose dissolved in 350mL water) as measured by 2D ultrasound and scintigraphy (n=14 healthy, young volunteers). (Am. J. Clin. Nutr. (1997;66:127-32), American Society for Nutrition).

Despite numerous advantages, 2D ultrasonographic assessment of gastric emptying is associated with some limitations. It is not a direct measure of gastric emptying but rather an assessment of changes in antral area (Holt *et al.*, 1980; Bolondi *et al.*, 1985; Holt *et al.*, 1986). Additionally, it does not take into account the full geometrical shape or distribution of the contents of the stomach (Gilja *et al.*, 2005).

6. 3D assessment of gastric emptying

Initially, assessment of gastric emptying with ultrasound was limited to the abovementioned 2D technique; however, 3D examinations of the stomach, including the emptying and distribution of its contents, have been developed with the increasing availability of suitable technology (Gilja *et al.*, 2005).

The concept was originally pioneered in the 1980s (Snyder *et al.*, 1986), and further developed by the Bergen group in Norway. 3D volume estimation of organs by ultrasound was originally only possible with a transducer mechanically tilted through 90° with a motor device whilst scanning continuously, with the ultrasonographic data transferred to a separate workstation for 3D reconstruction and processing (Hausken *et al.*, 1994; Gilja *et al.*, 1996a; Thune *et al.*, 1996; Gilja *et al.*, 1998). Obviously limited by the pre-determined scanning range and position of the sensor, a magnetometer based position and orientation measurement (POM) device was developed (Detmer *et al.*, 1994) providing precision mapping of points in space (Detmer *et al.*, 1994) and was validated as an accurate method of volume estimation (Hodges *et al.*, 1994; Matre *et al.*, 1999).

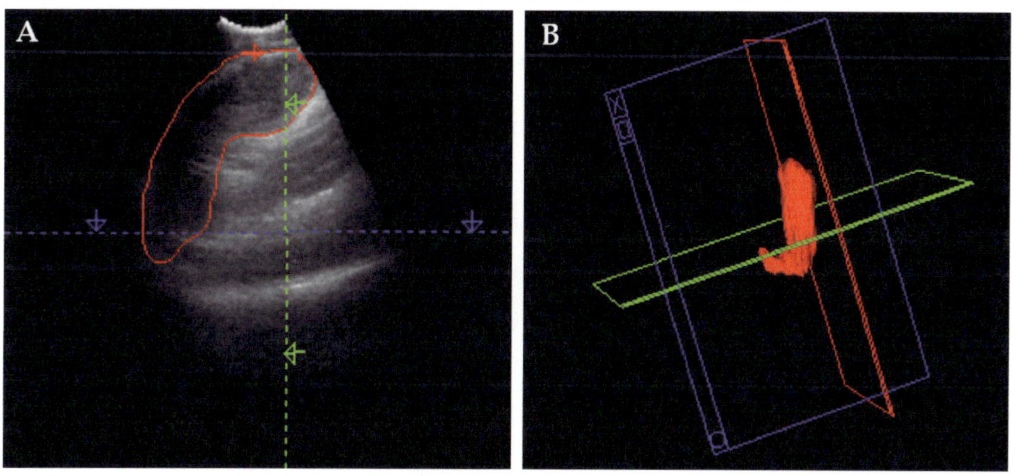

Fig. 4. 3D ultrasound to measure gastric emptying (A) a region of interest drawn around the stomach (B) reconstructed volumetric image of the stomach.

A series of sagittal slices are acquired with a continuous sweeping motion towards the midline, beginning with the transducer at the left subcostal margin, tilted cranially, to image the most proximal part of the stomach, through to the distal stomach and ceasing at the gastro-duodenal junction (Gilja *et al.*, 1997a; Gilja *et al.*, 2005). The resulting images can be analysed with specialised software (EchoPAC-3D) to provide 3D reconstruction and volume estimation (Martens *et al.*, 1997) (Figure 4), this software also enables intragastric distribution to be studied by dividing the stomach into proximal and/or distal volumes (Gilja *et al.*, 1997a).

Currently, 3D ultrasound to measure gastric emptying is restricted to work in the research setting. This method has been applied to stomach volumes and validated against scintigraphy in both the healthy elderly (Gentilcore *et al.*, 2006) and in patients with diabetic gastroparesis (Stevens *et al.*, 2011) (Figure 5 and 6).

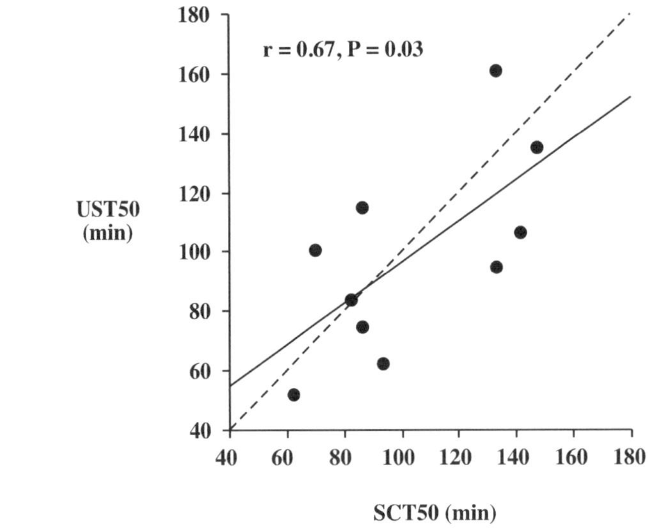

Fig. 5. Relationship between the gastric emptying half times ($T_{1/2}$) of a high-nutrient dextrose drink (75g dextrose dissolved in 300mL water) as measured by 3D ultrasound and scintigraphy (n=10 diabetic patients with gastroparesis). (Neurogastroenterol Motil (2011;23:220-e114)).

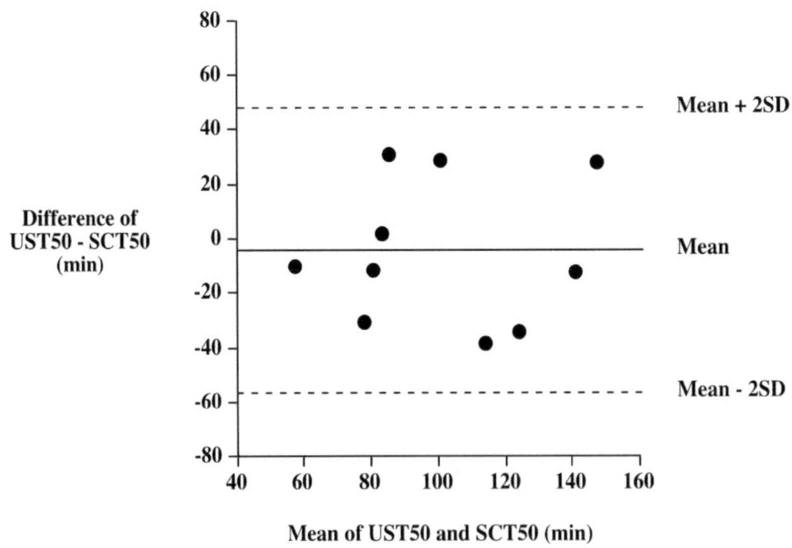

Fig. 6. Limits of agreement for scintigraphic (SCT50) and 3D ultrasonographic (UST50) 50 % emptying times (T50s) for the drink (75 g dextrose in 300 mL water) (n=10 diabetic patients with gastroparesis). (Neurogastroenterol Motil (2011;23:220-e114)).

3D ultrasound has also been shown to have higher accuracy and less variability than 2D ultrasound of the stomach (Gilja *et al.*, 1997a) and in a study with a fluid-filled barostat bag, has correlated well with true stomach volumes with low inter-observer variation (Tefera *et al.*, 2002).

3D ultrasound is limited by the complexities of scanning technique and technological availability. Additionally, difficulties in imaging due to the presence of intragastric gas may limit accuracy.

7. Measurement of antropyloroduoenal motility

Gastric emptying in humans is predominantly a pulsatile phenomenon in which the contents of the stomach move across the pylorus in response to either a local increase in the pressure between the antrum and duodenum caused by an increase in local antropyloric pressure waves (i.e., peristaltic flow), or non-peristaltic flow caused by differences in pressure between the distal antrum and duodenum (Berstad *et al.*, 1994; Gilja *et al.*, 2007).

Much information about gastric emptying can be obtained by evaluating the physical contractions of the antropylorodudodenal region. While manometric apparatus have been traditionally used to assess antropyloric pressure changes during these events, the technique is limited to assessment of lumen occlusive contractions (Gilja *et al.*, 2007). Following ingestion of a low nutrient soup with simultaneous ultrasound, approximately 45% of pyloric contractions which were visible on ultrasound images were not correlated to manometric pressure changes (Hveem *et al.*, 2001; Hausken *et al.*, 2002). While providing more comprehensive information about the timing and magnitude of antropyloric pressure contractions, ultrasound has the added benefit of also providing visual information about the movement of gastric contents across the pylorus in relation to individual peristaltic contractions (King *et al.*, 1984; Hausken *et al.*, 1992). Additionally, intubation with a manometric catheter is invasive, associated with significant patient discomfort, and is not always practical.

Ultrasongraphic measurement of antropylorodudodenal contractions, whilst beneficial in that it overcomes the limitations of manometry, is restricted in that it requires a well trained operator. Currently, use is restricted to the research setting (Gilja *et al.*, 2007).

8. Measurement of transpyloric flow

Ultrasonography can be used to both quantify and qualify the movement of the contents of the stomach across the pylorus, into the duodenum. This normal movement of the stomach contents into the duodenum is normally followed by a short period of duodenogastric reflux immediately prior to the closing of the pylorus (Berstad *et al.*, 1994; Hausken *et al.*, 2001; Gilja *et al.*, 2007).

Transpyloric imaging employs duplex ultrasonography (simultaneous Doppler and B-mode imaging) of the pylorus enabling the motion and velocity of gastric contents to be assessed (Hausken *et al.*, 1992; Berstad *et al.*, 1994; Hausken *et al.*, 1998a). Gastric emptying is said to occur when there is flow across the pylorus with a mean velocity of 10 cm/s or more, lasting for at least one second (Gilja *et al.*, 2007). Contraction of the antrum occurs when there is visible movement of the antral wall which propagates with time and is not caused by pulsation of nearby vessels or the adjacent intestine, or by respiration (Gilja *et al.*, 2007).

A technique involving 3D ultrasonography of transpyloric flow has been developed by Hausken et al. to assess flow during the abovementioned duodenogastric reflux period. This technique enables quantification of duodenogastric stroke volume (Hausken *et al.*, 2001). High intra and inter individual correlations of stroke volume have been shown (Hausken *et al.*, 2001).

Whilst there are substantial operational and technical demands of this type of ultrasound, the significant insight into the normal physiological movements involved in digestion it provides has proven invaluable in the research setting (King *et al.*, 1984; Hausken & Berstad, 1992; Hausken *et al.*, 1998a; Jones *et al.*, 2006). Transpyloric flow has been shown to be greater in a sitting position, compared to a supine position, with no effect on the overall emptying of a standardised drink consisting of 600mL of water and 75g of glucose (Jones *et al.*, 2006). Measurements of transpyloric flow have been shown to be decreased, along with the overall rate of gastric emptying, in older, when compared with young, subjects (O'Donovan *et al.*, 2005). In studies of patients with type 2 diabetes, with and without autonomic neuropathy, reduced transpyloric flow was shown (Kawagishi *et al.*, 1994). Additionally, altered movement of the contents of the stomach across the pylorus may be responsible for postprandial symptoms in patients with functional dyspepsia (Hausken *et al.*, 1998b).

9. Gastric strain rate imaging

The deformation of the gastric wall due to mechanical stress (strain) can be imaged with B-mode ultrasonography (Gilja *et al.*, 2002). Gastric strain is of interest for a number of reasons; mechanoreceptors respond to changes in stress in a muscular wall, not changes in pressure or volume so it allows these direct effects to be studied, it provides information on the elastic properties of the muscular walls of the stomach, it can differentiate phasic motions from passive changes in muscle tone (which is of particular importance in a research setting) and it allows the normal geometry of the stomach to be maintained while assessing these parameters (Gregersen *et al.*, 2002).

Gastric strain rate imaging (SRI) involves the recording of tissue velocity to obtain strain, and the strain rate is defined by the gradient of the velocity component of two points along the ultrasound beam (Gilja *et al.*, 2007; Ahmed *et al.*, 2009). SRI is able to distinguish between contraction of the circular and longitudinal muscle layers, even when not distinctly visible on the 2D ultrasound image (Gilja *et al.*, 2002).

Technically, continuous imaging is necessary and a small sample size (~2 mm) should be selected (Gilja *et al.*, 2007; Ahmed *et al.*, 2009). Cine imaging should be acquired over the antral lumen whenever a change in luminal cross-section or antral circularity is observed (Gilja *et al.*, 2007; Ahmed *et al.*, 2009).

SRI has been validated *in vivo* with a silicone phantom to mimic moving tissue (Matre *et al.*, 2003) and in an *in vitro* porcine model (Ahmed *et al.*, 2006). In a study involving the artificial distension of the antrum with a barostat device, there was a significant inverse correlation between balloon pressure and gastric strain (Gilja *et al.*, 2002).

The use of SRI has been applied in patients with functional dyspepsia (Ahmed *et al.*, 2008), and in these patients, divided into subgroups of 'epigastric pain syndrome' (EPS) and 'postprandial distress syndrome' (PDS), antral strain was shown to be higher in EPS patients, compared with PDS patients and normal controls, both in the fasting and postprandial state (Ahmed *et al.*, 2008; Ahmed *et al.*, 2009).

Due to the relatively novel nature of this type of imaging, and the requirement for a well trained operator, SRI imaging is still largely reserved for the research setting. Further studies would be required to assess potential clinical applications for this type of imaging.

10. Conclusion

Ultrasonography remains a safe and effective means by which the structure and function of the stomach can be assessed in an accurate and reproducible manner. Ultrasonography offers several advantages over other imaging modalities in that it is easy to perform, readily accessible, cheap and not associated with a radiation burden.

The techniques described in this chapter have been applied in a meaningful way in either the clinical or research setting, or in some cases, both. 2D ultrasonography of the stomach stands out as a simple and well-validated means by which antral area, proximal stomach accommodation and gastric emptying can be assessed, whereas 3D ultrasonography offers added information about the physiology of the stomach. New techniques involving the imaging of the flow of the stomach contents across the pylorus, motility of the pylorus, and the mechanical stress placed on the gastric wall, continue to be developed.

It should be recognised that for these techniques to be effective, they require the hand of a skilled, well trained operator, and are only applicable in situations where there is relevance or interest in the added information that ultrasonography of the stomach has to offer. Whilst at this time, this is often limited to the research setting, as these techniques are more widely adopted, clinical use will become more widespread.

Provided the limitations of each ultrasonographic technique discussed in this chapter are observed, ultrasound has the ability to provide significant anatomical and physiological information about the stomach and its contents in both the clinical and research setting.

11. References

Ahmed AB, Gilja OH, Gregersen H, Odegaard S & Matre K. (2006). In vitro strain measurement in the porcine antrum using ultrasound doppler strain rate imaging. *Ultrasound Med Biol* 32, 513-522.

Ahmed AB, Gilja OH, Hausken T, Gregersen H & Matre K. (2009). Strain measurement during antral contractions by ultrasound strain rate imaging: influence of erythromycin. *Neurogastroenterol Motil* 21, 170-179.

Ahmed AB, Matre K, Hausken T, Gregersen H & Gilja OH. (2008). T1326 ROME III Subgroups of Functional Dyspepsia Exhibit Different Characteristics of Antral Strain Measured By Strain Rate Imaging. *Gastroenterology* 134, A-531.

Azpiroz F & Malagelada JR. (1987). Gastric tone measured by an electronic barostat in health and postsurgical gastroparesis. *Gastroenterology* 92, 934-943.

Benini L, Brighenti F, Castellani G, Brentegani MT, Casiraghi MC, Ruzzenente O, Sembenini C, Pellegrini N, Caliari S, Porrini M & et al. (1994). Gastric emptying of solids is markedly delayed when meals are fried. *Dig Dis Sci* 39, 2288-2294.

Berstad A, Hausken T, Gilja OH, Thune N, Matre K & Odegaard S. (1994). Volume measurements of gastric antrum by 3-D ultrasonography and flow measurements through the pylorus by duplex technique. *Dig Dis Sci* 39, 97S-100S.

Bian RW, Lou QL, Gu LB, Kong AP, So WY, Ko GT, Ouyang XJ, Mo YZ, Ma RC, Chan JC & Chow CC. (2011). Delayed gastric emptying is related to cardiovascular autonomic neuropathy in Chinese patients with type 2 diabetes. *Acta Gastroenterol Belg* 74, 28-33.

Bolondi L, Bortolotti M, Santi V, Calletti T, Gaiani S & Labo G. (1985). Measurement of gastric emptying time by real-time ultrasonography. *Gastroenterology* 89, 752-759.

Bouvet L, Miquel A, Chassard D, Boselli E, Allaouchiche B & Benhamou D. (2009). Could a single standardized ultrasonographic measurement of antral area be of interest for assessing gastric contents? A preliminary report. *Eur J Anaesthesiol* 26, 1015-1019.

Brown BP, Schulze-Delrieu K, Schrier JE & Abu-Yousef MM. (1993). The configuration of the human gastroduodenal junction in the separate emptying of liquids and solids. *Gastroenterology* 105, 433-440.

Collins PJ, Horowitz M, Cook DJ, Harding PE & Shearman DJ. (1983). Gastric emptying in normal subjects--a reproducible technique using a single scintillation camera and computer system. *Gut* 24, 1117-1125.

Collins PJ, Houghton LA, Read NW, Horowitz M, Chatterton BE, Heddle R & Dent J. (1991). Role of the proximal and distal stomach in mixed solid and liquid meal emptying. *Gut* 32, 615-619.

Darwiche G, Almer LO, Bjorgell O, Cederholm C & Nilsson P. (1999). Measurement of gastric emptying by standardized real-time ultrasonography in healthy subjects and diabetic patients. *J Ultrasound Med* 18, 673-682.

De Schepper HU, Cremonini F, Chitkara D & Camilleri M. (2004). Assessment of gastric accommodation: overview and evaluation of current methods. *Neurogastroenterol Motil* 16, 275-285.

Detmer PR, Bashein G, Hodges T, Beach KW, Filer EP, Burns DH & Strandness DE, Jr. (1994). 3D ultrasonic image feature localization based on magnetic scanhead tracking: in vitro calibration and validation. *Ultrasound Med Biol* 20, 923-936.

Folvik G, Bjerke-Larssen T, Odegaard S, Hausken T, Gilja OH & Berstad A. (1999). Hydrosonography of the small intestine: comparison with radiologic barium study. *Scand J Gastroenterol* 34, 1247-1252.

Gentilcore D, Hausken T, Horowitz M & Jones KL. (2006). Measurements of gastric emptying of low- and high-nutrient liquids using 3D ultrasonography and scintigraphy in healthy subjects. *Neurogastroenterol Motil* 18, 1062-1068.

Gilja OH, Detmer PR, Jong JM, Leotta DF, Li XN, Beach KW, Martin R & Strandness DE, Jr. (1997a). Intragastric distribution and gastric emptying assessed by three-dimensional ultrasonography. *Gastroenterology* 113, 38-49.

Gilja OH, Hatlebakk JG, Odegaard S, Berstad A, Viola I, Giertsen C, Hausken T & Gregersen H. (2007). Advanced imaging and visualization in gastrointestinal disorders. *World J Gastroenterol* 13, 1408-1421.
Gilja OH, Hausken T, Bang CJ & Berstad A. (1997b). Effect of glyceryl trinitrate on gastric accommodation and symptoms in functional dyspepsia. *Dig Dis Sci* 42, 2124-2131.
Gilja OH, Hausken T, Odegaard S & Berstad A. (1995). Monitoring postprandial size of the proximal stomach by ultrasonography. *J Ultrasound Med* 14, 81-89.
Gilja OH, Hausken T, Odegaard S & Berstad A. (1996a). Three-dimensional ultrasonography of the gastric antrum in patients with functional dyspepsia. *Scand J Gastroenterol* 31, 847-855.
Gilja OH, Hausken T, Odegaard S & Berstad A. (2005). Ultrasonography and three-dimensional methods of the upper gastrointestinal tract. *Eur J Gastroenterol Hepatol* 17, 277-282.
Gilja OH, Hausken T, Olafsson S, Matre K & Odegaard S. (1998). In vitro evaluation of three-dimensional ultrasonography based on magnetic scanhead tracking. *Ultrasound Med Biol* 24, 1161-1167.
Gilja OH, Hausken T, Wilhelmsen I & Berstad A. (1996b). Impaired accommodation of proximal stomach to a meal in functional dyspepsia. *Dig Dis Sci* 41, 689-696.
Gilja OH, Heimdal A, Hausken T, Gregersen H, Matre K, Berstad A & Odegaard S. (2002). Strain during gastric contractions can be measured using Doppler ultrasonography. *Ultrasound Med Biol* 28, 1457-1465.
Gregersen H, Gilja OH, Hausken T, Heimdal A, Gao C, Matre K, Odegaard S & Berstad A. (2002). Mechanical properties in the human gastric antrum using B-mode ultrasonography and antral distension. *Am J Physiol Gastrointest Liver Physiol* 283, G368-375.
Hausken T & Berstad A. (1992). Wide gastric antrum in patients with non-ulcer dyspepsia. Effect of cisapride. *Scand J Gastroenterol* 27, 427-432.
Hausken T & Gilja OH. (2006). Functional Ultrasound of the Gastrointestinal Tract. *Ultrasound of the Gastrointestinal Tract* Springer.
Hausken T, Gilja OH, Odegaard S & Berstad A. (1998a). Flow across the human pylorus soon after ingestion of food, studied with duplex sonography. Effect of glyceryl trinitrate. *Scand J Gastroenterol* 33, 484-490.
Hausken T, Gilja OH, Undeland KA & Berstad A. (1998b). Timing of postprandial dyspeptic symptoms and transpyloric passage of gastric contents. *Scand J Gastroenterol* 33, 822-827.
Hausken T, Li XN, Goldman B, Leotta D, Odegaard S & Martin RW. (2001). Quantification of gastric emptying and duodenogastric reflux stroke volumes using three-dimensional guided digital color Doppler imaging. *Eur J Ultrasound* 13, 205-213.
Hausken T, Mundt M & Samsom M. (2002). Low antroduodenal pressure gradients are responsible for gastric emptying of a low-caloric liquid meal in humans. *Neurogastroenterol Motil* 14, 97-105.
Hausken T, Odegaard S, Matre K & Berstad A. (1992). Antroduodenal motility and movements of luminal contents studied by duplex sonography. *Gastroenterology* 102, 1583-1590.

Hausken T, Thune N, Matre K, Gilja OH, ØDegaard S & Berstad A. (1994). Volume estimation of the gastric antrum and the gallbladder in patients with non-ulcer dyspepsia and erosive prepyloric changes, using three-dimensional ultrasonography. *Neurogastroenterology & Motility* 6, 263-270.

Hodges TC, Detmer PR, Burns DH, Beach KW & Strandness DE, Jr. (1994). Ultrasonic three-dimensional reconstruction: in vitro and in vivo volume and area measurement. *Ultrasound Med Biol* 20, 719-729.

Holt S, Cervantes J, Wilkinson AA & Wallace JH. (1986). Measurement of gastric emptying rate in humans by real-time ultrasound. *Gastroenterology* 90, 918-923.

Holt S, McDicken WN, Anderson T, Stewart IC & Heading RC. (1980). Dynamic imaging of the stomach by real-time ultrasound--a method for the study of gastric motility. *Gut* 21, 597-601.

Hveem K, Jones KL, Chatterton BE & Horowitz M. (1996). Scintigraphic measurement of gastric emptying and ultrasonographic assessment of antral area: relation to appetite. *Gut* 38, 816-821.

Hveem K, Sun WM, Hebbard G, Horowitz M, Doran S & Dent J. (2001). Relationship between ultrasonically detected phasic antral contractions and antral pressure. *Am J Physiol Gastrointest Liver Physiol* 281, G95-101.

Jones KL, Doran SM, Hveem K, Bartholomeusz FD, Morley JE, Sun WM, Chatterton BE & Horowitz M. (1997). Relation between postprandial satiation and antral area in normal subjects. *Am J Clin Nutr* 66, 127-132.

Jones KL, O'Donovan D, Horowitz M, Russo A, Lei Y & Hausken T. (2006). Effects of posture on gastric emptying, transpyloric flow, and hunger after a glucose drink in healthy humans. *Dig Dis Sci* 51, 1331-1338.

Kawagishi T, Nishizawa Y, Okuno Y, Shimada H, Inaba M, Konishi T & Morii H. (1994). Antroduodenal motility and transpyloric fluid movement in patients with diabetes studied using duplex sonography. *Gastroenterology* 107, 403-409.

King PM, Adam RD, Pryde A, McDicken WN & Heading RC. (1984). Relationships of human antroduodenal motility and transpyloric fluid movement: non-invasive observations with real-time ultrasound. *Gut* 25, 1384-1391.

Lunding JA, Tefera S, Gilja OH, Hausken T, Bayati A, Rydholm H, Mattsson H & Berstad A. (2006). Rapid initial gastric emptying and hypersensitivity to gastric filling in functional dyspepsia: effects of duodenal lipids. *Scand J Gastroenterol* 41, 1028-1036.

Martens D, Hausken T, Gilja OH, Steen E, Alker H & Odegaard S. (1997). 3D processing of ultrasound images using a novel EchoPac-3D® software. *Ultrasound Med Biol* 23 (suppl 1), 136.

Matre K, Ahmed AB, Gregersen H, Heimdal A, Hausken T, Odegaard S & Gilja OH. (2003). In vitro evaluation of ultrasound Doppler strain rate imaging: modification for measurement in a slowly moving tissue phantom. *Ultrasound Med Biol* 29, 1725-1734.

Matre K, Stokke EM, Martens D & Gilja OH. (1999). In vitro volume estimation of kidneys using three-dimensional ultrasonography and a position sensor. *Eur J Ultrasound* 10, 65-73.

Moragas G, Azpiroz F, Pavia J & Malagelada JR. (1993). Relations among intragastric pressure, postcibal perception, and gastric emptying. *Am J Physiol* 264, G1112-1117.

Mundt MW, Hausken T & Samsom M. (2002). Effect of intragastric barostat bag on proximal and distal gastric accommodation in response to liquid meal. *Am J Physiol Gastrointest Liver Physiol* 283, G681-686.

Nylund K, Odegaard S, Hausken T, Folvik G, Lied GA, Viola I, Hauser H & Gilja OH. (2009). Sonography of the small intestine. *World J Gastroenterol* 15, 1319-1330.

O'Donovan D, Hausken T, Lei Y, Russo A, Keogh J, Horowitz M & Jones KL. (2005). Effect of aging on transpyloric flow, gastric emptying, and intragastric distribution in healthy humans--impact on glycemia. *Dig Dis Sci* 50, 671-676.

Parys V, Bruley des Varannes S, Ropert A, Roze C & Galmiche JP. (1993). [Use of an electronic barostat for measurement of motor response of the proximal stomach to feeding and different nervous stimuli in man]. *Gastroenterol Clin Biol* 17, 321-328.

Perlas A, Chan VW, Lupu CM, Mitsakakis N & Hanbidge A. (2009). Ultrasound assessment of gastric content and volume. *Anesthesiology* 111, 82-89.

Sheiner HJ. (1975). Gastric emptying tests in man. *Gut* 16, 235-247.

Snyder JE, Kisslo J & von Ramm O. (1986). Real-time orthogonal mode scanning of the heart. I. System design. *J Am Coll Cardiol* 7, 1279-1285.

Stevens JE, Gilja OH, Gentilcore D, Hausken T, Horowitz M & Jones KL. (2011). Measurement of gastric emptying of a high-nutrient liquid by 3D ultrasonography in diabetic gastroparesis. *Neurogastroenterol Motil* 23, 220-225, e113-224.

Sturm K, Parker B, Wishart J, Feinle-Bisset C, Jones KL, Chapman I & Horowitz M. (2004). Energy intake and appetite are related to antral area in healthy young and older subjects. *Am J Clin Nutr* 80, 656-667.

Szarka LA & Camilleri M. (2009). Methods for measurement of gastric motility. *Am J Physiol Gastrointest Liver Physiol* 296, G461-475.

Tarjan Z, Toth G, Gyorke T, Mester A, Karlinger K & Mako EK. (2000). Ultrasound in Crohn's disease of the small bowel. *Eur J Radiol* 35, 176-182.

Tefera S, Gilja OH, Hatlebakk JG & Berstad A. (2001). Gastric accommodation studied by ultrasonography in patients with reflux esophagitis. *Dig Dis Sci* 46, 618-625.

Tefera S, Gilja OH, Olafsdottir E, Hausken T, Hatlebakk JG & Berstad A. (2002). Intragastric maldistribution of a liquid meal in patients with reflux oesophagitis assessed by three dimensional ultrasonography. *Gut* 50, 153-158.

Thune N, Gilja OH, Hausken T & Matre K. (1996). A practical method for estimating enclosed volumes using 3D ultrasound. *European journal of ultrasound : official journal of the European Federation of Societies for Ultrasound in Medicine and Biology* 3, 83-92.

Undeland KA, Hausken T, Gilja OH, Aanderud S & Berstad A. (1998). Gastric meal accommodation studied by ultrasound in diabetes. Relation to vagal tone. *Scand J Gastroenterol* 33, 236-241.

Undeland KA, Hausken T, Svebak S, Aanderud S & Berstad A. (1996). Wide gastric antrum and low vagal tone in patients with diabetes mellitus type 1 compared to patients with functional dyspepsia and healthy individuals. *Dig Dis Sci* 41, 9-16.

van den Elzen BD, Bennink RJ, Wieringa RE, Tytgat GN & Boeckxstaens GE. (2003). Fundic accommodation assessed by SPECT scanning: comparison with the gastric barostat. *Gut* 52, 1548-1554.

Vantrappen G. (1994). Methods to study gastric emptying. *Dig Dis Sci* 39, 91S-94S.

Vasavid P, Chaiwatanarata T & Gonlachanvit S. (2010). The Reproducibility of Tc-Pertechnetate Single Photon Emission Computed Tomography (SPECT) for Measurement of Gastric Accommodation in Healthy Humans: Evaluation of the Test Results Performed at the Same Time and Different Time of the Day. *J Neurogastroenterol Motil* 16, 401-406.